BEHAVIORAL CASE
FORMULATION

BEHAVIORAL CASE FORMULATION

Edited by

Ira Daniel Turkat

University of North Carolina, Greensboro
Greensboro, North Carolina

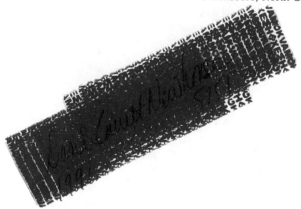

Plenum Press • New York and London

Library of Congress Cataloging in Publication Data

Main entry under title:

Behavioral case formulation.

Includes bibliographies and indexes.
1. Psychiatry—Case formulation.2. Behavioral assessment. I. Turkat, Ira Daniel.
RC473.C37B44   1985   616.89   85-24463
ISBN 0-306-42047-3

Acknowledgment is made for permission to reprint the following tables in this book:

Table 1, page 96 is from "Biofeedback and Headache: Methodological Issues" by H. E. Adams, P. J. Brantley, and K. Thompson in *Clinical Biofeedback: Efficacy and Mechanisms*, edited by L. White and B. Turskey. Copyright 1982 by Guilford Press, New York. Reprinted by permission.

Table 1, page 166 is from "An Empirical Study of the Issue of Sex Bias in the Diagnostic Criteria of DSM-III Axis II Personality Disorders" by F. Kass, R. L. Spitzer, and J. B. W. Williams, 1983, *American Psychologist, 38*. Copyright 1983 by the American Psychological Association. Adapted by permission of the author.

©1985 Plenum Press, New York
A Division of Plenum Publishing Corporation
233 Spring Street, New York, N.Y. 10013

Printed in the United States of America

For my loving family:
Justin, Holly, Derek, and Jaclyn

Contributors

Henry E. Adams, Department of Psychology, University of Georgia, Athens, Georgia

Phillip J. Brantley, Departments of Psychology and Family Medicine, Louisiana State University, Baton Rouge, Louisiana

Eleanor B. Callon, Department of Psychology, Louisiana State University, Baton Rouge, Louisiana

Alan R. King, Department of Psychology, Southern University, New Orleans, Louisiana

Stephen A. Maisto, Veterans Administration Medical Center, Alcohol Dependence Treatment Program, Davis Park, Providence, Rhode Island

Victor J. Malatesta, The Institute of Pennsylvania Hospital, University of Pennsylvania School of Medicine, Philadelphia, Pennsylvania

Patricia B. Sutker, Psychology Service, Veterans Administration Medical Center, Department of Psychiatry and Neurology, Tulane University School of Medicine, New Orleans, Louisiana

Ira Daniel Turkat, Department of Psychology, University of North Carolina at Greensboro, Greensboro, North Carolina

Joseph Wolpe, Department of Psychiatry, Temple University School of Medicine, Philadelphia, Pennsylvania

Foreword

In the opening chapter of this book, Wolpe and Turkat provide an admirable explanation of case formulation. It is the "idiographic adaptation of empirical procedures." Their explanation captures the essence of applied psychology, and its major challenge. How can we move from the empirical data, systematically gathered from many subjects under highly controlled conditions, to the problems presented by the particular case?

The transfer from one domain to the other is beset with difficulties, and as the editor remarks in his preface, graduate students commonly request help and guidance in traversing from laboratory to clinic. The possibility of successfully applying empirical findings to the particular case is implicit in clinical research, but frustrated students sometimes develop an unfortunate scepticism about the feasibility of bridging the gap. Collections of behavioral formulations of clinical cases can provide a valuable model and guide for students and practitioners, and the present volume is a rich and useful addition to the literature.

In their own ways, all of the contributors demonstrate the essential value of empirical data, the need for a structured approach to data collection, and the process of formulating case hypotheses. The case formulation process imposes a necessary discipline on the clinician's reasoning and actions, and generally leads to the construction of specific goals and thereby to specific outcome criteria. By contrast, the omission of a case formulation can leave the clinician, and the patient, with an amorphous blur that has no direction and can have no clean conclusion.

This collection is diverse, rich, and didactic, and is likely to prove of considerable value and interest to students and clinicians.

S. RACHMAN

Department of Psychology
University of British Columbia
Vancouver, British Columbia

Preface

One of the most frequent requests I receive from graduate students is for references on how to formulate a complex clinical case. Typically, after reading the recommended materials, the student returns to request more detailed accounts of how clinicians "think" about particular cases. The general lack of such materials in the behavior therapy literature led to the formation of the present volume.

Throughout much of the behavior therapy literature, one gets the impression that most cases seen present circumscribed and straightforward psychological problems. In my experience, such cases are rare. Accordingly, the present volume was designed to cover more complex problems such as sociopathy and paranoid personality. These disorders are rarely discussed in the behavior therapy literature but nonetheless seem to appear regularly in clinical settings. The cases presented in this book are descriptions of patients seen clinically by the editor or by the contributors.

Work on this text began while I was a faculty member at Vanderbilt University and took several years to complete. As the contributors would attest, the task I set out for them was atypical and often difficult. The complexities involved in articulating *how* one conceptualizes a case are numerous and may help to explain why there are so few sources available on case formulation. The fact that our current state of knowledge in psychopathology is rather limited further exacerbates the problem.

This book is intended to serve as a sourcebook for ideas on how to formulate and deal with complex psychopathological cases. Be it the practicing clinician or the student training to become one, the present text should be of immense value. In addition, the following pages are replete with novel clinical hypotheses, ripe for investigation.

I am greatly indebted to the Department of Psychology at the University of North Carolina at Greensboro for its support to help me complete this project. In addition to the resources allocated, the intellectual stimulation provided by my colleagues and graduate students fostered the completion of this book. Gratitude is also expressed to the many people at Vanderbilt University who aided me in this task and to the departments of psychology and medicine for their support. Most important, I am forever indebted to the professors who trained me as an undergraduate (University of Vermont), intern (Middlesex Hospital Medical School of the University of London), and graduate (University of Georgia) student.

IRA DANIEL TURKAT

Contents

3 CHRONIC HEADACHE 87

Case Formulations of Chronic Headaches 93

Henry E. Adams

4 ANTISOCIAL PERSONALITY DISORDER 111

Antisocial Personality Disorder: Assessment and Case Formulation 115

Patricia B. Sutker and Alan R. King

5 PARANOID PERSONALITY DISORDER 155

6 HISTRIONIC PERSONALITY 199

7 GERIATRIC ORGANIC SYNDROME 253

Introduction

IRA DANIEL TURKAT

Treatment of psychological problems has become a billion-dollar industry and lately everyone seems to want to get in on it. Thousands of students each year apply for doctoral training in clinical psychology; the majority of these graduates will seek applied jobs. Professional schools offering a doctor of psychology degree are springing up all over. Psychiatrists, social workers, counselors, psychiatric nurses, pastors, and so on hang out their shingles. Radio and television studios offer regularly scheduled programs on which individuals can talk to a psychologist. Self-help books for psychological problems continually make the best seller list. No matter what the problem, there is no shortage of individuals who claim to be able to treat it.

What does the scientific literature say about the efficacy of psychological intervention? In most respects, it depends on who is interpreting the literature. Some argue that without a doubt, psychotherapy is effective. Others feel that a third of those treated get better, a third remain the same, and a third get worse. Some argue that psychotherapy is purely an art and that science is irrelevant. And for those who believe that psychotherapy has an effect of some kind, there is disagreement as to why and how to get it. Some believe that the more techniques applied, the better the prognosis. Others believe that techniques are irrelevant and that the "effective ingredient" in psychotherapy is the development of a good relationship with the patient. Some believe that biofeedback is the answer; for others it is hypnosis or primal screaming. The bottom line is that billions are spent on psychological services on which there is considerable disagreement about efficacy, appropriateness, and rationale.

In their excellent review of the treatment outcome literature, Rachman and Wilson (1980) concluded that there was considerable scientific support for psychological intervention for a small group of disorders (e.g., simple phobia); other disorders were seen as having either little or no support although certain interventions appeared "promising." Five years later, I believe it is reasonable to conclude that there is strong scientific support for psychological intervention still only for a handful of disorders and that the vast majority of disorders have yet to be shown scientifically to be amenable to change.

Given our inability to modify the vast majority of behavior disorders we encounter clinically, how should we proceed? If we were to examine the history of behavioral treatment for anxiety (which has good scientific support) as an example, we would find that systematic desensitization stemmed directly from Wolpe's formulation of anxiety (1958). In his classic text, *Psychotherapy by Reciprocal Inhibition*, Wolpe (1958) outlined his view of anxiety, speculated on how anxiety developed, and tested his hypotheses in the laboratory. On the basis of this foundation, Wolpe derived systematic desensitization. Thus, without a formulation of anxiety itself, it is unlikely that Wolpe would have developed his now famous treatment procedure.

The lesson to be learned from Wolpe is that the development of effective procedures depends largely on a good formulation of the phenomenon targeted for change. Other applied fields have shown this to be so time and time again. For example, triple by-pass surgery could never have developed successfully without a solid understanding of the heart and the cardiovascular system. Similarly, the "cure" for the common cold still eludes us as we have yet fully to understand the common cold. It would appear that those psychologists and other mental health professionals who are concerned with treating behavior disorders which we have yet to understand could benefit greatly by an increased emphasis on developing good formulations of psychopathology.

Up to this point we have discussed the formulation–treatment issue on a broad level, but it is equally if not more pertinent to the everyday clinical case. How does the clinician assess the problems of the presenting case? How does the clinician choose an appropriate psychological intervention? All of these questions are integral to treatment of the individual case. If the clinician cannot properly formulate a case, is it reasonable to expect the clinician to be able to treat the case successfully?

Although the importance of case formulation seems so rudimentary, it is surprising how few sources on the subject are available in the literature. The problem is highlighted by the fact that definitions of what a case formulation is appear to be practically nonexistent. Furthermore, although numerous case studies are published each year in the literature, hardly any provide detailed information on the case formulation, how the clinician arrived at it, the data to support or refute it, and so on.

The present book was designed to serve as a beginning attempt to illustrate the process and mechanics of case formulation. In the first chapter, Wolpe and Turkat review one approach to case formulation in general and present actual case transcripts with detailed commentaries to illustrate the thinking behind the clinician's actions. The remaining chapters follow an atypical format. Each chapter is preceded by a presentation of a complex case, each experiencing problems that typically are not covered in the literature (e.g., paranoid personality, sociopathy, conversion reaction). The authors of each chapter then attempt to explain how they would go about formulating this case in light of current literature and their own clinical and/or research experience with similar cases.

I hope that the reader finds these chapters stimulating and useful.

REFERENCES

Rachman, S. J., & Wilson, G. T. (1980). *The effects of psychological therapy* (2nd ed.). New York: Pergamon Press.

Wolpe, J. (1958). *Psychotherapy by reciprocal inhibition.* Stanford: Stanford University Press.

1

Behavioral Formulation of Clinical Cases

JOSEPH WOLPE and IRA DANIEL TURKAT

The basic premise of this text is that maximally effective clinical intervention is dependent upon an accurate understanding of the factors that cause and maintain disordered behavior. Despite the presentation of this clinical position over two decades ago (Wolpe, 1958), professional obsession with treatment technology has predominated.

The present chapter will focus on the behavioral formulation of clinical phenomena that provides the framework for idiographic adaption of empirical procedures. Because of the dearth of such discussion in the literature, we will illustrate the strategies and tactics involved in the behavioral conceptualization of clinical phenomena. Step-by-step descriptions of the behavioral framework for formulating clinical cases will be provided, followed by a number of clinical examples.

Theoretical understanding is necessary but by itself is insufficient. For a thorough conceptual consideration the reader is referred to earlier publications (e.g., Wolpe, 1958, 1976, 1982).

JOSEPH WOLPE • Department of Psychiatry, Temple University School of Medicine and Medical College of Pennsylvania, Philadelpia, Pennsylvania 19122.   IRA DANIEL TURKAT • Department of Psychology, University of North Carolina at Greensboro, Greensboro, North Carolina 27412.

THE HUMAN EXPERIENCE

Every human being is born with certain behavior potentials and limitations; we can see iron objects but not through them; we can empathize with others but cannot read minds; we can lift books but not buildings. Yet humans differ considerably in many of these abilities.

Individual differences become quite apparent when nongenetic factors are considered. Two children are attacked by the same dog. Both are bitten on the left shin; both children bleed and cry. On subsequent exposure to the dog, one child runs away whereas the other plays with the animal. Thus, a uniform stimulus appears to generate diverse reactions.

How can such variation be explained? Investigation reveals that the mother of the first child reacted to the attack with tears and screams; the other comforted her child and stroked the animal with her child's hand. Although simple in nature, this example illustrates the relationship between an environmental event and subsequent behavioral differences in reaction to that event.

The development, maintenance, and modification of pathological behavior, although more complex, is viewed similarly. Each individual presents a unique environmental history and behavioral reaction to it. The process is constant (i.e., learning mechanisms), but it is the content of such experience that determines the nature of pathological behavior.

Accurate understanding of an individual's behavior requires an investigation of idiosyncrasies. Thus, behavioral conceptualization of the human experience depends on operational descriptions of the phenomena of interest. Behavior is categorized according to three basic response systems (Lang, 1971; Wolpe, 1973), namely, the cognitive-verbal (e.g., thoughts, images), autonomic-somatic (e.g., respiration rate, arterial dilation) and overt-motoric (e.g., walking, hand movement). Within each category, there is infinite variability in response parameters (e.g., type, frequency) between and within individuals. Similarly, environmental events (e.g., objects, others' behavior) are infinitely diverse as well. The complexity of behavior-environment interactions is illustrated by Wolpe (1982, p. 14) in his hypothesized network of simultaneous and successive stimulus–response relations, to which the reader is referred. For the behavioral clinician, the human experience becomes understandable through operational descriptions of idiosyncratic phenomena.

In the search for idiographic relations between environment and behavior the principle of determinism is assumed. In essence, behavior is viewed as the result of certain conditions; when these conditions are manipulated systematically, behavioral consistency is observed. Given a deterministic view of behavior, the task of the clinician is to identify the precise relationships between environment and behavior for a given patient.

THE FRAMEWORK OF BEHAVIORAL CASE FORMULATION

Meyer and Turkat (1979) have suggested that the process of behavioral analysis and therapy follows a three-phase progression. First, the patient is *interviewed* so that a formulation of the presenting problems can be developed. This is followed by *clinical experimentation* which aims to validate the formulation (cf. Turkat & Maisto, 1983). Finally, a *modification methodology* is devised from the formulation and is implemented and monitored for its efficacy. In the present chapter, we will focus on how one develops a behavioral formulation.

Throughout all phases of behavior analysis and therapy, the clinician has one goal in mind: to help the patient maximally improve the quality of life. In this regard, *the clinician must be able to determine which behaviors among an infinite repertoire should be modified and which methods are most suited to do so.* Accordingly, the clinician's ability to sift through the data is the most critical ingredient in conducting a behavioral analysis.

INTERVIEWING THE PATIENT

The purpose of interviewing the patient is to gain as much *relevant* information as possible toward elucidating precisely what habits need to be changed. The critical information must answer the following questions:

1. What are the problems this patient is experiencing?
2. Which of any of these are behavioral problems (i.e., are any physiologically based)?
3. If psychologically based, what are the functional relations between environment and behavior?
4. Why have these developed and persisted?
5. What factors can produce change?

Modification methods for producing long-lasting changes can only be devised if these questions receive accurate answers. Resistance and relapse are common consequences of poor case conceptualization (Wolpe, 1977).

Meyer and Turkat (1979; Turkat & Meyer, 1982) have argued that the goal of interviewing the patient is to develop a formulation, defined as a hypothesis which

1. relates all of the presenting complaints to one another,
2. explains why these difficulties have developed, and
3. provides predictions of the patient's behavior given any stimulus conditions.

Development of an efficacious treatment program is facilitated by an accurate predictive model. Points one and two above provide the data for developing such a model. Operating with these considerations in mind, behavioral interviewing is progressive in nature. Information is elicited in a logical and systematic way. One does not jump randomly from topic to topic; hypotheses are tested until satisfactorily accepted or rejected. Thus, the interviewer attempts to cover only information that is required to develop a formulation, although at times he or she may cast a "wider net." Most important, the clinician must have well-formulated hypotheses which direct the interview. If the clinician is unsure as to what information to seek, it is unlikely that the patient will get what he or she requires.

The steps by which the required information is elicited will vary in sequence from case to case (Wolpe, 1980; 1982). Nevertheless, there are certain steps which are universal ingredients of a behavioral analysis. These are specification of

1. all of the patient's problems,
2. the onset of each problem,
3. the development of each problem, and
4. the predisposing factors.

The first interview begins with a quick survey of the patient's appearance, dress, posture, and so on, searching for possible clues about the patient. In most cases, nothing special immediately emerges. Then one typically asks the general question, "What seems to be the problem?" Depending on the patient's response, the clinician focuses on the presenting complaint and its maintaining factors, then proceeds to the specification of other problems. There is no standard order. Hypotheses and data determine the sequence of events.

In examining the presenting problem (and all behavioral phenomena for that matter), the clinician keeps to the facts as much as possible.

Responses of interest are fleshed out to fill in the picture. The information should be as complete as possible; when a patient says, "I am anxious," the clinician should try to know exactly what is meant by that statement. Investigation of all affected responses is undertaken within each of the basic response systems. Parameters of each response are specified, such as intensity, frequency, and duration. Finally, the sequence of responding is delineated as well.

Hypothesized maintaining factors are established by precise delineation of antecedents and consequences. As Turkat (1979) has noted in the behavior analysis matrix, behavioral reactions as well as environmental events can serve as important antecedents and consequences.

Etiological parameters are elucidated by examining the onset of each behavior problem and then tracing the developmental history through the present. All changes in the phenomenon are examined. Strict attention is paid to the consistency among antecedents, behaviors, and consequences. Once the onset and developmental information is derived, a search for predisposing factors is undertaken. In essence, the clinician seeks to identify those environmental and genetic factors which have promoted the patient's vulnerability to develop the current difficulties given the "right" conditions.

Examination of each problem presented by the patient provides the basis for discovery of the relationship between complaints. The interrelationships illuminate the primary problem(s) (i.e., that which serves as the basis for all of the presenting complaints) and becomes the major target for treatment. Clinical examples are presented in subsequent portions of this chapter.

RELATING TO THE PATIENT

There is no question but that the way the therapist relates to the patient is critical in formulating and treating a particular case. Many have argued that the therapist should play a Rogerian role, reflecting back in summary form what the patient has said to indicate understanding and to demonstrate empathy (Goldfried, 1982; Lazarus & Fay, 1982; Meichenbaum & Gilmore, 1982). As argued elsewhere (Turkat, 1982; Turkat, 1983; Turkat & Brantley, 1981), such an approach is incompatible with that of behavioral case formulation. Unquestionably, one must be able to empathize with the patient if one is to be able to formulate the case. However, the question as to what demonstrable empathy is remains the basis of difference. We would argue that *accurate empathy is demonstrated when the therapist can accurately predict the patient's behavior.* This difference in demonstrating empathy can be seen in the following example:

PATIENT: I get very nervous when I leave the house by myself, I just
    feel as if I were going to pass out.
ROGERIAN BEHAVIORAL INTERVIEWER: It must be upsetting when this
    happens.
PATIENT: Oh yes, I just want to run away.

Here, the clinician has "demonstrated empathy" by providing a summary statement of how the patient must have felt during this situation. This can be compared with the response of the skilled behavior analytic interviewer.

PATIENT: I get very nervous when I leave the house by myself, I just
    feel as if I were going to pass out.
BEHAVIOR ANALYTIC INTERVIEWER: Do you also get this feeling of passing
    out in airplanes? (*patient nods*), trains? (*patient nods*), elevators?
    (*patient nods*), crowds? (*patient nods*), and if you *can* make it
    to a movie, you sit in the last row, the seat closest to the exit?
PATIENT: That's me, all right.

Here, the interviewer is testing hypotheses the validity of which demonstrates more accurate empathy than a simple pseudo-expression of understanding as advocated by Rogerian approaches. In this regard, for the behavior-analytic clinician, the relationship to the patient is a means to an end; a good relationship exists if the clinician has created an environment for the patient which enables him to get the information he needs to make accurate predictions. This does not necessarily require reflective summary statements as advocated by the Rogerian approach. In fact, such time in the interview may be wasted. *Nondirective interactions in the interview are incompatible with the directive interview style of behavior analysis, unless, of course, a specific hypothesis is being tested.* Guidelines for establishing the appropriate therapeutic climate can be found in Wolpe (1982).

CLINICAL ILLUSTRATIONS

In this section, our purpose is to illustrate and elaborate some of the practical indicants of the behavioral framework for developing a clinical formulation. It is essential for the reader to recognize that the framework for behavioral case formulation is not a standardized procedure. Rather, it consists of the methodological guidelines for idiographic behavior therapy. Standardized procedures, be they assessment-oriented or treatment-oriented, have little relevance to the clinical activity of behavioral case formulation.

The Initial Interaction

As we mentioned previously, the initial interview begins with a brief scrutiny of the patient's physical characteristics and mannerisms. While recording the patient's name, age, and so forth, close examination of the patient's behavior and style often provides clues to the basic problem. Whether the clinican immediately begins questioning relevant to the initial hypothesis or seeks basic introductory data is the therapist's perogative. In any case, the clinician attempts to use all of the available data to begin formulation of an initial hypothesis.

DR. TURKAT: Please come in and have a seat.
PATIENT: Thank you, Dr. Turkat.

The clinician notices that the patient is very neatly dressed and appears stiff in walk. When seated, the patient's posture is formal as well: she sits on the edge of the seat; her shoulders are straight and erect; her left knee is perfectly placed over the right; hands are clasped around both knees; hair is perfectly groomed; lipstick is fresh; and eye brows are evenly lined. This information is used to begin the hypothesis testing process.

The patient has provided clues which can lead to inductively reasoned hypotheses, such as: Is she generally cautious? If so, why? Does she present herself so formally and properly because she demands perfection in herself? Is she excessively concerned about how she appears to others? Is she afraid of criticism? Is she a compulsive individual? She is probably not a very impulsive person. Accordingly, the therapist begins the interview with a variety of hypotheses in mind.

DR. TURKAT: Let me get some general information before we begin. Your name?
PATIENT: Mrs. Alice Green. A-l-i-c-e G-r-e-e-n.
DR. TURKAT: Age?
PATIENT: Thirty-four and a half years old. I was born on the eleventh of May, 1947.

The patient has provided further preliminary data in line with some of the initial hypotheses. Her answers are stiff, formal, and detailed. On the basis of this initial information, the clinican adopts a preliminary hypothesis, namely, that the patient is a perfectionist. Accordingly, he expects her to be fearful of making mistakes, being criticized, failing. He further expects interpersonal difficulties and perhaps depression. With this beginning hypothesis, the clinician moves on with the inquiry.

DR. TURKAT: You seem to be very good at providing the appropriate details.
PATIENT: It's funny that you should mention that.
DR. TURKAT: Why?
PATIENT: Sometimes I think that I . . . well, it bothers the heck out of my husband.
DR. TURKAT: Tell me about that.

Further investigation revealed the initial hypothesis to be correct. Accordingly, the interview was conducted in an efficient manner aimed at validating the hypotheses derived from the initial interaction. However, it is important to recognize that not many cases can be so quickly and easily conceptualized; the initial hypothesis often proves incorrect. Hypotheses are tested to generate data and the information is used to confirm or dispute such hypotheses. Behavioral case formulation demands that all of the data must be accounted for by the formulation.

The Initial Complaint

Since the process of behavioral case formulation cannot proceed without specific hypotheses to direct the clinical investigation, the therapist seeks to develop a hypothesis as quickly as possible. When the initial interaction does not provide sufficient data for hypothesis creation, examination of the initial complaint usually does. Thus, the clinician typically asks the general question, "What seems to be the problem?" Depending upon the patient's response, subsequent inquiry may take various paths. Following a description of the initial complaint, the clinician either: (1) examines the onset of the problem, (2) investigates maintaining factors, or (3) examines other problems the patient may be experiencing. It is difficult to describe operationally the points at which one must decide which route to take. In any event, all three lines of inquiry are necessary in order to be able to develop a behavioral formulation of the patient's difficulties.

As we have emphasized, the clinician attempts to develop a predictive model of the patient's behavior. When discussion of the initial complaint is followed by an analysis of the problem's onset, this facilitates prediction of maintaining factors. Similarly, when discussion of the initial complaint is followed by an examination of maintaining factors or other current problems, etiological variables may be predictable. As one fits together a jigsaw puzzle, one has a better picture of where the remaining pieces might fit. In each example, the clinician is attempting to validate hypotheses concerning the precise cause–effect relationships. An example of this type of inquiry following statement of the initial complaint is provided.

DR. WOLPE: What's your first name?
PATIENT: Brenda.
DR. WOLPE: And your age?
PATIENT: Forty.
DR. WOLPE: What's your phone number?
PATIENT: 828–1171.
DR. WOLPE: Well, what's your problem?
PATIENT: A fear of passing out.

At this point, the clinician begins hypothesis testing. The patient reports "a fear of passing out." An important consideration is the extent to which stimulus and response generalization has occurred. The clinician might hypothesize that "passing out" is a variation of "losing control" and that other possible responses such as going insane or having a heart attack are part of the clinical complex. Hypothesized stimuli include all situations in which "losing control" might be evident. Examples include seeing others lose control, driving a car, and the like. Somewhere in the history, the patient will usually report one or several experiences related to passing out or losing control. The essential point is that all available information is used to develop a hypothesis of a cause–effect relationship the validity of which is subsequently examined. The present example continues with a focus on etiological information.

DR. WOLPE: How long have you had this fear?
PATIENT: Since I was seventeen.
DR. WOLPE: Have you ever passed out?
PATIENT: No. That's the silly thing. I never have.

If the case is to be formulated appropriately, then the etiology of the problem should be clear. Since the patient suggests that she has never passed out, then it is necessary to identify whether this problem was conditioned indirectly or whether further investigation will reveal a direct conditioning etiology (see Wolpe, 1982; Wolpe & Wolpe, 1981). In the former case, the patient may never have actually passed out but may have had parents who taught her that losing control or consciousness was dangerous. Another possibility is that she witnessed others suffer punishing consequences for passing out. If the patient did have a direct conditioning etiology for this problem, then she must have lost consciousness at least once and aversive consequences must have occurred. With these points in mind, the clinician examines the onset of the problem.

DR. WOLPE: Can you remember how this began?
PATIENT: Ah, the first incident, I know, was in church at an Easter service and I felt very dizzy and I left the service and after that I was just afraid that it would recur. I remember my parents took me to a family doctor, but they never really found anything wrong after a lot of testing. Finally, it was diagnosed that my tonsils were causing inner ear problems. I had the tonsils removed but continued to have that fear. I don't know.

Although the patient described the first incident of the problem, it was still unclear why a fear of losing consciousness developed. Would all individuals who get dizzy at an Easter service become phobic? Probably not. It is necessary to test hypothesis as to why the patient became dizzy in the first place.

DR. WOLPE: Does that mean you do not believe it was due to your tonsils?
PATIENT: Possibly.

A considerable number of agoraphobics, whose basic fear is of losing control, report a history of dizziness produced by inner ear problems (Meyer, 1979). Whether the onset of the present patient's difficulties stemmed directly from this experience remains an empirical question. In any event, an elaboration of the presenting complaint is pursued to develop hypotheses pertinent to etiological factors as well as to validate the initial hypothesis.

DR. WOLPE: Well, you say you continue to have fear of passing out? What do you actually mean by that?

PATIENT: Of losing consciousness.

It is imperative that the precise antecedents and behaviors be established. The clinician attempts to tease out the precise stimuli of relevance.

DR. WOLPE: All the time?
PATIENT: Uh–in new situations.
DR. WOLPE: Only in new situations?
PATIENT: Not wholly. If I'm in a room such as a church or a meeting, something like that, I always make sure I'm near a door.

This latter report is consistent with the initial hypothesis. In most cases wherein loss of control is feared, crowded rooms indicate a possibility of being trapped (or out of control). The anticipatory avoidance response is to stay by the exit.

DR. WOLPE: Even if it's not a new situation?
PATIENT: Yes—uh-huh.
DR. WOLPE: Well, then, does this mean that it's only new situations or public situations, like being in church?
PATIENT: Public—more public, I would say than new.
DR. WOLPE: You don't have a fear of passing out when you're at home?
PATIENT: No.
DR. WOLPE: What about when you're at the homes of your friends?
PATIENT: Uh—I play bridge at the homes of friends quite a bit and I would say that I'm sometimes uncomfortable.
DR. WOLPE: What are the times?
PATIENT: I don't know how to differentiate.
DR. WOLPE: Well, can you point to any circumstances that might occur at the homes of your friends that would make you uncomfortable?
PATIENT: Not really. No.

The reader should note how the therapist is methodically testing out various stimulus situations, trying to identify the precise antecedents. Since the patient reports difficulty in identifying the antecedents herself, the clinician must take a different tack. Here, the clinician switches to understanding the responses that occur when the fear is present. Here, at least, the patient can describe the sensations and cognitions she experiences which may lead to discovering the antecedents of relevance.

DR. WOLPE: Well, how do you imagine this passing out would happen?
PATIENT: Since I never have, it's hard to imagine, although occasionally
    I have a weak feeling and my knees start to shake a little bit. My
    hands perspire.

The patient unquestionably experiences autonomic arousal. Her
cognitions during these experiences may aid in understanding the feared
stimuli.

DR. WOLPE: And what do you think could happen after that?
PATIENT: I don't really know. I guess just drop over. I could be wrong
    but I've been doing a lot of thinking about how it could have
    started and I remember when I was five I had an eye operation.
    In those days the parents weren't allowed in the hospital and you
    weren't told about it beforehand. I remember being dropped off
    at the hospital very frightened, and a few days later a voice saying
    "That gown means you're going to have surgery." And then very
    vividly remembering the ether. And it's that feeling sometimes. I
    refused to have an anesthetic when I had my four children.

Several points should be made here. First, the patient described
a traumatic out-of-control experience at the age of five; she was unaware
of impending surgery and was without her parents (i.e., security).
Apparently, the terror of an unanticipated operation with no possible
escape was paired with the loss of consciousness from ether. Second,
subsequent avoidance of losing consciousness was reinforced during
four pregnancies. Finally, the reader should note that the latter response
was the type of information sought in the beginning of the interview.
Unfortunately, it did not immediately emerge. This exemplifies why
one should not rely implicitly on the patient's report; etiological information helps to clarify the consistency of the independent-dependent
variable relationships.

DR. WOLPE: Well, what was the effect on you when the voice said you
    were going to have to have ether?
PATIENT: He didn't say anything about ether. He just said "You're going
    to have an operation." I just remember total terror. In those days,
    there was no shot before you went up into the room. So, I don't
    know.

It now appeared that direct conditioning had occurred. The patient
was brought to a hospital for an operation without any understanding

as to why or what was to be involved. When told that an operation was to be performed, a five-year-old's natural response is to be frightened. This autonomic arousal was then paired with ether, forcing her to lose consciousness. This explanatory hypothesis is explored further for its validity.

DR. WOLPE: When they dropped you at the hospital they didn't tell you that you were going to have an operation?
PATIENT: No. No.
DR. WOLPE: Do you remember the anesthetic?
PATIENT: Yes.
DR. WOLPE: You say when the boy told you, you had total terror.
PATIENT: Well, maybe not so much when the boy told me. It was getting on that cart.
DR. WOLPE: I see. He told you just before.
PATIENT: Yes—when they brought in the surgical gown.
DR. WOLPE: I see. So, when did you have the total terror?
PATIENT: Being in the room, I remember bottles on the wall, or something like that and then being told to breathe into something.
DR. WOLPE: Did you struggle?
PATIENT: I don't know.

To test the hypothesis that this earlier experience relates to the present difficulty, the patient is asked to comment on the similarities.

DR. WOLPE: You said that a feeling that you recall from that time is in some way similar to the feeling that you have now?
PATIENT: Uh-huh.
DR. WOLPE: In what respect?
PATIENT: Just a feeling of a slight dizziness. Sounds getting louder maybe.
DR. WOLPE: Uh-huh. You said a few minutes ago that sometimes you have a kind of, well, dimming reaction. You say your knees shake, your hands perspire; do you feel giddy? Dizzy?
PATIENT: Not too giddy.
DR. WOLPE: Well, you said three things. What is the third thing you said? Knees shake, hands perspire—
PATIENT: I don't think I would say—I probably have never been that giddy.
DR. WOLPE: What are the feelings that you have?
PATIENT: A light-headed feeling—yes.
DR. WOLPE: Does that have some similarity to this terror experience when you were five? Or what?

PATIENT: Pardon me?

DR. WOLPE: What is the similarity? Where do you see the similarity between the present fear and what happened when you were five?

PATIENT: The light-headed feeling, and, as I say, it's just a feeling of things going up and down. I don't know how to explain that.

DR. WOLPE: Things going up and down? Do you mean the world seems to go up and down?

PATIENT: It doesn't tilt or slide. I don't know how to really explain it.

The patient demonstrates difficulty in expressing her reactions. It is incumbent upon the therapist to collect the data he or she requires, by providing an example for comparison:

DR. WOLPE: You know, something that children often do is, they sort of spin themselves around and around. Then they sit on the floor and the world seems to—

PATIENT: It may be slightly like that, but not to that extent.

DR. WOLPE: But it's something of that sort?

PATIENT: Yes.

The clinician seems confident of the relationship between the present fear and the operation at age 5. A developmental trace is undertaken.

DR. WOLPE: Did you have any other fearful experiences?

PATIENT: I don't believe so.

DR. WOLPE: Well, after the age of six, between the ages of 6 and 17, did you have any fearful experiences?

PATIENT: No. I would say not.

DR. WOLPE: Okay. On this occasion when you were 17 you had dizziness at the Easter service. Have you ever had dizziness again?

PATIENT: Well, in just some of these situations.

DR. WOLPE: You mean public situations.

PATIENT: Yes.

DR. WOLPE: You mean if you were going say, into a crowded room, you would become dizzy?

PATIENT: Yes. Not if I'm near a door. You know, the easy escape route!

DR. WOLPE: Well, when you become dizzy, is it that you then think that you may lose consciousness?

PATIENT: Yes.

DR. WOLPE: Do you feel fearful without feeling dizzy?

PATIENT: Oh, yes. Yes. Every morning when I think of my schedule for the day. It's so silly.

To validate further the initial hypothesis, the therapist predicts the content of the patient's thinking about her daily schedule and pursues current parameters.

DR. WOLPE: Well, when you think of your schedule for the day, what are you thinking about? The possible situations that may in a sense endanger you?

PATIENT: Exactly. And after I get through the first one or two safely, then usually the rest of the day is good.

DR. WOLPE: Can you suggest what there is about a crowd situation that makes it particularly dangerous from this point of view?

PATIENT: Just no way of ready escape. I don't know.

DR. WOLPE: You said that you had refused to have anesthetics at other times? Have you never had an anesthetic since the age of 17?

PATIENT: I don't believe so. No.

DR. WOLPE: And you've never been unconscious at all?

PATIENT: No.

DR. WOLPE: So that means that nobody has seen you in a state of unconsciousness?

PATIENT: No.

The clinician now has a general understanding of the anxiety response and how it may have developed through direct conditioning. Given this understanding, the clinician returns to an examination of the stimuli which currently elicit the anxiety.

DR. WOLPE: But somebody has seen you in a state of sleep? Is that right?

PATIENT: Yes. That's natural.

DR. WOLPE: That's okay?

PATIENT: Yes.

DR. WOLPE: Well, these crowd situations, or fearful situations, are there any other fearful situations?

PATIENT: Sometimes driving, car-pooling with neighbors, when I'm taking the children places—I'm fine in the car alone, but in our neighborhood—we live in the car—taking children to all activities.

DR. WOLPE: Does that also at times make for dizziness or not?

PATIENT: The trembling and sweaty hands, but no, I wouldn't say dizziness.

DR. WOLPE: Well, in those situations, do you ever have a fear that you might lose consciousness?

PATIENT: Yes.

DR. WOLPE: Any other situations?

PATIENT: We belong to a swim club and I have to go when my five-year-old wants to go in the deeper water. I have to be with him. I'm out there with a lot of people, diving around me, and that—

DR. WOLPE: That makes you feel afraid?

PATIENT: Uh-huh.

DR. WOLPE: Well, do you then also think you might lose consciousness?

PATIENT: Yes—there again.

At this point, the clinician must determine the degree to which any anxiety might serve as a conditioned stimulus for possible impending loss of consciousness or control.

DR. WOLPE: Sometimes a person has anxiety due to, you know, what you might call legitimate causes. Has that happened to you?

PATIENT: Yes.

DR. WOLPE: Give me an example.

PATIENT: Well, a serious illness in the family, something like that.

DR. WOLPE: Well, when that happens you appear anxious too?

PATIENT: Yes, but maybe no more anxious than normal.

DR. WOLPE: Yes, but when you feel anxious, under those circumstances, do you have the same feeling of hands sweating, trembling, etc.?

PATIENT: Well, if it's a real crisis, no—maybe when it's over, but I seem to be able to handle it.

DR. WOLPE: Okay. Then you say you begin to get trembling and sweaty. Well, when that happens, do you have any fear that you might lose consciousness?

PATIENT: Yes.

DR. WOLPE: You do—even then?

PATIENT: Oh, no, not then. It's more of a relief-type thing.

It is clear that not all anxiety-related situations will lead to fear of passing out. The stimuli of relevance are being narrowed down.

DR. WOLPE: Okay. So, when somebody's ill, there's something rather special in regard to that. But there are other kinds of fearful situations, like possibly the fear of being late for an appointment.

PATIENT: Oh, I'm compulsive. I'm always five minutes early.

The patient describes herself as generally being compulsive. It is important to determine whether she was trained to be like this by her parents and whether this predisposed her to develop the fear of passing out as a result of the hospital experience at age five. Another possibility is that the "compulsive" behavior is a consequence of attempts to avoid stimuli which could lead to the sensations of passing out (e.g., anxiety about being late for an appointment). Furthermore, she may not really be compulsive. These aspects must be explained if the case is to be formulated in full.

DR. WOLPE: Well, supposing circumstances compelled you to be late. Would you become anxious?

PATIENT: Yes. But not with a fear.

DR. WOLPE: Then you wouldn't have a fear?

PATIENT: No. I don't think so.

DR. WOLPE: What is the difference between the anxiety that you have about being late and the anxiety that you have in a crowd? I mean the difference in the feeling.

PATIENT: I sometimes think if I'm afraid of being late, I'm so concerned about that, that I forget to be anxious about it. All my energies are concentrated on getting there on time.

DR. WOLPE: What about the kind of anxiety you might have if there was danger? You know the situation, for example, say you are in a boat in a storm. Something of that sort. Has that every happened to you?

PATIENT: No. I don't think I've ever been in a very dangerous situation.

DR. WOLPE: So, this fear of passing out is the only important problem in your life.

PATIENT: Yes. I would say so.

DR. WOLPE: If that was taken away—

PATIENT: That would be wonderful.

DR. WOLPE: Your life would be quite importantly different?

PATIENT: Yes.

DR. WOLPE: Let me get some of your background.

PATIENT: Okay.

The problem presented by the patient is straightforward and the primary target of treatment is established. To gather the specifics of etiology which might aid in validating the stimuli hypothesized to be involved, the therapist begins to investigate possible predisposing factors.

The reader should note that the interview was directive and empathetic. Hypotheses were continuously tested. The precise antecedents of responses were investigated. Several predictions proved to be accurate.

Pursuit of Hypotheses

At any stage during the assessment and treatment of an individual case, the clinician must be certain that his or her particular hypotheses are valid. In certain instances, contradictory data may emerge. In such cases, it is incumbent upon the therapist to decide if the hypothesis is correct and the data are invalid or if the hypothesis must be modified. Patients often present contradictory data, purposely or inadvertently. When an hypothesis has considerable data to support it in the face of newly emerging inconsistent data, the hypothesis should be pursued. The therapist should attempt to understand why a discrepancy exists. Often the discrepancy is due to not asking the right questions. On the other hand, when the data are consistently contrary to the therapist's prediction, the hypothesis should be abandoned.

Many tactics are available for pursuing a hypothesis that might resolve the discrepancy. Patients often respond to an idiosyncratic stimulus and not the antecedent of interest (i.e., intended basis of the question) provided by the clinician. At times, asking the question in a different way or returning to the question at a later point in the interview provides the expected response after all (Wolpe, 1980). In certain cases, the therapist frankly explains the hypothesis–data discrepancy to the patient and asks for clarification. An example is presented below.

DR. TURKAT: Okay, now, you are going to have to help me. You tell me that you are attracted to both men and women. We have examined your sexual history in detail and I cannot identify one instance where you have had sexual experiences or even fantasies involving women. Your first orgasm occurred at the oral stimulation of your cousin, Robert. You continued to have this relationship with him for two months during your summer vacation at your aunt's. You masturbated to this fantasy for some time. You met Jack and have now lived with him sexually and no one else. You have not indicated any experiences with females, any masturbating fantasies about females, or any instances where you seemed sexually aroused to a female. I cannot understand why you say that you are sexually attracted to women.

PATIENT: Well, I don't know. I just am.

The clinician checks to see if he has missed any direct conditioning experiences.

DR. TURKAT: Can you give me one example where you either had a sexual encounter with a woman, masturbatory experience with a woman involved, or experienced an erection in the presence of a woman?

PATIENT: Let me think. Well, kind of. Last week I saw a lady at the library and I thought that she was attractive. I even felt as if it would be great to be with her.

Again, it is critical to determine whether direct conditioning occurred or not.

DR. TURKAT: Okay. Did you feel or notice any physical changes such as erection or otherwise in her presence or afterwards?

PATIENT: No.

DR. TURKAT: Anything at all?

PATIENT: No, just this thought that it would be nice to be with her.

DR. TURKAT: Did you imagine what this would be like or how it would be if it occurred?

PATIENT: No.

At this point it is clear that no direct conditioning occurred. It is necessary to explain what this patient meant by "feeling attracted" to this woman.

DR. TURKAT: Earlier you told me that last week when you visited your parents you felt guilty that you did not have a girlfriend like your older brother. Did this occur on the same day?

PATIENT: I think so. Yes it did, I remember.

DR. TURKAT: Now, Blake. Very often I see patients with similar problems. They are attracted only to males but would *like* to be attracted to females, even though they aren't sexually aroused by them. Often, they think they are attracted to females because they *want* to be, even though they aren't actually attracted. Is this what you mean when you say you are sexually attracted to females?

PATIENT: You've hit it on the head.

The above example is common when working with homosexual males who claim to be bisexual (see Tollison & Adams, 1979). If the interview does not resolve the hypothesis–data discrepancy, one may test the patient's sexual responses to various stimuli by monitoring sexual arousal by strain gauge and polygraph. The essential point is that contradictory data must be accounted for. Thus, tenable hypotheses must be pursued until a clear relationship emerges. The clinician must be careful, however, not to bulldoze the patient to "fall in line" with the therapist's hypothesis. Otherwise, treatment is bound to be misdirected.

The reader should recognize that the examination of hypotheses is not limited to information from the patient. Significant others may sometimes have to be interviewed. Certain records perhaps should be obtained. At times, the therapist may have to change settings when seeing the patient or visit the patient in his or her natural setting. The methods employed depend on the nature of questions being asked. As an example of pursuing a hypothesis beyond the level of discussion, we join Wolpe in a subsequent session with Brenda. At this point, the clinician is interested in testing a hypothesis about the chain of events regarding the anxiety Brenda feels which leads to dizziness.

DR. WOLPE: How do you feel right now?
PATIENT: Fairly relaxed.
DR. WOLPE: Well, I like to quantify communication and if I say to you, "How do you feel," and you say, "Quite calm, or pretty nervous" or something like this, this gives me information, but it's very imprecise. We can improve communication by using figures—in this way. Think of the worst anxiety you ever had, a state of panic and call that 100; then think of being absolutely calm—that's 0, so you have a kind of scale. Now, on that scale, how would you rate yourself at this moment?

The therapist has introduced the Subjective Unit of Discomfort (SUD) Scale (see Wolpe, 1973) to facilitate accurate communication about experienced anxiety. He then shapes the patient to use the scale by means of going over events in the patient's life.

PATIENT: About 50.
DR. WOLPE: Okay. When you came in here was it any different?
PATIENT: Yes, about 80 I would say.
DR. WOLPE: And this morning when you were at home?
PATIENT: Ninety.
DR. WOLPE: Why was it so high this morning?
PATIENT: Well, just thinking of the trip down. I had to take my son to nursery school this morning and then come here.

DR. WOLPE: When you arrived here, though, you say it was 80.

PATIENT: Yes.

DR. WOLPE: Why was it that high?

PATIENT: I guess because I waited in that small room so long this morning in the office.

This is consistent with being trapped and therefore losing control. Note the therapist asking "why" questions as tests of prediction.

DR. WOLPE: In the future, come straight here.

PATIENT: Okay.

DR. WOLPE: Now, you are 50. What do you think is making you 50 right now? Let me start in a different way. On an average day, what is the range of anxiety through which you go?

PATIENT: I guess most mornings it's about 80, then by afternoon it's down to 50 and by dinner not too bad, 20.

DR. WOLPE: Twenty. Do you ever go down to 0?

PATIENT: Yes. I suppose so.

DR. WOLPE: Well, why do you think it goes down on a whole lot like this in the course of a day?

PATIENT: Well, the silly things I worry about—nothing has happened.

DR. WOLPE: I think I know what you mean by this, but I'm not entirely sure, so would you just tell me what you mean by silly things?

Again, the therapist takes precautions to avoid miscommunication by asking the patient to define what she means by her global statement.

PATIENT: Well, chauffeuring children here and there and shopping, meetings.

DR. WOLPE: Are you not sure of your capability of doing these things? Is that part of it?

PATIENT: I don't think so.

DR. WOLPE: Or is it perhaps that you think you may become dizzy?

PATIENT: Yes—that's it.

DR. WOLPE: That's there all the time?

PATIENT: Yes.

DR. WOLPE: So, that means you are better in the evening because by then the threats are behind you.

PATIENT: Yes, It's a sense of relief in the evening.

DR. WOLPE: If you were to go away on a holiday and had no particular burdens at all?

PATIENT: I'm absolutely okay. We were just in Miami at a convention. Absolutely fine.

We may note the series of predictions made by the therapist which were confirmed.

DR. WOLPE: Quite calm, down to about 0.
PATIENT: Except for one, just one experience, it was just fine, you know.

Given the basic formulation of this case, the therapist would predict that the one experience was related to being trapped or losing control. Rather than stating this, the therapist keeps it in mind, expecting it to emerge.

DR. WOLPE: What was the experience?
PATIENT: Well, the wives were to go to a luncheon and fashion show. There were maybe a thousand women at the convention along with their husbands, and the luncheon was to start at 12:00. I went down to the lobby to get in line to go into the luncheon and by 12:15 the doors still hadn't opened and there were a thousand women all jammed together. I just left. That was the only time.
DR. WOLPE: Otherwise you were really happy and relaxed.
PATIENT: Right.

The hypothesized stimuli (e.g., trapped, control) are confirmed; there is no need to go over this in detail with the patient.

DR. WOLPE: Now, as you're sitting here, is your mind on things that are going to happen later on today?
PATIENT: No.
DR. WOLPE: So is there anything else that can be making you tense while you're sitting here?
PATIENT: I don't think so.
DR. WOLPE: Is your score going down?
PATIENT: I would say so.

The patient is becoming more relaxed and presents a good opportunity to test the hypothesis concerning dizziness mentioned earlier. The SUD scale is still used.

DR. WOLPE: Now there's one thing that I want to test out with you. First of all, when your score was 90 this morning, did you get dizzy at all?

PATIENT: No.

DR. WOLPE: When you were in that crowd in Miami, did you get dizzy?

PATIENT: No.

DR. WOLPE: What was your score?

PATIENT: Oh, 100, I guess.

DR. WOLPE: 100 means you were as anxious as you can get.

PATIENT: Oh no, 90, because I have gotten a little bit dizzier on occasions maybe.

DR. WOLPE: Then this morning there was a 90, or do you want to reevaluate it?

PATIENT: Eighty, I guess.

DR. WOLPE: And when you arrived here?

PATIENT: That would be 80 too.

DR. WOLPE: Do you become dizzy when you are at 100?

PATIENT: Uh-huh.

DR. WOLPE: Now I would like to do a test with you because that may tell us what it is about anxiety that makes you dizzy. What I would like you to do is to get comfortable, just sit back comfortably. I want you to breathe very rapidly like this (*breathes rapidly*) Deeply and rapidly. I'm going to time you. When a person does this, various sensations and experiences can happen. I want you to report to me every feeling that you have. Just report it quickly and then go on breathing that same way.

(*Patient breathes*)

DR. WOLPE: Faster.

PATIENT: I may be a little bit dizzy now.

DR. WOLPE: Go on.

PATIENT: (*Keeps breathing*) Rapid heart beat. (*keeps breathing*) Dizzier.

DR. WOLPE: Go on.

PATIENT: (*Keeps breathing*) I'd better not smoke anymore.

DR. WOLPE: Go on.

PATIENT: My knees are a little trembly.

DR. WOLPE: Go on.

PATIENT: Dizzier.

DR. WOLPE: Go on. Faster.

PATIENT: Not too much change anymore.

DR. WOLPE: Well is it anything like your dizziness?

PATIENT: Yes. Like 100 almost.

DR. WOLPE: Do you feel anxious?

PATIENT: Surprisingly not too. No.

DR. WOLPE: There's no reason why you should because nothing is happening here to make you feel anxious, but what is important here is that we have shown how you get dizzy. If we went on like this for 5 minutes you would be very dizzy. You see, when you're anxious, and especially when you're very anxious, various things happen in your body. Your heart beats faster, your hands sweat and you breathe faster.

PATIENT: Oh.

DR. WOLPE: Breathing faster has the effect of washing out carbon dioxide from your bloodstream. Though we all get rid of carbon dioxide, our blood chemistry requires a certain amount. One result of getting rid of a little too much carbon dioxide is that you get dizzy. Knowing this gives us a way of controlling the dizziness. You can stop the dizziness by not allowing yourself to overbreathe—quite simply by keeping your mouth firmly shut in the situations where you became anxious. It's impossible to overbreathe if your mouth is shut.

Etiology

Throughout this chapter, we have emphasized that behavior therpay is an idiographic approach to maladaptive behavior which is based on learning mechanisms. As such, the etiology of problematic behavior provides the core for developing a behavioral formulation and subsequent use of a modification methodology. In earlier publications (Meyer & Turkat, 1979; Turkat & Meyer, 1982; Wolpe, 1958; 1973), etiological inquiry was considered to address predisposing factors, trace the problem from onset to present (development), and establish current parameters (maintenance). Predisposing factors will be addressed in the next section.

Behavior therapists have recognized for some time that the cause and maintenance of disordered behavior may differ. However, causative factors not only provide insight into current parameters (Wolpe, 1958, 1980) but facilitate the clinician's ability to make predictions. The animal literature has shown that previous behavior is often an excellent predictor of future behavior (Morse & Kelleher, 1977). Such data are consistent with the assumptions of behavioral analysis.

Examination of the onset, course, and maintenance of disordered behavior involves a variety of steps. These may be listed as follows:

1. An operational account of the very first occurrence of the presenting problem
2. An exhaustive specification of the precise independent and dependent variables

3. Observation of the consistency and/or change in such variables during the course of the problem's development
4. Delineation of current independent and dependent variable relationships
5. Completion of steps 1 through 4 for each and every problem the patient presents or is perceived to experience

In beginning the etiological inquiry, the patient is generally asked, "When did this problem first occur?" The clinician then shapes the patient to articulate the relevant information. The precise antecedents and their effects on behavior are delineated. The response systems affected and the unique molecular responses (e.g., elevated heart rate, cognitive label of event) are operationalized as well. The consequences of such experiences are examined, and then a thorough chronological tracking to the present is undertaken. Potential predisposing factors (see subsequent section) are investigated in light of the presented data.

In order to develop a behavioral formulation, the clinician must understand the development and maintenance of the patient's behavioral repetoire. The data must make sense. Thus, the presented history should seem appropriate to the patient's current complaints. For example, if the patient presents a phobia of specific stimulus, somewhere in the history the patient will usually recall episodes in which the current stimulus was directly (or indirectly) paired with autonomic arousal and motor avoidances.

Predisposing Factors

In conceptualizing the etiology of disordered behavior, one should be able to explain why one patient develops a clinical disorder and another does not, given exposure to the same stimulus situation. The concept of *predisposing factors* facilitates explaining such individual differences. Wolpe (1958) has defined a predisposing factor as "any factor that facilitates the acquisition of [neurotic] behavior in a subject exposed to [characteristic] precipitating conditions" (p. 76; our parentheses). In other words, predisposing factors promote a patient's susceptibility to develop a specific problem, given certain conditions.

The definition of predisposing factors given above implies that absence of such factors reduces the individual's susceptibility to develop a particular problem. The above definition does *not* suggest that predisposing factors are *essential* for developing a particular behavior problem; such factors only *facilitate* the acquisition of behavior. In utilizing the concept of predisposing factors to conceptualize behavior etiology, *the behavioral formulation specifies the particular relevant predisposing conditions.* Illustrations will follow.

Wolpe (1958; 1973; 1980) has identified a variety of areas which have common predisposing (and, for that matter, precipitating) conditions for many behavior disorders. Such background information includes early family life, parental and sibling characteristics and interaction styles, religious training, educational experiences, social relations, sexual experiences, and other variables (Wolpe, 1982). Although examination of all of this information may not always prove relevant, one cannot formulate a case appropriately without explaining etiology. Thus, one must hypothesize certain predisposing factors.

During the clinical interview, the search for predisposing conditons follows specification of current parameters, problem onset, and development. The preliminary formulation which is based on such information directs the search for specific predisposing conditions. For example, the socially inept individual is likely to have had parental models for such behavior (i.e., vicarious conditioning), promoting a lack of opportunity to acquire appropriate skills (operant conditioning) and, perhaps, traumatic consequences such as social rejection resulting in the present social anxiety (classical conditioning) problem. Another example is the case of Mrs. R. (see Turkat & Meyer, 1982). This individual presented an incapacitating vomit phobia. Etiological inquiry revealed that the patient had been exposed to vomiting situations without any anxiety during early childhood. At the same time, however, the patient was an only child, her mother died when she was three, and Mrs. R. was raised by a perfectionistic father who criticized her constantly. As early as age 3, she reported experiences indicating a fear of the father's criticism but no fear of vomiting. At age 5, she joined her father on a road trip and they stopped along the highway to get a drink. For some reason, the drink she had was spoiled and she vomited. Her father reacted with anger and ordered her not to vomit again, particularly in his car. The patient began to fear vomiting and to perform avoidance responses. This developed into an incapacitating phobia as an adult. It appeared that her original hypersensitivity to criticism predisposed her to develop a fear of *any unpredictable stimulus which led to criticism.* Thus, the vomiting phobia might not have developed had she not developed the original sensitivity to criticism. Her treatment involved not only the vomiting-related stimuli but criticism exposures as well (see Turkat & Meyer, 1982).

The above illustration points up the necessity of formulating the etiology of behavioral problems including predisposing factors if an effective modification program is to be developed.

Presenting the Formulation

In certain cases it is useful to present the formulation to the patient. Although not always necessary, doing so can solidify the clinician's confidence in it. The clinician attempts to relate all the data provided, explain why the current difficulties developed, and provide predictions based on this information. Typically, the presentation begins with an introductory statement such as "Given the information with which you have provided me, I want to give you my view of what the problems are and why they developed." A description of the current problems is provided and then a discussion of predisposing factors, etiology, and current parameters ensues. The patient's unique history is described so that he can understand the formulation. He is invited to comment on, evaluate, and confirm or refute all aspects of the formulation.

It should be remembered that presentation of the formulation has been preceded by earlier shaping of the patient's conceptualization of his problems and their development. Further, as various operational descriptions have been obtained, the clinician often interprets these and reflects this understanding back (note: this should not be confused with standard Rogerian reflection statements) seeking confirmation. Thus, the patient has typically been "shaped" toward the clinician's understanding of his dilemma and the formal presentation ties all the data together.

The following illustration of a presented formulation involves the case of a seventeen-year-old insulin-dependent diabetic female who was referred because of "inexplicable hyperglycemic episodes." Many diabetics respond to psychological stress with increased presence of glucose in the blood (among other responses), and this appeared to contribute to the patient's problems with carbohydrate metabolism status. Additionally, the patient was hypersensitive to criticism resulting in text anxiety, overconcern with others' scrutiny and opinions of her, tension headaches, and depression. She described her parents as over-protective, demanding, exceptionally critical, and perfectionistic.

DR. TURKAT: Okay, let's recap. I want to see if I understand you very well. As we go along, comment as to whether I am right, wrong, or whatever. Okay?

PATIENT: Fine.

DR. TURKAT: Right. Okay. You're seventeen now. You feel anxious in many situations where others' opinions of you are important such as taking tests, interacting with your friends at school, dating, making errors in front of your parents, and so forth. You experience tension headaches and the doctors are concerned about your diabetes, the sugars being high.

PATIENT: That's right.

DR. TURKAT: There's no doubt that your mom has had and continues to have great influence on you. She is a very, very perfectionistic kind of person. Very concerned about what people think of her and her family, and also she has very high standards about how you and your brothers should behave. She taught you as a kid that you should always present a good image to people, always be very concerned about what they think of you, people should always like you, right?

PATIENT: Yes. She wants us all to put on a good image.

DR. TURKAT: So as a little kid you start developing the idea that you have to do things to make people really like you and thus, anytime any little indication that you're not doing the right thing or you're not making a good impression makes you very upset. Your mother is particularly like this and has taught you to be like her in this regard. Even as a young child, you indicated having this sensitivity and shyness around other people, particularly your parent's friends and other authority figures such as teachers. Then at age nine you become diabetic and, given this background and training that "I should always do things right and good" and "people should like me," you interpret this as "I must have done something wrong and I'm being punished, I'm not being a good person." Then you get a little older, puberty, junior high school, where peers and friends become very important to you, and here's a perfect place to become even more concerned about doing the right thing, so you generally try to be very good to your friends and you really want them to like you very much. You start having to take tests and you worry, "Will I do the right thing? Will I prepare very well? Will I blow this exam? What will my teacher think of me?" You can stop me at any point and comment.

PATIENT: I know; it's all right so far.

DR. TURKAT: Okay. You become a very, very sensitive little girl so that feedback from anyone that you're not doing things right upsets you. You cry, get depressed, and you start getting headaches, from tension. The tension you get is so constant because you're always thinking "Am I doing the right thing? Am I being a good person? Am I doing the things I'm supposed to"? And, you get on yourself practically all the time. Therefore, you're continuously on the lookout for any sign that you've made a mess of it, and as soon as it happens you overreact and get extremely upset, right?

PATIENT: Yes.

DR. TURKAT: Okay. So when you are criticized or expect to be, you become anxious, leave the situation or avoid it, and then see yourself as being a terrible, inept person. Thus, you come home from school each day, you do your chores, your mom criticizes your performance, and you run up to your room. You then stay there, trying to avoid further criticism. But you think about how inept you are, what others such as your friends and the guys you've dated think of you. Naturally, you get depressed. Well?

PATIENT: It's true.

DR. TURKAT: Okay. Your parents are concerned about protecting you, and you very often resent this because their standards for you to do everything perfectly and right are so high. So when you make a mistake, you get upset by it and anticipate what they are going to think of you, right?

PATIENT: (Nods head)

DR. TURKAT: Having such stress, that is all, this criticism of a girl who is very fearful of criticism could help explain why your blood glucose is so high. As you know, emotions affect diabetes. But sometimes, when you run up to your room after your parents criticize you, you eat a bunch of candy bars. Of course, you're not going to let them know you did it because you're afraid they will get angry that you did something like that. So it's really quite clear if you look at your history why you developed this way, what all the problems are, their relationship. What do you think about all that?

PATIENT: What's to say?

DR. TURKAT: You must have some thoughts.

PATIENT: It's true.

DR. TURKAT: Does what I've said make sense?

PATIENT: (Nods head)

DR. TURKAT: What aspects about it are true and are not?

PATIENT: (Smiles)

DR. TURKAT: Well, was there anything I said that wasn't right?

PATIENT: You understand me.

DR. TURKAT: Now the question is, what do we do? On the basis of this understanding it seems that the basic thing that's causing all these difficulties is your excessive concern about what everyone is thinking of you. So if you somehow learned how not to care or take as dearly as you do people's reactions then you probably wouldn't get upset so much, your headaches would probably go, and your sugar would come back down. I would expect you to be

not so depressed because you would not be upset all the time.
Now, what's the possibility of doing that? There are procedures
that can be used to help you to become less sensitive or, in essence,
desensitized to criticism.

Given the patient's agreement on the relationship among the presented problems and their etiology, a discussion of treatment indicants
and predictions of efficacy is then provided.

The reader should note that the style of conversation was conducted in words that the patient might have used. The data she provided
were employed in presenting the clinician's understanding. Continual
checking for confirmation and reiteration of points helped to be certain
the patient was clear on the formulation. The relationship between
complaints was made clear and the primary problem was illuminated
as the major treatment target. Finally, the formulation provided the
necessary framework for developing clinical predictions.

The novice to behavioral case formulation often asks "What if the
patient doesn't agree?" If the patient disagrees, this is very useful information. Clearly, the formulation is in need of modification and discrepancies must be resolved. In practice, it is relatively rare for this to
occur because the operational analysis of the patient's problems and
history (which is required in order to develop a formulation) has already
been discussed. The patient has been prepared throughout the interview
to perceive the clinician's understanding. The typical patient reaction
is one of agreement, relief, and optimism because understanding one's
problems elicits expectations that something can be done (this of course
does not mean that insight will change the problem). Because of the
emphasis on learning, the patient can feel that he or she is normal and
not crazy.

CONCLUSION

Throughout this chapter we have argued that the practice of behavior therapy is an idiographic approach to clinical phenomena based on
scientific principles. Before one can test a hypothesis in the laboratory,
one must first be able to specify the relevant independent and dependent variables in precise detail. In the clinical arena, one must do the
same in order to develop an appropriate intervention methodology.
Thus, the major prerequisite for successful treatment is an accurate
understanding of the patient's problems.

The framework for behavioral case formulation demands that the clinician "put himself on the line" by continually creating and evaluating specific testable hypotheses concerning the patient's dilemma. Given the complexity of life and the idiosyncratic nature of problems presented by patients, successful clinical intervention depends largely on the ingenuity and skill of the clinician. It is our hope that the present chapter will facilitate successful outcomes in the clinical practice of behavior therapy.

REFERENCES

Goldfried, M. R. (1982). Resistance and clinical behavior therapy. In P. L. Wachtel (Ed.), *Resistance: Psychodynamic and behavioral approaches.* New York: Plenum Press.

Lang, P. J. (1976). The application of psychophysiological methods to the study of psychotherapy and behavior modification. In A. E. Bergin & S. L. Garfield (Eds.), *Handbook of psychotherapy and behavior change: An empirical analysis.* New York: Wiley.

Lazarus, A. A., & Fay, A. (1982). Resistance or rationalization? A cognitive-behavioral perspective. In P. L. Wachtel (Ed.), *Resistance: Psychodynamic and behavioral approaches.* New York: Plenum Press.

Meichenbaum, D., & Gilmore, J. B. (1982). Resistance from a cognitive-behavioral perspective. In P. L. Wachtel (Ed.), *Resistance: Psychodynamic and behavioral approaches.* New York: Plenum Press.

Meyer, V. (1979). Personal communication to IDT, London.

Meyer, V., & Turkat, I. D. (1979). Behavioral analysis of clinical cases. *Journal of Behavioral Assessment, 1,* 259–270.

Morse, W. H., & Kelleher, R. T. (1977). Determinants of reinforcement and punishment. In W. K. Homg & J. E. R. Staddon (Eds.), *Handbook of operant behavior.* Englewood Cliffs, NJ: Prentice-Hall.

Tollison, C. D., & Adams, H. E. (1979). *Sexual disorders: Treatment, theory and research.* New York: Gardner Press.

Turkat, I. D. (1979). The behavior analysis matrix. *Scandinavian Journal of Behavior Therapy, 8,* 187–189.

Turkat, I. D. (1982). Behavior-analytic considerations of alternative clinical approaches. In P. L. Wachtel (Ed.), *Resistance: Psychodynamic and behavioral approaches.* New York: Plenum Press.

Turkat, I. D. (1983). The behavioral interview. In A. R. Ciminro, K. S. Calhoun, & H. E. Adams (Eds.), *Handbook of behavioral assessment* (2nd ed.). New York: Wiley Interscience.

Turkat, I. D., & Brantley, P. J. (1981). On the therapeutic relationship in behavior therapy. *The Behavior Therapist, 4,* 16–17.

Turkat, I. D., & Maisto, S. A. (1983). Application of the experimental method to the formulation and modification of personality disorders. In D. H. Barlow (Ed.), *Behavioral treatment of adult disorders.* New York: Guilford Press.

Turkat, I. D., & Meyer, V. (1982). The behavior-analytic approach. In P. L. Wachtel (Ed.), *Resistance: Psychodynamic and behavioral approaches.* New York: Plenum Press.

Wolpe, J. (1958). *Psychotherapy by reciprocal inhibition.* Stanford, CA.: Stanford University Press.

Wolpe, J. (1973). *The practice of behavior therapy* (2nd ed.). New York: Pergamon.

Wolpe, J. (1976). *Theme and variation: A behavior therapy casebook.* New York: Pergamon.

Wolpe, J. (1977). Inadequate behavior analysis: The achilles heel of outcome research in behavior therapy. *Journal of Behavior Therapy and Experimental Psychiatry, 8,* 1–3.

Wolpe, J. (1980). Behavioral analysis and therapeutic strategy. In A. Goldstein & E. B. Foa (Eds.), *Handbook of behavioral interventions.* New York: Wiley.

Wolpe, J. (1982). *The practice of behavior therapy* (3rd ed.). New York: Pergamon Press.

Wolpe, J., & Wolpe, D. (1981). *Our useless fears.* Boston: Houghton Mifflin.

2

ALCOHOL ABUSE

The Case of Mr. S.

Mr. S. was a married 33-year-old Caucasian residing in a major city in the southeast United States. He had recently been fired from his job as a clerk in a large office supply outlet. He had been married for eight years and was the father of a five-year-old girl.

The Referral

The patient was referred by a physician from a primary care center at a major teaching hospital. The physician was concerned about the patient's depression.

Physical Appearance

Mr. S. was five feet eight inches tall. He was approximately 25 pounds overweight. His hair was black, moderate in length, and combed across the frontal area. The patient wore a thick, untrimmed beard which covered most of his face. He wore a buttoned-down flannel shirt, blue-jeans, and work boots to the interview.

Presenting Complaints

The patient began the interview by stating that he had been depressed for quite some time and unclear as to which events to attribute this to. He indicated that many things had gone wrong for him over the past few years. He expressed concern that he might not be able to present the "logical sequence" of events.

The patient reported that at present he was feeling apathetic, having little appetite, sleeping excessively, and having a general desire to do nothing. This worried him greatly. Mr. S. reported that he had been drinking heavily (whiskey) for the past few weeks and was now trying to get this under control.

Mr. S. reported that he had lost his job about a month before. He found this perplexing. The patient indicated that he was always the first one at work each day and among the last to leave. He reported that he was a very hard, meticulous, and dedicated worker, albeit sometimes late in completing tasks. The patient was shocked to learn that he had been fired because of his employer's perception of him as being unhappy there. The employer stated that he always seemed to have a "mean look" about him and that his behavior was disturbing to the other workers. Mr. S. indicated that he felt that he was always "smiling." More disturbing to the patient was the employer's rationale for his termination. Mr. S. viewed himself as a "solid" worker and could not see how he was negatively affecting the other employees. The employer described him as "too serious, stubborn, rational, and just plain unhappy." Mr. S. could understand the comment about rationality (which he was proud of) but felt that he was happy at work.

The patient reported that he was currently in the process of divorcing his wife. He stated that he had a clear rationale, namely, that his wife had refused to engage in sex with him for the past four years. He evaluated their first six months of marriage as sexually satisfying, but then his wife became inorgasmic, culminating in total abstinence. Mr. S. reported that she refused ever to discuss her lack of sexual interest in him. Additionally, he could not identify any reasons as to why she had become like this. Mr. S. indicated that his wife would never discuss things and her "irrationality drove me crazy." He also stated that she was not meticulous in her housekeeping and her carelessness bothered him greatly. He would take on these tasks to be sure they were done correctly.

During the second year of marriage, the patient began to drink whiskey at night, a habit which often led to arguments with his wife. Sometimes he would just drink by himself until he fell asleep on the sofa. He reported that his drinking "would come and go in spurts."

Mr. S. stated that divorce was out of the question at first since they were both of the Mormom faith and because of his belief that it was their "duty" to make the marriage work. As a father, he reported that he always tried to be moral and to do the "right thing." Mr. S. indicated that he tried to follow the procedures he read in a book on "How to be a good parent." He stated that he intended to support his family even though separated (and, at present, financially unable) and that his daughter "belonged" with her mother.

About three months ago, the patient had been drinking at home one night and decided to go to his office to finish a task. There, one of the secretaries had been working late. He reported that he was taken by surprise when she came on to him and they began to have sex. Unfortunately, he was unable to perform. He became depressed about it. In subsequent interactions with this woman, he could never tell whether she wanted to have sex with him again or not. In addition to feeling guilty, he felt inept sexually and socially.

The patient reported having no close friends. Prior to his marriage, he had had a few short-term relationships with females. In each case, he was accused of being too formal and unable to relate emotionally. He stated a desire to have a close intimate partner who could understand him and to develop a circle of friends. However, he felt that he first needed to gain stable employment where he could be productive.

Parents

The patient described his parents as devout followers of the Mormon faith. His father was an accountant. He recalled him as a very rational, fair, and orderly individual. The mother was described as a "saint." She kept an extremely clean and organized home. The patient laughed when he described the "inventory lists" his mother kept regarding the status of canned foods, toilet paper, and so forth in the house.

Mr. S. did not recall that his parents had many close friends but they did have many acquaintances. These were primarily from their church.

Interview Behavior

Throughout the interview, the patient was serious, stiff, and formal. He seemed excessively concerned with presenting information in clear-cut logical form. He apologized when switching topics without warning.

In describing the various events, Mr. S. showed little variation in affect. He appeared to have a stern look about him. When asked deliberately to smile, it appeared difficult for him to do.

Generally, he was very cooperative throughout the interview and seemed motivated to find a clear-cut logical approach to resolve his difficulties.

2

Behavioral Formulation of Cases Involving Alcohol Abuse

STEPHEN A. MAISTO

INTRODUCTION

The purpose of this chapter is to describe a behavioral formulation of a case of alcohol problems. Because there is disagreement among researchers and clinicians about the definition of alcohol problems, the chapter will begin with a discussion of the Diagnostic and Statistical Manual (DSM-III; American Psychiatric Association, 1980) diagnostic criteria for this disorder. This discussion will be followed by an overview of the general behavioral approach to the etiology and treatment of alcohol problems. A review of definition and the behavioral model of alcohol problems will provide the background for description of a general approach to formulating such cases. This general approach will then be applied to the formulation of an actual case.

Alcohol problems are complex and have been the subject of much speculation during the twentieth century about their etiology and treatment. This lively debate has involved both the scientific and nonscientific communities, and as a consequence consensus among them has been difficult to achieve. For example, there is still disagreement about

STEPHEN A. MAISTO • Veterans Administration Medical Center, Alcohol Dependence Treatment Program, Davis Park, Providence, Rhode Island, 02908.

such basic questions as a formal definition of alcohol-related disorders and about the label to apply to such behaviors. Many terms have been proposed, including alcoholism, alcohol dependence, alcohol abuse, and problem drinking.[1] As a result, confusion can be avoided only by clearly stating definitions and assumptions.

The formal definition of alcohol problems provided in the DSM-III will be used in this chapter. Although there are some difficulties with this definition, such as ambiguity of several terms, it has the important advantage of capturing the complexity of alcohol-related disorders. In this respect, DSM-III appears useful for classifying alcohol problems. According to this diagnostic system, alcohol problems are one type of "substance use disorders." Three distinctions are made to describe human consumption of various substances, such as alcohol, marijuana, or heroin: *substance use, substance abuse,* and *substance dependence.* Use is defined as an *absence* of evidence of substance abuse or dependence. In the case of alcohol, abuse is defined according to three criteria, including pattern of pathological use, social or occupational dysfunction caused by pathological use, and duration. Pathological use of alcohol is not easy to specify, since what is called pathological often depends on setting and cultural variables. However, according to DSM-III a variety of patterns of alcohol use may meet the criterion for pathology. These include a need for daily use of alcohol for adequate functioning, an inability to reduce or to stop drinking, blackouts (amnesic periods for events occurring while intoxicated, even though the individual is fully conscious during their occurrence), and continued drinking despite the presence of a physical disorder that is exacerbated by alcohol (DSM-III, 1980, p. 169).

Impairment in social or occupational functioning is typically what compels an individual to enter treatment. Such impairment may span the array of social settings which may be disrupted by drinking alcohol. For example, an individual may considerably disrupt his or her family by spending more income on alcohol than on meeting financial obligations. Another example is that occupational functioning may be impaired by excessive absences due to severe hangovers. Some events cause disruption in several areas. For instance, an individual may be arrested for driving under the influence (DUI) of alcohol. This event not only results in involvement with the legal system, but may also involve considerable financial cost (especially in cases of multiple

---

[1]The vast majority of authors in the literature have not distinguished among these terms. Therefore, for ease of discussion the labels are used interchangeably in this chapter except where noted.

offenders) and large daily inconvenience due to suspension or revocation of driver's license. Suffice it to say that alcohol may be associated with an assortment of negative social consequences for the individual that vary with the characteristics of his or her social environment. Finally, duration is the third criterion for alcohol abuse. In this regard, signs of disturbance should be present for at least one month. The disturbance does not have to be continuous to meet criterion, but the individual's behavior should form an "apparent pattern" of alcohol-related disturbance. For example, the individual may miss four days of work during a month because he or she is hung over from heavy drinking. However, between drinking occasions there may be no signs of occupational impairment.

Alcohol dependence is considered a more extreme form of alcohol abuse. It is important to note that dependence is often referred to in the literature as alcoholism. There are two criteria for dependence. First, the individual must show either a pattern of pathological use or impairment in social or occupational functioning, as defined above. Second, there must be evidence of either *tolerance* to or *physical dependence* on alcohol. Tolerance is the more difficult criterion to apply because, except in extreme cases, it is difficult to specify. Tolerance simply means that, as a consequence of using a drug, a higher dose is required to achieve the same effects that were formerly experienced at lower doses, or that a given dose of the drug has less effect than it once did. (Kalant, LeBlanc, & Gibbons, 1971, provide an excellent review of tolerance to alcohol. Maisto, Henry, Sobell, & Sobell, 1978, discuss the implications of tolerance for the treatment of alcohol dependence, and this subject was later discussed by Cappell, 1981.) As can be surmised from this definition, identifying changes in tolerance that may be clinically significant depend on what "effects" are being considered as well as having some tolerance "reference point" in order to allow comparison of present level of tolerance. To compound these problems, there are large individual differences in initial level of tolerance and in its development.

The physical dependence criterion is easier to assess because it is based on a well-specified operational definition. An individual is said to be physically dependent on alcohol if, upon its withdrawal (Victor & Adams, 1953) or upon a drop in the level of alcohol in the blood (Mello, 1972), he or she shows a clearly defined pattern of physiological symptoms. (In this sense, physical dependence is circularly defined, since it is not defined independent of its operations.) These symptoms vary in type and severity but have been clearly specified and related directly to a decrease of the blood alcohol level.

In summary, alcohol abuse and dependence are complex disorders that may involve many aspects of the individual's functioning. Therefore, treatment rarely is limited to drinking behavior but also must concern physical, psychological, social, and environmental factors that are related to it.

Behavioral Approach to Alcohol Abuse and Dependence

Although application of the behavioral approach to alcohol problems is viewed by some as a recent development, behavioral principles were used in alcohol treatment programs in the United States over 40 years ago. In this regard, classical conditioning procedures were applied to modify the abusive drinker's taste for alcohol from (assumed to be) positive to negative (see Rachman & Teasdale, 1969). Both electrical and chemical aversion have been applied in treatment. According to the standard classical conditioning procedures, electrical aversion involves pairing electric shock with, for example, the smell and taste of the individual's preferred alcoholic beverages. In chemical aversion, feelings of nausea and eventual vomiting are paired with the sensory properties of alcoholic beverages. Drugs such as emetine or apomorphine are typically used to induce the required nausea. In both the chemical and electrical approaches, it is assumed that alcohol will acquire aversive properties by pairing it with the aversive unconditioned stimuli.

As is apparent from this description, classical conditioning procedures are used to alter the sensory qualities of alcohol so that its consumption becomes aversive, resulting in abstention from alcohol. It is important to note, however, that classical conditioning was applied as a technique focusing on the individual's drinking response. Furthermore, classical conditioning procedures generally were not part of a behavioral statement of the etiology, maintenance, and treatment of abusive drinking. The most popular early behavioral approach that addressed these questions was based on drive reduction theory and called the tension reduction hypothesis (Conger, 1956). According to this theory, excessive drinking is based in the use of alcohol for its tension (drive)-reducing properties. Reinforcement of drinking occurs through drive reduction which strengthens the response and makes it more likely when future tension states are aroused. This cycle continues to the eventual development of abusive drinking.

Although the tension reduction hypothesis was one of the first behavioral attempts to explain the development and maintenance of excessive alcohol consumption, the restrictions in its scope are apparent. Later research (see Adesso, 1980) showed the deficiencies in such an approach and has led to current behavioral models (Miller, 1976). The current behavioral approach includes the assumption that drinking is a voluntary response that has definable antecedents and consequences that contribute to its development and maintenance. Furthermore, consistent with the DSM-III, the antecedents and consequences of drinking are viewed as multidimensional (Pattison, Sobell, & Sobell, 1977). Therefore, antecedents may include psychological, social, physiological, and environmental factors, as may the consequences of drinking. Some behavioral researchers and clinicians have supplemented this model by incorporating cognitive factors as mediators of alcohol consumption (Maisto, Connors, & Sachs, 1981; Marlatt & Rohsenow, 1980; Wilson, 1977). For example, a particular setting may elicit an expectation about the effects of alcohol which mediates the individual's drinking in that setting.

In summary, therefore, behavioral approaches have evolved from narrow conceptions of alcohol abuse that focused on precise aspects of the drinking response to broader, multivariant models. This current behavioral approach will be applied in the present discussion.

General Approach to Assessment and Treatment of Alcohol Problems

It follows from the behavioral approach to alcohol abuse that the first steps in developing a treatment plan are to discover the antecedents and consequences that are associated with and maintain current problem behaviors and then to examine the acquisition of those same behaviors. This information is typically obtained in a *behavioral assessment* (e.g., Hersen & Bellack, 1981; Nathan & Lipscomb, 1979) of the individual during the initial interviews. Application of this approach to alcohol abuse typically comprises several important dimensions of the interview. These include data gathering relevant to the individual's current drinking and other problems that he or she reports and to the development (etiology) of these problems. Also important are informal observations of the patient during the interview that can provide the clinician with additional information about the patient's problems and about the most efficacious way of conducting an interview. Finally, on the basis of these data-gathering efforts the clinician should be able to make an informed statement about the patient's motivation and prospects for change.

DATA GATHERING RELEVANT TO CURRENT DRINKING

Functional Analysis of Drinking

Understanding of the patient's current drinking rests upon a full, systematic description of the behavior, its antecedents, and its consequences. The procedure of obtaining such information has been called a "functional analysis" of drinking behavior (Sobell, Sobell, & Sheahan, 1975). The goal of a functional analysis is to specify the constellation of factors that are correlated with a high probability of abusive drinking.

Consistent with current social learning models of alcohol abuse, there is an attempt to define a combination of factors instead of looking for one antecedent that precedes all of the individual's abusive drinking. Sobell and Sobell (1981) have categorized the sets of factors that may comprise drinking antecedents as the *drinking setting*. These may include, first, *biological factors* such as genetic endowment, state of health, physical limitations, and immediate physiological state. Psychological factors also contribute to the drinking setting and include variables such as the individual's mood state, learning history, response tendencies, beliefs about alcohol, and information-processing style. Finally, *environmental factors* consist of characteristics of the physical setting, presence of others, alcohol availability, others' expectations (of the individual) and their behavior, and alcohol-related cues. Therefore, alcohol consumption must be viewed in the *total context* of the individual's psychological and physiological characteristics and of the environment in which drinking occurs.

It is important to note that this description is based on a *concept* of the setting as consisting of an interaction between the person and the external environment. The idea that the person and the environment together define settings is a relatively recent addition to social learning theory (see, e.g., Bandura, 1977; Mischel, 1973), although it has been prominent in general personality theory for some time (e.g., Endler, 1980). In this regard, a functional analysis requires obtaining and using information that provides as complete an understanding of the individual as possible and the contexts in which he or she drinks. Of course, obtaining such data is the goal of the initial interview, as will be seen below.

Sobell and Sobell (1981) noted another important feature of setting factors. A brief review of these factors shows that some of them are invariant (such as genetic endowment), some are stable but modifiable (such as response tendencies), and some are situation-specific (such as the presence of others and access to alcohol). In practice, therefore, once characteristics of the individual are understood, a functional analysis consists of collecting data on the variety of contexts in which the individual is likely to drink.

A final important point is that knowledge of the influence of various setting factors is based on a large body of experimental studies of human drinking behavior (e.g., Adesso, 1980; Maisto, Connors, & Sachs, 1981; Marlatt & Rohsenow, 1980) as well as studies in natural settings, such as taverns (Kessler & Gomberg, 1975; Reid, 1978; Rosenbluth, Lawson & Nathan, 1978). However, no assumptions are made about which factors are generally more influential than others. Rather, the factors that in combination are most important are determined for *individual* patients.

For each setting delineated the clinician must determine the frequency with which the patient drinks alcohol and the quantity of alcohol that is consumed. These data, of course, are the bases of estimating the likelihood of drinking in a given setting and the *risk* (of negative consequences) associated with such drinking. Perhaps not so obvious as the need to collect data on the frequency and quantity of drinking in a stimulus setting is the need to establish the frequency with which the individual engages in a nondrinking response. This information places the drinking behavior in a more balanced context and allows a better evaluation of the extent and quality of the nondrinking coping behaviors that the patient brings to treatment.

In the case of alcohol problems, it is also essential to collect information about the patient's present and past drinking that goes beyond specific settings. In this regard, in order to construct a diagnosis and treatment plan several types of data are needed that center on typical quantities of alcohol that are consumed regularly, typical and atypical drinking patterns (such as daily, weekends only, with specific groups of people at certain times); indices of tolerance to alcohol (e.g., highest quantity of alcohol ever consumed on one occasion, highest blood alcohol concentration ever reached, and history of the alcohol withdrawal syndrome). This information is needed for diagnosing the individual, since the DSM-III criteria for alcohol dependence include evidence of a history of the alcohol withdrawal syndrome (see above). Furthermore, these data aid the development of treatment plans by providing information to answer such questions as the appropriateness of different drinking outcome goals (i.e., abstinence or moderate drinking; see Maisto, Henry, Sobell, & Sobell, 1978; Miller & Caddy, 1977) and the degree to which the individual's daily activities revolve around alcohol.

The final aspect of a functional analysis of drinking behavior is the consequences for drinking and not drinking in a given setting.

Consistent with the multivariate approach to alcohol problems presented in this chapter, the consequences for drinking span several domains, including physiological effects, psychological effects, personal effects, social/interpersonal effects, and environmental effects (Sobell & Sobell, 1981). The physiological effects of drinking alcohol relate to the pharmacological action of the drug and may include such consequences as central nervous sytem depressant action and impairment in cognitive function. The psychological consequences of drinking alcohol, long held to be central to abusive drinking (e.g., Conger, 1956) may include an alteration in mood and perception of self (Hull, 1981). Some of the personal consequences of drinking for the individual may be in the areas of job, financial resources, and legal involvement. Drinking may also affect elements in the individual's social environment, such as family, peers, and colleagues. Finally, an individual's drinking in a physical setting may serve to alter that setting in one or more ways.

It is important to remember that the presence, magnitude, and type of consequences that the individual experiences as a result of drinking are dependent on where and how much alcohol is consumed. Therefore, the alcohol-related problems that an individual reports cannot be taken out of that context. In addition, consequences vary temporally from relatively short-term to relatively long-term in relation to the behavior. Indeed, one traditional tenet of the behavioral approach to alcohol dependence was that individuals continue to abuse alcohol in the face of serious aversive consequences because such consequences are typically farther removed from the behavior and control it less than the shorter-term typically positive consequences (Bandura, 1969). Interestingly, however, there are few if any experimental demonstrations of such differential control in human drinking behavior. Finally, a well-rounded behavioral assessment requires that the clinician evaluate the same consequences for *not* drinking in a setting as he or she does for drinking.

Summary. The purpose of this section was to describe a behavioral approach to the assessment of drinking behavior. A behavioral assessment was described as consisting of evaluating general patterns of alcohol consumption as well as a functional analysis of drinking which involves delineation of the specific antecedents and consequences of drinking and not drinking. The patient's drinking was presented as the first behavior requiring the clinician's attention because it is generally the predominant problem in individuals who are treated for alcohol problems. Furthermore, as will be discussed below, an understanding of the patient's drinking often provides invaluable leads for understanding other problems that he or she reports.

Obtaining Drinking-Related Data

Measurement Requirements. A fundamental characteristic of behavioral assessments is the fact that independent and dependent variables are specified and operationalized. In the context of assessing alcohol problems this feature can be clearly illlustrated in doing a functional analysis of the individual's drinking. For example, the patient may report that when he or she is anxious, drinking to intoxication occurs. The first problem is to specify what the patient means by "anxious." In order to answer this question the patient may be asked, for example, what type of physiological changes accompany that state (e.g., hands sweating, rapid heart rate). Or the clinician may ask the patient to assign some number ranging from 0 to 100 to anxious states, if typical arousal equals, say, 50. In these ways the clinician may assure that he or she understands this element of the drinking setting. Similarly, "drinking to intoxication" is not a precise description of the quantity of alcohol that the person tends to drink when anxious. Rather, the clinician may have to ask the patient to specify what is meant by intoxication (e.g., correlated physical, psychological, and behavioral cues). Furthermore, if intoxication is operationalized, the quantity of consumption should then be specified. Therefore, the patient may report "a lot of" beer, but the clinician must probe further to achieve a precise definition of "a lot" in terms of quantities of beverage alcohol, such as two six-packs of 12-ounce beers. These same requirements should be applied to describing the consequences of drinking. The point of specifying the independent-dependent variable relationships is to assure that the clinician has as accurate a representation of the patient's behavior as possible that can be used for designing further clinical tests and treatment interventions as needed (Meyer & Turkat, 1979). Another important feature of behavioral assessments is to collect continuous data from the patient whenever possible. In this regard, such indices provide for more sensitive measures than, for example, nominal scaled data. Another advantage is that continuous measures are most sensitive to measuring the effects of an intervention (Maisto & Cooper, 1980; Sobell, 1978). For example, for many years the major criterion in alcohol treatment outcome studies was abstinence, and the patient was measured as being either abstinent or not. Not only does this approach eliminate a large amount of useful data that could be gathered, but it also produces an extremely conservative measure of treatment effectiveness.

The final aspect of behavioral assessments is to use validated measures of phenomena whenever possible, which means that measures should have demonstrated reliability and validity. Therefore, the criteria for behavioral assessments are entirely consistent with those of any type of scientific measurement: the use of validated procedures to measure variables that have been clearly and precisely operationalized.

Methods of Measurement. As in the measurement of a number of behavioral and psychological disorders, assessment of drinking and related behaviors is complicated by the absence of a generally agreed upon, "fool-proof" method of measurement. As a result, clinicians should use as many different ways of measuring phenomena as appropriate (Sobell & Sobell, 1980). Because each method of measurement has its own strengths and weaknesses, the clinician must evaluate the data according to the consistency among individual measures (Foy, Rychtarik, & Prue, 1981; Sobell & Sobell, 1980). During the last 15 years several different methods of measuring drinking and related behaviors have been developed.

Self-Reports. Patients' self-reports are the oldest and cheapest method of measuring their drinking behavior. Until recently self-reports were typically the only method that both clinicians and clinical researchers used to measure drinking and related behaviors. Because of their low cost and relative ease of collection, patients' self-reports are still the most prevalent way of obtaining information about drinking behavior.

Unfortunately, the validity of self-reports is always suspect and open to question. This problem is compounded when the reporters are alcohol abusers. In this regard, the drinking-related information that is desired often relates to a period long past, so that self-reports are vulnerable to an imperfect memory. Furthermore, alcoholics are typically assumed to lie about their drinking. For example, Block (1980) asserted that "denial is a characteristic of patients suffering from alcoholism" (p. 54). If Block's assertion were universally correct, and many in the field agree with him, most of the present and past clinical research with alcohol abusers would be next to useless. Fortunately, however, recent research has shown that sober alcoholics do give reliable and valid self-reports about their drinking in clinical or research settings in which confidentiality of the data are assured (e.g., Maisto & Cooper, 1980; Sobell, Sobell, & VanderSpek, 1978).

Recent evidence for the utility of self-reports in specific settings has contributed to the development of several validated methods of collecting drinking data. Two outstanding examples include the time-line calendar technique (Sobell, Maisto, Sobell, & Cooper, 1979), in which the subject uses a calendar as an aid to report his or her daily drinking behavior over a specific period. Another self-report data collection method prominent among behavioral clinicians is Marlatt's (1975) Drinking Profile Questionnaire, which is designed to obtain detailed information on the antecedents and consequences of drinking. It is important to note that both of these techniques follow the standards for behavioral assessment in that measures are specified, operationalized, and validated. For information on other types of drinking self-report inventories see Foy *et al.* (1981).

Breath Tests. Alcohol research was aided substantially by invention of precise techniques to measure blood alcohol content (a direct measure of the level of *physiological* intoxication) by breath analysis, based on the known ratio between the amount of alcohol in the blood and the amount in alveolar air. Although breath analysis has had its greatest effects on basic research, it has also influenced clinical research. For example, it has become possible to assess quickly a patient's level of intoxication in clinical settings. This is critical for both clinical and research reasons, since alcohol abusers who have a high degree of tolerance to alcohol can often drink substantial amounts of alcohol and still appear sober (Maisto, Henry, Sobell, & Sobell, 1978; Sobell, Sobell & VanderSpek, 1978).

An important advance in the measurement of alcohol consumption in clinical research projects occurred with the introduction of portable breath testing devices (See Sobell & Sobell, 1975). These devices make it possible to obtain, either in the clinic or in the natural environment, a fairly accurate measure of the individual's acute intoxication. Therefore, breath testing devices have been an important advance in obtaining objective, precise measures of the individual's drinking. However, it is important to note that, unlike self-reports, breath testing can be used only to measure *acute* intoxication.

Liver-Function Tests. Another method developed to measure *recent heavy* drinking is by blood test to assess hepatic functioning. In this regard, it has been shown that some biochemical markers (e.g., mean cell volume, CMV; gamma-glutamyl transpepsidase, γ-GT) tend to correlate (there is a high degree of individual variability) with recent, extremely heavy levels of alcohol consumption. It is important to note the emphasis on *recent*, because if the individual is abstinent for about three weeks or more the levels of these biochemical markers return to normal (Sobell & Sobell, 1981). Furthermore, the markers can be elevated with hepatic dysfunction unrelated to drinking. Therefore, liver function tests should be viewed as an objective measure of probable recent, heavy drinking, but not as an absolute criterion of such drinking.

Official Records. Official records of agencies such as hospitals, community mental health centers, and law enforcement departments can be an invaluable complement to other measures of patients' functioning (Maisto & Maisto, 1983). In this regard, such records have been used most frequently by substance abuse clinicians and researchers to corroborate patients' self-reports of events such as alcohol-related arrests and hospitalizations. Therefore, although imperfect in validity, official records may be used as an inexpensive, relatively easy way to obtain additional data on patients' alcohol-related dysfunction.

Behavioral Observations. Several behavioral measures of drinking behavior in alcoholic and nonalcoholic subjects have been reported. These include, for example, the taste test introduced by Marlatt, Demming, and Reid (1973) as an unobtrusive test of alcohol consumption. A number of studies have involved measuring various aspects of drinking behavior through requiring the individual to make simple operant responses in order to obtain alcohol under different contingencies (e.g., Mendelson & Mello, 1966; Miller, Hersen, Eisler, & Hilsman, 1974; Nathan, Titler, Lowenstein, Solomon, & Rossi, 1970). Finally, several researchers have observed alcoholic subjects' use of alcohol in experimental bars (e.g., Schaefer, Sobell, & Mills, 1971).

Although direct behavioral measures of alcohol consumption are an excellent way to acquire an understanding of *how* the alcoholic approaches and uses alcohol in specific settings, they have been applied far more often in research than in clinical settings (with a few notable exceptions; see Miller, Hersen, Eisler, & Elkin, 1974; Sobell & Sobell, 1973). This differential application is probably due to the expense and time involved in arranging some of the procedures (e.g., operant behavior recording equipment and building a simulated bar). More importantly, there are severe restrictions in administering alcohol to individuals who have been diagnosed as alcoholic, whether for purposes of research or of treatment. For example, medical personnel and facilities are always required. Finally, in the vast majority of treatment settings, administering alcohol to alcoholics would not even be considered, regardless of the facilities that were available.

Reports of Significant Others. Another excellent measure of the patient's past and present drinking that has shown to be reliable (Maisto, Sobell, & Sobell, 1979, 1982) is the reports of collateral informants or "significant others" regarding the patient's behavior. The major advantages in using colaterals is that they can corroborate patients' own reports as well as provide a different perspective on the patient's behavior (Ersner-Hershfield, Sobell, & Sobell, 1980). Of course, if collaterals are used, the patient must be so informed. Furthermore, defensiveness in the patient may be reduced to a minimum if he or she is told that collaterals are being contacted in order to obtain as complete representation of the patient's health as possible (Ersner-Hershfield et al., 1980).

Informal Observations. The final way to assess the individual's drinking behavior, especially when evaluating abusive drinking, is informal observations during the interviews. In this regard, various discriminable cues may be present during the initial interview that suggest strongly that the patient has an alcohol problem. The presence of such cues can lead to an initial hypothesis about the patient's problems that can be tested further by using any of the techniques (for examining the drinking aspects of the problem) discussed above. Ernser-Hershfield et al. (1980, p. 245) have listed some of the cues that might indicate an alcohol problem and that can be observed in the initial interview. These include the odor of alcohol on the breath; unexplained bruises, abrasions, and lacerations; cigarette burns on the fingertips; puffy appearance to the skin; and blood alcohol content of .15% (mg alcohol/100 ml blood) or higher without evidence of intoxication. Other signs may include complaints of depression, irritability, nervousness, insomnia, or sexual problems. Patients may be using alcohol to alleviate these symptoms, which also may be indicants of alcohol withdrawal. It is important to note that these cues can be used in clinical settings to obtain an initial hypothesis about the severity of the patient's alcohol problem or, if the patient does not acknowledge such problems, to cue the interviewer that the patient may be withholding information.

Summary. A number of methods have been developed to measure the individual's drinking behavior. These measures differ according to the period of drinking (past, current) that they are designed to assess, their degree of objectivity (self-reports, blood alcohol level), and kinds of strengths and weaknesses regarding validity. Therefore, the clinician should attempt in as many different ways as possible to measure the variables of interest and to make decisions about the validity of his or her data according to the consistency or convergence among measures.

Other Common Areas of Dysfunction

By definition of the disorders alcohol abuse and alcohol dependence, patients so diagnosed will have complications in other areas of their lives that are somehow associated with drinking. Therefore,

regardless of whether dysfunction in other areas is cause or consequence of alcohol consumption, it is essential that assessment of the
extent of such dysfunction is made. The criteria for these assessments
are the same as those discussed for drinking: variables should be specified, operationalized, and measured with reliability and validity.

As indicated earlier, abusive drinking interacts with patients'
physical, psychological, and social functioning. Alcohol abuse is associated with disorders of a number of biological systems (see American
Medical Association, 1977, and National Council on Alcoholism, 1972,
for a detailed discussion). Furthermore, the clinician must also evaluate
for a history of alcohol withdrawal symptoms, including psychomotor
agitation, blackouts, gastritis, seizures or convulsions, alcohol-related
auditory and visual hallucinations, and delirium tremens. Assessment
of social dysfunction should span areas such as job, family, peers, and
legal involvement. Therefore, interviewers should probe for information such as days of work missed due to drinking, frequent marital
discord and arguments with friends, amount of money spent each week
on alcohol, and involvement with the police for reasons such as driving
under the influence of alcohol. The psychological problems most commonly correlated with alcohol abuse include cognitive impairment (see
Parsons & Leber, 1982, for a review), depression, manic depression,
obsessive compulsive disorder, and antisocial personality disorder
(National Council on Alcoholism, 1972; Pickens & Heston, 1979).

There are several different sources of data to assess patients' functioning in these areas. As with the measurement of drinking, patients'
self-reports are most frequently used to assess areas of social functioning. Fortunately, a number of studies have shown (see Maisto & Cooper,
1980; Sobell & Sobell, 1985, for reviews) that these reports are highly
correlated with other methods of measurement, including official records (e.g., police, hospital, motor vehicle) and the reports of significant
others. Because of the variety of physical complications correlated with
abusive drinking, a medical history should be taken from each patient
as a minimum requirement, including a history of use of prescribed
and nonprescribed drugs (Bissell, 1980). Such a medical history would
inform the clinician of the need for further medical examination as well
as provide data for formulating treatment plans, especially as regards
appropriate drinking outcome goals. Finally, further probing of psychological functioning is made possible by using appropriate standardized neuropsychological and psychiatric tests (see, e.g., Owen &
Butcher, 1979; Parsons & Leber, 1982).

An important point to remember in assessing alcohol problems
concerns cases in which other psychopathologies appear to be present.

In this regard, the clinician should distinguish between primary and secondary disorders when assigning diagnoses. In a primary diagnosis of alcohol abuse, other psychopathologies that are identified are judged to be a consequence of abusive drinking. In contrast, when a secondary diagnosis of alcohol abuse or dependence is made in conjunction with a diagnosis of some other psychopathology, it is judged that the pathology preceded any abusive drinking. This distinction is not only essential for technical accuracy in diagnosing the patient but is crucial for developing treatment interventions. Furthermore, it reemphasizes that alcohol use and abuse cannot be isolated from the rest of the individual's behavior.

Amount of Detail in Assessments. It should be apparent that assessment of alcohol problems is a complex task because of the correlation between abusive drinking and an array of other areas of functioning. This may lead to the conclusion that much detail is required in assessments. Although it may sometimes occur that assessment of a case is extremely detailed and covers a wide range of factors, the goal is not to obtain mounds of data *per se*. Rather, the goal in assessment is to obtain as much data as necessary to afford the clinician a thorough understanding of the case and enable him or her to make a formulation that leads to effective treatment interventions.

Summary. The purpose of this section was to survey the primary types of data that are gathered in a behavioral assessment of alcohol abuse. Because abusive drinking is a disorder that affects patients' total health, the content of the data is not limited to drinking behavior but expands to physical, psychological, and social functioning. For each area examined, different measurement techniques have been developed, each with its own strengths and weaknesses. Therefore, clinicians should attempt to use multiple methods to measure patient functioning and examine the data for their consistency. With such an approach clinicians may achieve more confidence in their formulations of the case and therefore in the design of treatment interventions.

Development of Alcohol Problems

Alcohol use and abuse are associated with a variety of social and cultural variables (e.g., Cahalan & Cisin, 1976; Stivers, 1976). Therefore, trends in the patterns of alcohol use are apparent as a function of group and cultural membership. However, the clinician is necessarily most concerned with how individuals within sociocultural categories differ in their use of alcohol and the consequences of such use. Accordingly, the major etiological problem for the clinician is to explain the process leading to differential patterns of alcohol use. Collecting etiological data appears to be essential to understanding present drinking patterns and their maintenance. For example, if psychopathologies other than drinking are currently manifested, the only way to understand how they interact with drinking is to do a historical assessment. As discussed earlier in this paper, the behavioral clinician takes the approach that the behaviors comprising an alcohol-related diagnosis are more or less (e.g., depending on inherited characteristics) learned according to the general principles of classical and operant conditioning and modeling. Therefore, an investigation of etiology is accomplished through analysis of the environmental events that contributed to the development of alcohol drinking and related behaviors.

There are a number of excellent reviews of the etiological factors that would be of most importance to the behavioral clinician (see, e.g., Akers, 1977; Bandura, 1969; Goodwin, 1980; Tarter & Schneider, 1976; Zucker, 1979), and the reader may consult these sources for more detailed discussion than is possible here. The etiological variables on which behavioral clinicians would tend to focus include the family, peers, "macroenvironment," and individual resources.

The Family. A highly reliable finding that has been noted literally for thousands of years is that alcoholism tends to run in families. This, of course, implicated both genetic and environmental variables that may contribute to the development of alcohol problems. In this regard, the genetic hypothesis has been given a recent resurgence after lying dormant for the previous 25 years (see Goodwin, 1980). Although there are many problems with the available literature, it does appear that genetic predisposition accounts for some proportion of the variance in alcohol abuse, especially in its more extreme forms. However, "what" is transmitted is still unknown; speculations have included a constitution that produces extremely rewarding physiological effects of alcohol (such as deep relaxation) and a biochemical anomaly that produces "loss of control" drinking in the individual following ingestion of small quantities of alcohol. Regardless of the contribution of genetic factors, however, the behavioral clinician works with the characteristics of the patient who comes to treatment and attempts to discover how those characteristics interacted with environmental factors to determine current drinking. Therefore, the question becomes how the family "teaches" the individual to drink in a particular way.

The major conditioning process examined in evaluation of the contribution of the patient's family to his or her drinking is modeling. This is necessarily the case because knowledge about alcohol has been shown to be acquired long before individuals do any drinking themselves. The major facets of the parents' behavior (or that of other adults in authority) that the child models include quantity and frequency of consumption; the sorts of occasions on which consumption is considered appropriate and to what degree; and the functions of alcohol, for instance to reduce stress, to celebrate an event, to enhance self-perception of power, to ease socializing. Furthermore, parents' drinking behavior inevitably reflects attitudes toward alcohol and the value that is placed on it. Finally, it is often overlooked that parents who model the use of alcohol as a generalized coping response are less frequently modeling more adaptive coping behaviors.

Peers. When the individual reaches the age of young adolescence it appears that the peer group may be the most important single influence on the development of drinking patterns, replacing the family in that function. Early adolescence is the period when young Americans have their first direct drinking experience (see, e.g., a recent national survey reported by Rachal, Hubbard, Guess, Maisto, Cavanaugh, Waddell, & Benrud, 1980).

Therefore, the peer group is influential not only as a source of modeling but in affecting the individual in his or her own decisions to drink. Some of the factors that have been identified to be of etiological importance include the quantity and frequency of peers' alcohol consumption, their attitudes toward drinking, the proportion of peer group activities involving alcohol, and the amount of "pressure" to drink that peers exert on the individual.

Availability. A macroenvironmental factor that may be of etiological significance is the availability of alcohol. In this regard, such factors as the number and distribution of beverage alcohol retail outlets, the price of alcoholic beverages, and minimum drinking age laws may influence the establishment of patterns of drinking and settings in which it is done.

Individual Resources. Throughout the history of developing alcohol problems it is assumed that the individual is influenced by and influences the drinking-related environment. Therefore, the clinician should be alerted to individual characteristics that may affect etiological course, such as chronically high anxiety level, social skills deficits, and distorted beliefs about alcohol.

Summary. Consistent with the theme of this chapter, this brief overview of some important etiological factors in alcohol abuse shows it to be a disorder that has multiple and complex determinants. Bandura (1969) provided a hypothetical scenario of the development of alcoholism from a social learning perspective. Bandura's model relied heavily on the individual's modeling parents who used alcohol as a generalized response to stress. Then, by the time the individual began drinking, this function of alcohol was well learned and used. With continued drinking, individuals tend to drink in a wider array of environments which, in time, become associated with use of alcohol as a stress reducer. In this way alcohol takes on the properties of a generalized coping response, which is highly conducive to excessive consumption.

Although Bandura's (1969) scenario is consistent with a social learning approach, clinicians should be aware of the variety of etiological factors that are possible by different combinations of developmental factors. Therefore, it is of little surprise that there are individual differences among alcohol abusers in how they became problem drinkers. For this reason, clinicians should assess etiology for individual cases and not assume a general pattern. The etiological factors discussed above, therefore, may be used as a guide to case assessment of how abusive drinking developed to present patterns.

COLLECTING ETIOLOGICAL DATA IN THE CLINIC

As with any behavior disorder, tracing the etiology of alcohol-related disorders is not a simple task. The clinician, for the most part, is limited to the patient's self-reports of events that may have occurred many years past. In some cases it may be possible to seek corroborative data from significant others or official records, but these also are tarnished by serious threats to validity. However, the clinician can continually check for the internal consistency of the data as well as consistency across data sources if more than one is used.

Interview Observations

Earlier in this chapter a number of physical cues that suggest the patient may have alcohol problems were discussed. A number of other factors may suggest a hypothesis of an alcohol-related disorder. For example, during the course of the initial interview it may appear that alcohol is a running theme in many of the patient's leisure time activities. That is, the patient's life may appear to revolve around alcohol. Additionally, when the patient is not drinking, he or she may spend a considerable amount of time anticipating the first drink of the day. A correlate of this clinical picture is that the patient appears to spend a considerable portion of his or her income on purchasing alcoholic beverages.

A hypothesis of possible alcohol problems is also suggested by social and demographic information that is easily obtained from the patient. These factors have been discussed by Baekeland and Lundwall (1977) and are indications of a high risk for alcohol problems. They include sporadic attendance at work, particularly in days following holidays or weekends, and a poor driving record, especially a relatively high number of automobile accidents and DUI arrests (see also Maisto, Sobell, Zelhart, Connors, & Cooper, 1979). Furthermore, certain occupations may alert the clinician to the possibility of alcohol problems, including bartenders, cooks and restaurant workers, longshoremen and stevedores, musicians, housepainters, and policemen (Baekeland & Lundwall, 1977, p. 165).

As mentioned earlier, the complex of psychological problems that the patient presents must be considered in assessing for alcohol problems. These problems most commonly include depression, manic depression, antisocial personality disorder, and obsessive compulsive personality disorder. In formulating the case the central job for the clinician is whether these (and other possible) psychopathologies are primary or secondary to alcohol abuse. In this regard, there are a few useful ways to collect information that could help decide among hypotheses. One clue that immediately suggests a hypothesis that the patient's abusive drinking is secondary to psychopathology is the patient's sex. Alcohol problems are more often reactions to psychological distress in women than in men. The clinician can also look into the patient's developmental history to assess his or her functioning before the onset of abusive drinking. Evidence for psychopathology prior to use or abuse of alcohol is not only essential for an adequate formulation of the case but also has important implications for treatment (e.g., Schuckit, 1979). Finally, the clinician may also collect information from the patient on his or her current functioning when not using alcohol. If psychological problems are secondary to heavy use of alcohol, such symptoms should be alleviated after a short period of abstinence. However, if abstinence reveals enhanced levels of distress or inability to cope with life problems, it would suggest that alcohol abuse may be secondary to other psychopathologies.

Interview Style. Most of the literature on styles of relating to alcoholic patients has been written from the psychodynamic perspective, and several authors have described common personality characteristics among alcoholics that have implications for relating to them in a therapeutic setting. The most outstanding of these is sensitivity to rejection. Baekeland and Lundwall (1977) noted that such sensitivity is due to feelings of inferiority and worthlessness, fear of new situations that present challenges, especially relationships that make personal demands, ambivalence, denial, and low frustration tolerance. Blane

(1977) argued that because of these characteristics "it is generally accepted that the therapist must assume an active role in building a relationship with the alcoholic" (p. 113). Although such generalizations may be useful to the clinician in initial generation of hypotheses about a patient, they should not predetermine subsequent clinician–patient interactions. Rather, the clinician should use the interview as a method of collecting data about a patient in order to develop a case formulation and to test it. This formulation should determine the way in which the clinician relates to the patient, and not generalizations about the "alcoholic personality."

Motivation to Change. Alcoholics have the reputation among clinicians for showing a lack of motivation to change their behavior and, as a corollary, to deny their drinking problems. This purported lack of motivation is seen by many to be based in the personality traits described above that are "typical" of the alcoholic. As a consequence of their seeming lack of motivation, it is assumed that alcoholics present a poor prognosis for treatment success, which makes them undesirable cases to therapists. (However, it is interesting to note that clinicians' global impressions of patient motivation to change are not correlated with treatment outcome [Rossi & Filstead, 1976].) Relatedly, Blane (1977) adds, "Alcoholics, in common with other persons having behavioral and impulsive disorders, display a variety of relationship styles which many therapists view as countertherapeutic, manipulative, and hard to work with in a therapeutic setting" (p. 148).

The therapist may be able to obtain a relatively quick initial assessment of the alcoholic's motivation to change and acknowledgement of problems with alcohol. For example, in the middle of an assessment demonstrating regular, heavy use of alcohol and associated social dysfunction, the patient may be asked how long he or she has had alcohol problems. It is not uncommon for patients to say that they do not believe that they do have a problem. In such cases the alcohol-related negative events that have been experienced are attributed to external agents such as spouse, employers, and law enforcement agencies who seem intent on apprehending the patient when others are permitted to go free for the same behavior. Predictably, these and other resistance statements are more common among patients who are not entirely voluntary admissions to treatment, such as court referrals. However, patient resistance has been reported by numerous therapists in many different treatment settings.

The problem of lack of motivation among alcoholic patients has led many therapists to conclude that patients must be confronted in order to advance treatment. Confrontation, in this context, means forcing the patient to "confess" to his or her problems with alcohol. However, Brill (1981) notes that many substance abusers initiate treatment with the intention to challenge the therapist at every opportunity, almost daring rejection and then expecting it to happen eventually. Another reason that confrontation tactics, if *unrefined* and used *indiscriminantly*, are not likely to advance treatment is that no attempt is made to assess the stimuli controlling the patient's lack of motivation. That is, the perceived need to confront derives from the patient's lack of motivation, which is used as an explanation of his or her behavior instead of merely a description of it.

From a behavioral viewpoint, patient behaviors that are described as unmotivated must be understood as any other behaviors if treatment is to progress. Therefore, it is necessary to probe for the factors that control the patient's apparent lack of interest in changing his or her behavior. For example, Sobell and Sobell (1981) suggested that the patient may not appear motivated because of an inaccurate perception of setting events and unanticipated behavioral consequences. Therefore, patients may incorrectly perceive the consequences for different behaviors. They may also be unaware of different behavioral options that could be followed in different situations. Consistent with this idea, it is important to analyze with the patient the current consequences of drinking or not drinking alcohol in different quantities and settings as well as for achieving future goals (Block, 1980; Schuckit, 1979; Ersner-Hershfield, Sobell & Sobell, 1980). The clinician is in a potentially influential position to accomplish this task because, as Schuckit notes, he or she has the ability to help with whatever crisis is most important to the patient at the moment (frequently what brings the patient to treatment). Furthermore, Blane (1977) noted that the same traits that may underlie the patient's apparent lack of motivation often can work to the therapist's advantage if the patient is shaped to see incentives to change. In this regard, early in treatment patients often endow therapists with almost magical powers and influence that can be turned to therapeutic advantage if it is made clear that the patient has ultimate responsibility for his or her progress in treatment.

General Prognosis of Alcoholism Treatment

A recent review of the alcoholism treatment outcome literature covered many studies conducted over about 23 years and involving diverse patient populations admitted to different types of treatment programs in diverse settings (Emrick, 1974, 1975). This extensive review was the basis of several conclusions regarding the prognosis of patients admitted to alcoholism treatment. First, it appears that at follow-up assessment clinicians can expect about one-quarter to one-third of their patients to be abstinent and two-thirds to be at least improved in their drinking. The clinician can also expect to find that patients with certain psychological, social, and drinking history characteristics might do better than others, although the relationships are weak. Finally, Emrick's review informs the clinician that what intervention is used does not make too much difference in the patient's posttreatment functioning, just so long as the patient is exposed to some kind of intervention.

These essential findings were corroborated in a national study of alcoholism treatment outcome (Armor, Polich, & Stambul, 1978). It appears, therefore, that the average patient admitted to treatment for alcohol problems has a good chance for improved functioning, just as long as he or she stays in treatment for a reasonable amount of time. Such a conclusion would not appear to offer the clinician much incentive for carefully planning treatment interventions based on a well-established empirical base. However, it is important to be aware of some of the factors that may explain the data on alcoholism treatment effects. Part of the explanation lies in the difficulties that generally plague the scientific evaluation of psychological treatments, including problems in assigning patients randomly to different treatment interventions, in deciding on outcome criteria and their measurement, and in using a no-treatment control comparison. However, another part of the explanation, and a major assumption of this chapter, concerns poor conceptualization of cases. Most importantly, treatment interventions typically are not derived from case formulations that synthesize clinical data. If such steps are taken, then it would seem to be far more likely that the type of treatment intervention would affect behavior change and its maintenance.

Clinical Experimentation

In nonresearch treatment settings it is not essential to design and conduct clinical experimentation in every case. For example, on the basis of one or two sessions with the patient the clinician may have a high degree of confidence in his or her formulation of the case. Furthermore, for various reasons it may be necessary to begin a treatment intervention as soon as possible. In such a situation it would be appropriate to delete clinical experiments. However, in other cases clinical experimentation may be extremely useful in developing a formulation and testing it. In this regard, when clinical experiments are used they are designed to meet the data requirements of individual cases. Therefore, it is difficult to cite generalities about conducting experiments when working with certain patient classifications. The only generality that can safely be espoused is that the clinician attempts to follow the scientific method in making observations to develop a hypothesis (formulation) and then collects new data to test that hypothesis. The results of such tests are used to reevaluate the initial hypothesis (Meyer & Turkat, 1979).

Clinical Experimentation with Alcohol Abusers. The discussion of conducting clinical experimentation with alcohol abusers will focus on cases in which alcohol abuse is the primary problem instead of a secondary problem. There are two reasons for taking this approach. First, the topic of this chapter is alcohol problems, and this disorder should be prominent in illustrations. Furthermore, the discussions presented in other chapters of this book cover questions that would likely be asked in cases involving alcohol abuse as one secondary problem. However, this distinction is only one of content since the same general methodological approach underlies all cases.

The review presented earlier showed that the clinician may use a number of different validated data sources for assessing alcohol abuse cases. Of course, these same measures can be applied to problems of clinical experimentation. Since clinical experimentation is designed separately for each case, application to alcohol abusers will be illustrated by presenting hypothetical questions and formulations that could arise in treating this patient population. In addition, an illustration will be presented separately for each of various types of measures. In this regard, it is important to remember that this approach is being taken for ease of discussion. In practice, data sources would be used as available and combined to meet the clinician's needs.

Significant Others. As noted earlier, reports of significant others have been shown to be useful in the evaluation of alcohol abusers. Such reports may be a primary data source in validating formulations concerning the relationship between patient drinking behavior and the behavior of significant others. For example, an hypothesis might be that the patient responds with an urge to drink, and often does so, following arguments with his or her spouse. It is further hypothesized that a strong maintaining factor of the patient's drinking is that the spouse reacts to it with anger (which may lead to further arguing, and so forth). These hypotheses suggest that if the patient and spouse were observed discussing a particularly sensitive topic, such as household budget, the clinician should observe various tactics by each person that lead to ill feeling instead of resolution, and the patient should report increased urges to drink. Furthermore, the spouse could be interviewed about the typical ways in which he or she responds to the patient's drinking. Of course, this contrived example is only one of an almost unlimited number of hypotheses in which significant others are the most direct source of data.

Analogue and in Vivo *Observations.* Before describing situations in which analogue and *in vivo* observations could be used, several cautionary notes should be made. First, these methods of data are rarely collected in clinical settings because in many settings where alcoholics are treated administration of alcohol for any reason is strictly prohibited. In addition, measures that involve providing the patient with an opportunity to consume alcohol are limited only to those individuals whose health would not be threatened in any way by drinking. In settings where alcohol is administered for treatment purposes a typical requirement is that medical personnel, including a physician, be readily accessible.

Despite the serious limitations to administering alcohol to alcoholics in clinical settings, there have been a number of research reports suggesting that if alcohol can be used for treatment purposes clinicians' attempts at treatment may be helped substantially. By far the analogue study has been the most frequently used method to examine the drinking behavior of alcoholics (e.g., Marlatt, Demming, & Reid, 1973; Miller, Hersen, Eisler, & Hilsman, 1974). In such studies, a situation that is hypothesized to affect drinking is simulated in the laboratory in order to test hypotheses. A particularly useful measure of drinking behavior for application to the clinical setting is the taste test, which is an unobtrusive measure of alcohol consumption (Marlatt *et al.*, 1973). In this test, the subject is asked to rate alcoholic beverages on a number of taste dimensions, such as bitterness. However, these ratings are merely a way to observe the topography and quantity of the subject's ad lib drinking.

With such a measure, many hypotheses about the patient's drinking may be tested. For example, a formulation might be that the patient drinks excessively because alcohol is used as a generalized way of coping with interpersonal stress. This hypothesis can be tested by observing the patient in the taste test under conditions of no stress, noninterpersonal stress, and interpersonal stress. If the formulation is correct, then the patient should drink the most alcohol following conditions of interpersonal stress.

In vivo observations, despite their potential strength, would seem to have limited application in the clinical setting. The major exception to this is if the clinician desires to measure the patient's responses to alcohol *per se*. However, in the majority of circumstances, the strength of *in vivo* observations would be in their allowing direct observation of the patient drinking in situations where it typically occurs, such as taverns and at home. The limitations in conducting such assessment stem from having to observe the patient; that is, the observation loses much of its "natural" character if the clinician is obviously making observations. It could be argued that observations could be made surreptitiously, as in the bar studies mentioned earlier, but this could raise serious ethical problems.

Physiological Recording. There would seem to be much opportunity to use physiological recording equipment to test a number of hypotheses about the relationship between arousal level and drinking. For example, an intriguing interpretation of the construct of "craving" for alcohol was developed by Hodgson, Rankin, and Stockwell (1979). Craving has been assumed by many therapists and researchers to be the source of loss-of-control drinking that is often reported by alcoholics. However, Hodgson *et al.* conceptualized craving as consisting in large part of negative arousal that is avoided or escaped by drinking. The clinician may use this idea in testing case formulations. For example, it may be hypothesized that the patient drinks in specific situations, but not others, because he or she experiences a craving in those situations. It follows that if these situations were simulated in the clinic, and they can be as simple as the presence of a particular kind of beverage alcohol, the patient should show increased physiological arousal compared to baseline levels. On the other hand, in specified "noncraving" situations, the patient's level of physiological arousal should not change substantially from baseline.

Questionnaires and Other Psychological Tests. These standardized self-report measures may be applied in a variety of circumstances. For example, the analogue test described above was used to test the formulation that the patient drinks excessively as a way of coping with interpersonal stress. This hypothesis predicts that if such a patient responded to a series of items concerning assertiveness in drinking-related situations he or she would be evaluated as unassertive compared to nonalcoholic drinkers or to alcoholics who do not use alcohol as a way of coping with interpersonal stress. In this regard, Watson, Maisto, and Rosenberg (1982) have developed a standardized scale to assess alcohol-related assertion that could be used. Another formulation that might be tested by the use of psychological tests is that excessive drinking is used in response to depression. This suggests that, for example, the patient would have an elevated score on the MMPI depression scale.

Self-Monitoring Data. Self-monitoring of drinking behavior is perhaps best seen not in the context of a specific formulation but, more generally, as a way to aid hypothesis generation and testing. Drinking behavior is particularly amenable to self-monitoring because its components are relatively easy to observe and record. In fact, self-monitoring has been included in a number of clinical studies (see, e.g., Sobell & Sobell, 1973). A behavioral analysis of drinking requires that the patient record as specifically as possible the antecedents and consequences of drinking behavior for a given time. If records are kept faithfully, the data are invaluable in developing hypotheses about cases and in providing measures for testing those hypotheses.

Summary and Conclusions. In this discussion of clinical experimentation several hypothetical examples were used to show that many measurement opportunities exist for the clinician who wants to develop and validate empirically his or her alcohol abuse case formulations. The measures reviewed included reports of significant others, analogue and *in vivo* observations, physiological recording, standardized questionnaires and psychological tests, and self-monitoring data. Importantly, the clinician should not feel that his or her clinical experimentation is limited to the use of these or any other set of measures. Rather, what measures are used depends on their logical applicability (given the formulation), accessibility, and validation.

It is also important to note that in clinical experimentation conclusions may be reached only on a *pattern* of findings. Specifically, the clinician must look for consistency within and across measures in testing hypotheses. Although this approach is also a good one to take in more typical research settings, its importance is accented in the clinical setting because the experimenter is limited to one case and often imperfect control comparisons. Therefore, although this discussion of clinical experimentation generally treated each of a series of measures separately, in practice multiple tests and measures would have been used in conducting clinical experimentation.

The clinician may discover inconsistencies when reviewing his or her pattern of results. Several different factors could account for such discrepancies, including a poor case formulation, insensitive tests of a formulation, or inaccurate data in developing a formulation. When one is faced with discrepant data, the reasonable first question to ask is whether the information on which the formulation is based is accurate. The patient may be shown discrepancies in the data, and the clinician could attempt to shape the patient to help resolve them by appropriate, usually more detailed questioning about some aspect of the patient's behavior. If this does not solve the problem, significant others might be consulted. If this process results in a new or modified formulation it will be tested as was the original formulation. On the other hand, further probing may suggest that the original formulation was correct but not tested under the most sensitive conditions. The clinician would then seek to devise new or refined tests.

BEHAVIORAL FORMULATION OF THE CASE OF MR. S.

The purpose of this section is to apply the information presented thus far on alcohol use and abuse to the formulation of the case of Mr. S., who was described earlier in this book.

Complaints

Mr. S. described four major complaints: (1) depression, (2) loss of employment by firing, (3) marital problems culminating in current divorce proceedings, and (4) heavy use of alcohol that was associated with marital and other interpersonal problems. Mr. S.'s current primary complaint appears to be depression, which he presents with apathy, poor appetite, excessive sleep, and a lack of motivation to do much of anything.

Maintaining Factors

In this case it is perhaps easiest to discuss the factors that are involved in the etiology and maintenance of Mr. S.'s problem behavior by presenting the DSM-III diagnosis of his case. It is important to note that the diagnosis is used as a convenient way to summarize the distinctive features of the case, and not with the intent to disregard specific behaviors.

The primary diagnosis is compulsive personality disorder. The DSM-III (p. 327) criteria for this diagnosis are that at least four of the following characterize current and long-term functioning and cause either significant impairment in social or occupational functioning or subjective distress:

1. Restricted ability to express warm and tender emotion, for example, the individual is unduly conventional, serious and formal, and stingy
2. Perfectionism that interferes with the ability to grasp "the big picture," preoccupation with trivial details, rules, order, organizatin, schedules, and lists
3. Insistence that others submit to his or her way of doing things, and lack of awareness of the feeling elicited by this behavior;

for instance, a husband stubbornly insists that his wife complete errands for him regardless of her plans

4. Excessive devotion to work and productivity to the exclusion of pleasure and the value of interpersonal relationships
5. Indecisiveness: decision making is either avoided, postponed, or protracted perhaps because of an inordinate fear of making a mistake; for example, the individual cannot finish assignments on time because of ruminating about priorities

Mr. S.'s behavior clearly meets these diagnostic criteria. His inability to express emotions was evident in the interview and apparently has a long history. For example, during the interview Mr. S. was extremely serious and formal and when asked to smile he found it difficult to do so. Furthermore, the major reason Mr. S. lost his job, according to his employer, was his overly serious, stern style of interacting with others and never appearing happy. Finally, Mr. S.'s heterosexual and heterosocial relationships, including his marriage, were characterized by his inability to interact informally and to express his emotions. These aspects of his behavior appear to have impaired all of these relationships.

Mr. S. also appeared to be preoccupied with order. Several times during the interview he mentioned that being "rational" was important to him, and what had angered him most about the absence of sexual relations between his wife and him was her lack of rational explanation for this problem. Furthermore, his standards for a clean house were very high, and his wife's failure to meet them bothered him so much that he assumed those responsibilities himself so that they would be done "right." (This assuming of others' responsibilities because of their failure to meet standards of perfection is yet another criterion of the compulsive personality disorder.) A preoccupation with order and detail was also evident in Mr. S.'s job performance. His style of interacting during the interview was consistent with these historical data. In this regard, it seemed most important to him to present his history clearly and logically. Furthermore, Mr. S. was eager for the therapist to provide a logical approach to treatment.

Finally, Mr. S.'s history also contains evidence that work and productivity are extremely important to him. For example, though he purportedly desired a circle of close friends, his first thoughts were once again finding employment so he "could be productive." This desire to be productive, however, is combined with extremely high performance standards so that tasks often are not completed on time. Mr. S. showed this behavior on the job.

These data suggest, therefore, that the appropriate primary diagnosis for Mr. S. is compulsive personality disorder. However, one of Mr. S.'s presenting problems was heavy drinking of alcohol. It seems appropriate in this case to assign to Mr. S.'s case a secondary diagnosis of alcohol abuse. Although a detailed drinking history was not collected, this appears to be an accurate secondary diagnosis, according to DSM-III criteria. In this regard, Mr. S.'s drinking appears to meet the criterion of "pathological use" in that he is drinking heavily and has been trying to control his intake. This pattern follows Mr. S.'s past history of drinking in spurts to the point of passing out from intoxication. Furthermore, his pattern of pathological intake clearly has been evident for longer than the one-month minimum. Most importantly, Mr. S.'s drinking seems to have exacerbated his marital problems. For example, he reported that when he was living with his wife his nighttime drinking of whiskey often led to arguments. In addition, the more recent event of failure to perform sexually with a secretary at work may have been due in part to the impairing effects of alcohol on sexual performance. This event was significant to Mr. S.'s present complaints because this failure made him feel socially and sexually inept.

Alcohol abuse was listed as the secondary diagnosis because it appears to have been a result of problems related to the primary diagnosis of compulsive personality disorder. Mr. S.'s history indicates that his abusive drinking began during the second year of his marriage when he and his wife were already having frequent and serious arguments. Therefore, the data presented suggested that alcohol abuse originated as a reaction to a more primary set of problems.

The diagnostic summary of Mr. S.'s presenting problems and history emphasizes the high importance to this patient of perfection in personal conduct and in work performance. This suggests why Mr. S. currently shows symptoms of depression. Simply, Mr. S. has experienced two recent traumatic events that are inconsistent with his personal conduct standards. He is currently being divorced from his wife, which is morally inimical to him. Besides this failure in duty to make his marriage work, Mr. S.'s unemployment makes him currently unable to fulfill another duty of supporting his child. In addition, Mr. S. attempted to have sexual relations with one of the secretaries at work while he was still married, which was also inconsistent with his standards of moral conduct. The upshot of these events is that Mr. S. is probably engaging in many self-punishing statements that evoke guilt, a correlate of depression.

Mr. S. also recently lost a major source of reinforcement, work performance that is considered productive. It is possible that being fired from his job was the most serious blow to Mr. S., since his preoccupation with work and productivity ran through his professional and personal life. A major correlate of major loss of reinforcement that is not replaced is depressive affect.

Finally, the secondary diagnosis of alcohol abuse is based on an interpretation of the case data that alcohol is used to cope with depressive and other negative affects. For example, Mr. S. apparently started abusing alcohol when he and his wife were having serious arguments. He is currently drinking heavily during a period of depression that he does not seem to understand or know how to ameliorate more adaptively.

Predisposition and Development

Mr. S. came from a home where the Mormon religion's strict moral code was practiced. His father was an accountant whom Mr. S. described as rational, fair, and orderly. Mr. S. in describing his mother called her a "saint" who also seemed to value orderliness. This characteristic was manifested in her highly organized, meticulously clean housekeeping. She also kept inventory lists of items in the home, a trait which Mr. S. seemed to remember fondly. Furthermore, Mr. S.'s parents had few close friends, although they appeared to have a number of acquaintances who were associated with the Mormon Church.

If it is accepted that modeling is a strong determinant of the development of behavior, Mr. S.'s childhood home seems to be a place where it would almost be natural to learn behaviors comprising the compulsive personality disorder diagnosis. Both of Mr. S.'s parents displayed extreme orderliness, and the father's behavior stood out as fair and rational. Thus Mr. S. was continually exposed to these characteristics as a child. Furthermore, his parents' acting in this way implies that they reinforced these same behaviors in others, particularly their son. Therefore, the contingencies were present to provide incentives for Mr. S. to enact the behavior that he had observed in his parents. Furthermore, Mr. S. seems to have incorporated traits like rationality and extreme organization of details as behavioral ideals. For example, he highly regarded his own rationality and, when describing his mother's keeping of home inventory lists, he referred to her as a saint.

Mr. S.'s strict moral standards also seem to be a result of his childhood family environment. Both parents were committed to the Mormon religion and its moral strictures. In addition, the other adult models available to Mr. S. were also Mormons, since his parents' acquaintances were through the church.

According to these historical data, therefore, Mr. S. observed adults whose approach to life was rational instead of emotional, and who seemed to value order and organization. The primary adult models of Mr. S.'s childhood demonstrated and reinforced only a limited range of behaviors, which strongly affected his behavioral patterns in interactions outside of the home. Furthermore, modeling a strict religious moral code probably resulted in stringent judgments of Mr. S.'s own and others' behavior. It is also likely the primary influence in the development of Mr. S.'s perfectionistic standards.

Another important feature of Mr. S.'s childhood was the lack of opportunity for him to observe the expression of feelings. Mr. S.'s parents did not appear to be demonstrative toward each other. Furthermore, they had few close friends, so Mr. S. had little chance to observe ways of interacting in such relationships. Therefore, Mr. S. lacked a model or an incentive for expressing emotion or for responding to others' emotions. Apparently this was a primary determinant of Mr. S.'s current problems in these same behaviors.

Formulation

It is hypothesized that the predominance of Mr. S.'s presenting complaints can be explained by his learning to be indiscriminantly rational and by his lack of training in experiencing and expressing his own emotions and in perceiving emotions in others. Furthermore, because he was overtly rational and could not be emotional Mr. S.'s behavior was rigid. These deficits appear to underlie Mr. S.'s primary complaint of depression. In this regard, Mr. S. lost his job because of his affective demeanor and because of his failure to observe that he made the other employees uncomfortable at work. Much of the difficulty in Mr. S.'s marriage seems to be due to his failure to express positive emotion toward his wife and to read her feelings so that sexual relations were impaired and eventually ceased. For example, it is likely that Mr. S. often initiated sex at inauspicious times and persisted despite his wife's showing her displeasure. Conversely, he probably often failed to perceive occasions when his wife may have desired to have sex. Or, even if he did happen to perceive her desire he may not have responded if sex were not in his plans for the moment. It also follows from this formulation that Mr. S.'s approach to sexual encounters with his wife were rarely spontaneous and were perfunctory in manner and lacking in emotion to an unusual degree. This further raises the possibility that it did not take long for Mr. S.'s wife to habituate to him sexually. Mr. S.'s reactions to his sexual problems in marriage were, predictably, rational rather than emotional. It drove him "crazy" because his wife would not discuss sex rationally.

Mr. S. was also insensitive to his wife about nonsexual matters, which probably exacerbated their marital strife. For example, he assumed some of her responsibilities (e.g., housework) because of her failure to meet his overly high standards and failed to appreciate that such behavior might result in his wife's displeasure. Furthermore, Mr. S.'s insensitivity to and lack of intimacy with his wife may be viewed as a repetition, to a more serious degree, of earlier heterosexual relationships. Therefore, these ways of interacting with women seem to have been characteristic of Mr. S. for some time. The question might be raised of why Mr. S. ever was married, given his personality. According to the present formulation, it would be predicted that Mr. S. saw marriage solely in nonemotional terms, such as the belief that it is the responsibility of adults to marry and to raise a family in the proper way.

The negative effects (e.g., guilt, feelings of incompetence) of the failed sexual encounter between Mr. S. and a secretary at work were also magnified by Mr. S.'s social skills deficits. In this regard, he was faced with an event that involved emotional responses and he did not have the skills to express himself or to perceive how the secretary was feeling. Therefore, although the failed sexual encounter disturbed Mr. S., he neither did nor said anything about it. In general, if a social event has nonrational, emotional elements to it Mr. S. could be expected to be less than adequate. This analysis suggests that Mr. S. would have few, if any, close friends of either sex, since such relationships require the expression of emotion and appropriate response. Furthermore, it would be predicted that others would tend to view Mr. S. as a poor candidate for a close friend, since he would often appear to act incongruously with the emotional aspects of settings and since he would tend to extinguish others' expression of feelings by not responding to them. The diagnosis that was assigned to Mr. S. also indicates that these behavior patterns had long characterized his social life. Thus one would hypothesize that in childhood and adolescence Mr. S. did little socializing with peers and seldom engaged in behavior that might be construed as play and had no specific goal. It would also be expected that Mr. S. would recall his youth in terms of productive activities and of goals achieved rather than in terms of good times or of enjoyable events with others.

Finally, the present formulation explains that Mr. S.'s heavy drinking is related to the occurrence of negative affect like anger and depression. Since these are nonrational responses, Mr. S. lacks the skills

to cope with them effectively and thus uses alcohol to escape from
them.

Interview and Clinical Experimentation Strategies

Interview. According to the formulation of this case, it appears
that the interviewer should attempt to discuss the development of
Mr. S.'s problems, his current problems, and their treatment as *rationally* and *objectively* as possible. Although this approach is generally
appropriate, it seems particularly important in this case. Mr. S. feels
most comfortable and responds best to a rational approach to any problem or topic. Furthermore, because of Mr. S.'s extremely high moral
standards the therapist must assure that no imputations of "bad" behavior are made to this patient. Finally, Mr. S.'s primary diagnosis suggests
that he would be highly motivated to provide as accurate retrospective
self-reports as possible if the therapist reinforces him for providing
precise data to assist in a "rational" objective approach to his case.

Although it would be important for the interviewer to appear
rational and objective, there should be no hesitation to test hypotheses
about Mr. S.'s social and emotional deficits. Questions should be asked,
for example, that require Mr. S. to report how he and others *felt* about
specific events or to express for the clinician various positive and negative affects. If such questions were asked, then the clinician could
make comparisons between Mr. S.'s responses to questions about rational
and emotional subjects. For instance, it would be predicted that Mr. S.
would take longer to respond and to show more discomfort when asked
about an emotional subject than about one that is rational. Naturally,
questions about emotional topics could be woven into the interview in
a logical, rational way to achieve the goal of testing and retesting the
formulation's accuracy.

It would appear desirable to obtain some additional historical data
from Mr. S. before designing a treatment plan. Most outstanding is the
need for further data on Mr. S.'s drinking history and current patterns.
Such data were only minimally supplied in the initial interview and
are essential to confirming the initial hypothesis that Mr. S. uses alcohol
to cope with negative affect. In this regard, the present formulation
should be used to guide the clinician in collecting the required developmental data. For example, it would be hypothesized that Mr. S.'s first
encounter with alcohol was associated with much guilt. It is highly
likely that Mr. S. drank for the first time when he was an adolescent
and was influenced by his peers. Perhaps he drank with them on a

challenge or as a way to be accepted by them, since he found it difficult to win their acceptance in other ways. However, since Mr. S.'s parents were highly moralistic Mormons and probably viewed drinking at best as a complete waste of time, it is certain that Mr. S. drank alcohol for the first time with much trepidation about possible consequences if he were discovered. While drinking, Mr. S. learned that alcohol is associated with euphoric feelings and maybe even felt more at ease being with other boys his age. Despite the fact that (or maybe because) this and other early drinking events were not discovered by his parents, Mr. S. probably felt extremely guilty about using alcohol. Of course, these feelings were not expressed or handled effectively. It may be hypothesized, therefore, that Mr. S. learned that alcohol consumption is pleasant but is followed, for him, by negative feelings such as guilt and self-deprecation. Importantly, it would be expected that Mr. S. would presently feel this same way, since he still identifies drinking as an act that wastes time and that causes him to relinguish control over his behavior. This would be expected to create a cycle of negative affect–drink–negative affect–drink to Mr. S.'s drinking pattern. Therefore, according to the formulation, Mr. S. would be expected to have learned to use alcohol to escape from negative feelings that he cannot deal with in more adaptive ways. Furthermore, as discussed earlier, while testing this hypothesis about the variables controlling Mr. S.'s drinking, the clinician should thoroughly assess the social, environmental, and other psychological factors that may be correlated with the patient's drinking.

Another problem area wherein further data are needed concerns Mr. S.'s interactions with peers and other individuals outside of the home during childhood and adolescence. The available interview data suggested that Mr. S. modeled a specific style of interaction from his parents, as well as lacked models for expressing and responding to affect. As noted above, it would be hypothesized that this style of interaction resulted, first, in his not initiating many contacts with peers and, second, when he did make acquaintances, in his inability to turn them into close friendships. It is likely that Mr. S. reserved little time for leisure activities with friends, and when he was around people they would not tend to be attracted to his rigid, nonemotional style. Furthermore, since Mr. S. had deficits in expressing emotions and in perceiving others' feelings, intimacy with others would have been aversive to him and therefore likely to be avoided or escaped. The formulation also predicts that Mr. S. was often puzzled about social events. For example, if asked why a certain relationship terminated or why other people did not pursue his nor he their friendship, he would appear genuinely at a loss for an answer. According to Mr. S., he always is courteous to others and always does the "right thing" socially. He may further report that he has frequently done favors for others or has helped them in their work but that it apparently did not make much difference to them.

Clinical Experimentation

Clinical experimentation should be concerned with two general features of this case. First, the primary diagnosis of compulsive personality disorder is clear but it is based predominantly on one data source, Mr. S.'s self-reports of past and current events. This diagnosis was supported by some of Mr. S.'s behavior during the initial interview, such as his concern about presenting information logically and his difficulty in smiling when asked to. However, the diagnosis would be more strongly validated by converging evidence from other data sources. For example, one hypothesis is that a compulsive personality would score as more field-dependent on a test of cognitive style because of attention to minor details to the extent of failing to see "the big picture." Mr. S.'s high needs for planning, order, and organization also suggest that in a test of creativity, such as the Remote Associations Test (Mednick & Mednick, 1967), that requires discerning unusual or novel associations among stimuli, he would score below average.

The therapist could obtain as many tests to validate the diagnosis as is judged desirable or necessary. The major points, however, are that diagnoses are merely verbal summaries of behavioral observations and facilitate treatment only to the degree that they are based on valid data. Since there is no one measure in the clinical setting that has universal validity, the therapist can be most confident in his or her diagnosis if it is based on converging pieces of information.

If the primary diagnosis is confirmed, then confirmation of the secondary diagnosis of alcohol abuse is appropriate. As noted above, for this case the first step would be to obtain a more detailed functional analysis of Mr. S.'s drinking behavior. If these self-report data confirm the initial hypotheses, then behavioral data, if they can be obtained, would be extremely useful. For example, an analogue study could be contrived to test the quantity of Mr. S.'s alcohol consumption under conditions of neutral and (induced) negative affect (measured by self-report and if possible by physiological arousal). It would also be useful, and feasible according to Mr. S.'s diagnosis, to ask him to self-monitor his daily drinking behavior, including details on its antecedents and consequences. These self-recording data should reveal a high correlation between negative affect and drinking.

The next aspect of clinical experimentation is to test predictions that derive from the case formulation. As with validation of the diagnosis, the possible approaches are defined only by imagination and resources. It is important to note that tests do not have to be highly complex and technically sophisticated to be powerful. Indeed, in a clinical setting they often cannot be. Rather, the objective is to demonstrate empirically or to confirm, according to scientific criteria, the implications of the clinician's formulation. In applying these principles to Mr. S., a basic prediction is that he would score as differentially assertive and distressed on self-report and behavioral (role-play) tests of social skills as a function of whether situations involved expression of feelings or of objective, logical information. For example, if he were required to express displeasure in reaction to another person's actions, Mr. S. should have difficulty and report considerable discomfort. He should react similarly if he were required to compliment a person on some aspect of his or her behavior or appearance and would become uneasy if given compliments. In contrast, Mr. S. should show relatively little difficulty and discomfort when instructed to be assertive in situations involving, for example, someone stepping in front of him on a line or in informing a colleague that his or her report contained statistical errors.

Relatedly, the Alcohol Assertion Inventory (AAI; Watson *et al.*, 1982) could be used in testing more specific hypotheses about Mr. S.'s use of alcohol. The AAI includes intrapersonal and interpersonal settings involving alcohol use, and respondents are required to estimate the probability that they would drink in these settings, as well as to report the degree of discomfort that they would experience if they were in the settings. According to the present formulation, events that involve affect or its expression should be those in which Mr. S. reports the most discomfort. These should be the same settings in which Mr. S. reports a higher likelihood of drinking. Furthermore, if facilities are available, Mr. S.'s reports could be validated behaviorally by use of the "taste test" analogue that was described earlier.

It has been mentioned several times that the formulation includes the hypothesis that Mr. S. is deficient in recognizing affect in others. This could be tested, for example, by a task involving identifying emotions in others from their facial expressions. It would be predicted that Mr. S. would take longer to complete such a task and would label facial expressions of emotion differently than would an appropriate control group. The clinician would use the results of these and other possible tests of the formulation to determine whether additional data are necessary for its confirmation or the validity of the formulation should be questioned.

Use of the Formulation in the Design and Conduct of Treatment

A major benefit of the experimental approach to clinical cases is that hypotheses (formulations) to explain the patient's presenting problems lead to specific strategies for design and implementation of treatment. This can be clearly demonstrated in the case of Mr. S.

Accuracy of Self-Reports. In most cases the clinician's diagnoses, formulations, design of treatment, and evaluation of its effectiveness rest in large part on the patient's self-reports. Therefore, it is essential that the clinician do what he or she can to obtain as accurate data as possible. In the case of Mr. S., it is predicted that his self-report data would not be tainted by intentional misreporting or denial. There are several reasons for this hypothesis. First, Mr. S. places a high value on order and details. Thus, it is reinforcing for him to report such data accurately and he would respond to the clinician's praise for doing so. Furthermore, Mr. S. was cooperative during the interview and expressed concern that he present events correctly and in logical order. Of course, this prediction should be validated if possible. For instance, it might be possible to check Mr. S.'s recent employment records to verify his account of events at his last job that led to his dismissal.

Resistance. Based on the diagnosis and formulation of Mr. S.'s case, the clinician can expect several possible points of resistance in treatment. First, Mr. S. is likely to be resistant if he believes that the clinician is unjustly "blaming" him for his present behavioral and psychological difficulties. This follows from assessment of Mr. S. as having perfectionistic work and moral standards and therefore being susceptible to punishing feelings of inadequacy and guilt. Relatedly, since Mr. S. values rational and logical approaches to human behavior, the clinician should make particular effort to present his or her early analyses of the case in this way. However, over time it will be essential for the clinician to introduce nonrational, emotional interactions into treatment if Mr. S. is to make progress. Importantly, the clinician may expect that Mr. S. will show at least initial resistance at this time.

Another point derived from the case formulation is that the clinician should be explicit in the meaning of various statements. In this regard, since it appears that Mr. S. is deficient in appropriately attending to various social cues, what may appear as resistance could be based in misperceptions of what the clinician is saying. To compound the problem Mr. S. may have difficulty in expressing to the clinician any failure to understand therapeutic events. This could be due either to embarrassment at admitting a lack of understanding or to a behavioral deficit in expressing the problem. It follows from this general analysis of the case that the clinician should make clear, explicit statements to Mr. S. at all times and explain his problems to him as one possible logical outcome of his learning history. Similarly, means of alleviating his problems should be presented clearly using specific techniques to alter the problem behaviors that have developed.

Treatment Goals. In the case of Mr. S. the major treatment goals are: (a) reemployment in a satisfactory position; (b) achievement of rewarding social relationships; (c) reduction in depressive affect; and (d) reduction in drinking to a nonproblem level, which may be defined as either abstinence or moderate drinking.

The formulation suggests that the primary way to achieve these goals is to train Mr. S. in different dimensions of social skills. Specifically, Mr. S. has to learn how to (a) gauge more accurately others' behaviors (and feelings), (b) permit himself to react emotionally, and (c) express these emotional reactions appropriately. However, there are not any behavioral techniques that could be applied with confidence to achieve this set of goals. Some of the general social skills training techniques that have been developed (e.g., Lange & Jakubowski, 1976; Rimm & Masters, 1979) or some modification of them could be applied in treating Mr. S. Unfortunately, an extremely important aspect of Mr. S.'s treatment, training him in social perception and cognition (Arkowitz, 1981), has received scant attention from behavioral clinical researchers. Morrison and Bellack (1981) defined social perception skills as consisting of (a) knowledge of social mores, (b) knowledge of the meaning of various response cues, (c) attention to relevant aspects of an interaction, (d) information-processing ability, and (e) the ability to predict and evaluate interpersonal consequences.

The formulation also suggests that the clinician should simultaneously train Mr. S. in making alternative responses to drinking alcohol when he experiences negative affect (e.g., Miller, 1979). These may include, for example, activities such as relaxation, jogging, or meditation. The specific behavior (or behaviors) that is chosen is suited to the individual case; the objective is to provide the patient with behavioral skills that will compete successfully with drinking behavior.

Determining when to terminate treatment is never a simple matter. However, from the formulation of Mr. S. it appears clear that treatment should be terminated when objective outcome criteria have been attained (a generally good approach). In this regard, the drinking outcome would be based on a criterion that was designated by both the clinician and the patient. For Mr. S., it appears appropriate that the drinking outcome could include moderate drinking, since he does not have a history of either chronic abusive drinking or physical dependence on alcohol. Whatever goal is chosen, earlier sections of this chapter showed that a number of measures of drinking behavior that may be applied to the clinical setting have been developed to determine whether the outcome criterion has been reached.

Achievement of successful employment may be assessed directly both through Mr. S.'s self-report and through employer interview. Practically, progress in social relationships would require clear operationalization and would rely primarily on Mr. S.'s self-report. However, the popularity among behavioral clinicians of social skills training procedures has led to advances in assessment in this area (e.g., Arkowitz, 1981). Furthermore, if appropriate, it may be possible to interview the individuals whom Mr. S. identifies as his friends. Finally, there are a variety of methods that have been developed to evaluate depression (Rehm, 1981).

Motivation to Change. The case formulation suggests that Mr. S.is highly motivated to change and to cooperate with the therapist as long as the approach to treatment is logical and objective. There was ample behavioral evidence during the interview to support this hypothesis, as already discussed. Furthermore, Mr. S. does not seem to be denying any aspects of his drinking behavior and acknowledges that it is a problem for him. Fortunately, his drinking problem does not appear to be severe. The prognosis, therefore, is a qualified "promising." It is qualified because the source of Mr. S.'s current problems is a pattern of behavior that was acquired in early childhood and has been elaborated since then with little competition from more adaptive behaviors. Furthermore, the behavioral treatment techniques for the social skills deficits that Mr. S. presents have not been well developed. Therefore, although the necessary ingredient of motivation to change is present, Mr. S. (and the clinician) will have to sustain it through long periods of difficult work in order to achieve his treatment goals.

GENERAL SUMMARY

The purpose of this chapter was to describe behavioral formulations of cases of alcohol problems. A general approach to these cases was discussed, including data obtained in the initial interviews, interaction between patient and therapist during sessions, general prognosis, and strategies of clinical experimentation. It was shown that although cases of alcohol abuse are often complex and compounded by other psychopathologies, they can be approached empirically because of the number of validated data collection procedures that have been developed. Finally, many points reviewed in the general approach were illustrated in a complex case that was assigned a primary diagnosis of compulsive personality disorder and a secondary diagnosis of alcohol abuse. This example showed that it is feasible and productive to apply the experimental method to complex cases of alcohol abuse.

REFERENCES

Adesso, V. J. (1980). Experimental studies of human drinking behavior. In H. Rigter & J. Crabbe, Jr. (Eds.), *Alcohol tolerance and dependence*. New York: North-Holland Biomedical Press.

Akers, R. L. (1977). *Deviant behavior: A social learning approach*. Belmont, CA: Wadsworth.

American Medical Association. (1977). *Manual on alcoholism* (3rd ed.). Chicago: American Medical Association.

American Psychiatric Association. (1980). *Diagnostic and statistical manual of mental disorders* (3rd ed.). Washington, DC: American Psychiatric Association.

Arkowitz, H. (1981). Assessment of social skills. In M. Hersen & A. S. Bellack (Eds.), *Behavioral assessment: A practical handbook* (2nd ed.). New York: Pergamon Press.

Armor, D. J., Polich, J. M., & Stambul, H. B. (1978). *Alcoholism and treatment*. New York: Wiley Interscience.

Baekeland, F., & Lundwall, L. K. (1977). Engaging the alcoholic in treatment and keeping him there. In B. Kissin & H. Begleiter (Eds.), *The biology of alcoholism* (Vol. 5). New York: Plenum Press.

Bandura, A. (1969). *Principles of behavior modification*. New York: Holt, Rinehart, & Winston.

Bandura, A. (1977). *Social learning theory*. Englewood Cliffs, NJ: Prentice-Hall.

Bissell, L. (1980). Diagnosis and recognition. In S. E. Gitlow & H. S. Peyser (Eds.), *Alcoholism: A practical guide to treatment*. New York: Grune & Stratton.

Blane, H. T. (1977). Psychotherapeutic approach. In B. Kissin & H. Begleiter (Eds.), *The biology of alcoholism* (Vol. 5). New York: Plenum Press.

Block, M. A. (1980). Motivating the alcoholic patient. In S. E. Gitlow & H. S. Peyser (Eds.), *Alcoholism: A practical guide to treatment*. New York: Grune & Stratton.

Brill, L. (1981). *The clinical treatment of substance abusers*. New York: The Free Press.

Cahalan, D., & Cisin, I. H. (1976). Epidemiological and social factors associated with drinking problems. In R. E. Tarter & A. Sugerman (Eds.), *Alcoholism: Interdisciplinary approaches to an enduring problem*. Reading, MA: Addison-Wesley.

Cappell, H. (1981). Tolerance to ethanol and treatment of its abuse: Some fundamental issues. *Addictive Behaviors, 6,* 197–204.

Conger, J. J. (1956). Alcoholism: Theory, problem and challenge. II. Reinforcement theory and dynamics of alcoholism. *Quarterly Journal of Studies on Alcohol, 17,* 291–324.

Emrick, C. D. (1974). A review of psychologically oriented treatment of alcoholism. I. The use and interrelationships of outcome criteria and drinking behavior following treatment. *Quarterly Journal of Studies on Alcohol, 35,* 523–549.

Emrick, C. D. (1975). A review of psychologically oriented treatment of alcoholism. II. The relative effectiveness of different treatment approaches and the effectiveness of treatment versus no treatment. *Journal of Studies on Alcohol, 36,* 88–108.

Endler, N. S., & Magnusson, D. (1976). Toward an interactional psychology of personality. *Psychological Bulletin, 83,* 956–974.

Ersner-Hershfield, S., Sobell, M. B., & Sobell, L. C. (1980). Interviewing and identifying persons with alcohol problems. In M. Juspe, J. E. Nieberding, & B. D. Cohen (Eds.), *Handbook of psychological factors in health care: A practitioner's text in health care psychology.* Lexington, MA: Lexington Books.

Foy, D. W., Rychtarik, R. G., & Prue, D. M. (1981). Assessment of appetitive disorders. In M. Hersen & A. S. Bellack (Eds.), *Behavioral assessment: A practical handbook* (2nd ed.). New York: Pergamon Press.

Goodwin, D. W. (1980). The genetics of alcoholism. *Substance and Alcohol Actions/Misuse, 1,* 101–117.

Hersen, M., & Bellack, A. S. (Eds.). (1981). *Behavioral assessment: A practical handbook* (2nd ed.). New York: Pergamon Press.

Hodgson, R., Rankin, H., & Stockwell, T. (1979). Alcohol dependence and the priming effect. *Behavior Research & Therapy, 17,* 379–387.

Hull, J. G. (1981). A self-awareness model of the causes and effects of alcohol consumption. *Journal of Abnormal Psychology, 90,* 586–600.

Kalant, H., LeBlanc, A. E., & Gibbins, R. J. (1971). Tolerance to, and dependence on, ethanol. In Y. Israel & J. Mardones (Eds.), *Biological bases of alcoholism.* New York: John Wiley.

Kessler, M. & Gomberg, C. (1974). Observations of barroom drinking: Methodology and preliminary results. *Quarterly Journal of Studies on Alcohol, 35,* 1392–1396.

Lange, A. J. & Jakubowski, P. (1976). Responsible assertive behavior. Champaign, IL: Research Press.

Maisto, S. A., & Cooper, A. M. (1980). A historical perspective on alcohol and drug abuse treatment outcome research. In L. C. Sobell, M. B. Sobell, & E. Ward (Eds.), *Evaluating alcohol and drug abuse treatment effectiveness.* New York: Pergamon Press.

Maisto, S. A., & Maisto, C. A. (1983). Institutional measures in treatment outcome evaluation. In M. J. Lambert, E. R. Christensen, & S. S. DeJulio (Eds.), *The measurement of psychotherapy outcomes in research and evaluation.* New York: Wiley.

Maisto, S. A., Henry, R. R., Sobell, M. B., & Sobell, L. C. (1978). Implications of acquired changes in tolerance for the treatment of alcohol problems. *Addictive Behaviors, 3,* 51–56.

Maisto, S. A., Sobell, L. C., & Sobell, M. B. (1979). Comparison of alcoholics' self-reports of drinking behavior with reports of collateral informants. *Journal of Consulting and Clinical Psychology, 47,* 106–112.

Maisto, S. A., Sobell, L. C., Zelhart, P. F., Connors, G. J., & Cooper, T. (1979). Driving records of persons convicted of driving under the influence of alcohol. *Journal of Studies on Alcohol, 40,* 70–77.

Maisto, S. A., Connors, G. J., & Sachs, P. R. (1981). Expectation as a mediator in alcohol intoxication: A reference level model. *Cognitive Therapy and Research, 5,* 1–18.

Maisto, S. A., Sobell, M. B., & Sobell, L. C. (1982). Reliability of self-reports of low ethanol consumption by problem drinkers over 18 months of follow-up. *Drug and Alcohol Dependence, 9,* 273–278.

Marlatt, G. A. (1975). The drinking profile: A questionnaire for the behavioral assessment of alcoholism. In E. J. Mash & L. G. Terdal (Eds.), *Behavior therapy assessment: Diagnosis and Evaluation*. New York: Springer.

Marlatt, G. A., & Rohsenow, D. G. (1980). Cognitive processes in alcohol use: Expectancy and the balanced placebo design. In N. K. Mello (Ed.), *Advances in substance abuse: Behavioral and biological research*. Greenwich, CT: JAI Press.

Marlatt, G. A., Demming, B., & Reid, J. B. (1973). Loss of control drinking in alcoholics: An experimental analogue. *Journal of Abnormal Psychology, 81*, 233–241.

Mednick, S. A., & Mednick, M. (1967). *Remote associates test manual*. New York: Psychological Corporation.

Mello, N. K. (1972). Behavioral studies of alcoholism. In B. Kissin & H. Begleiter (Eds.), *The biology of alcoholism*. New York: Plenum Press.

Mendelson, J. H., & Mello, N. K. (1966). Experimental analysis of drinking behavior of chronic alcoholics. *Annals of the New York Academy of Sciences, 133*, 828–845.

Meyer, V., & Turkat, I. D. (1979). Behavioral analysis of clinical cases. *Journal of Behavioral Assessment, 1*, 259–270.

Miller, P. M. (1976). *Behavioral treatment of alcoholism*. New York: Pergamon Press.

Miller, P. M. (1979). Behavioral strategies for reducing drinking among young adults. In M. E. Chafetz & H. T. Blane (Eds.), *Youth, alcohol, and social policy*. New York: Plenum Press.

Miller, P. M., Hersen, M., Eisler, R. M. & Elkin, T. E. (1974). A retrospective analysis of alcohol consumption on laboratory tasks as related to therapeutic outcome. *Behavior Research & Therapy, 12*, 73–76.

Miller, P. M., Hersen, M., Eisler, R. M., & Hilsman, G. (1974). Effects of social stress on operant drinking of alcoholics and social drinkers. *Behavior Research & Therapy, 12*, 67–72.

Miller, W. R., & Caddy, G. R. (1977). Abstinence and controlled drinking in the treatment of problem drinkers. *Journal of Studies on Alcohol, 38*, 986–1003.

Mischel, W. (1973). Toward a cognitive social learning reconceptualization of personality. *Psychological Review, 80*, 252–283.

Morrison, R. L., & Bellack, A. (1981). The role of social perception in social skills. *Behavior Therapy.*

Nathan, P. E., & Lipscomb, T. R. (1979). Behavior therapy and behavior modification in the treatment of alcoholism. In J. H. Mendelson & N. K. Mello (Eds.), *The diagnosis and treatment of alcoholism*. New York: McGraw-Hill.

Nathan, P. E., Titler, N. A., Lowenstein, L. M., Solomon, P., & Rossi, A. M. (1970). Behavioral analysis of chronic alcoholism. *Archives of General Psychiatry, 22*, 419–430.

National Council on Alcoholism, Criteria Committee. (1972). Criteria for the diagnosis of alcoholism. *Americal Journal of Psychiatry, 129*, 127–135.

Owen, P. L., & Butcher, J. N. (1979). Personality factors in problem drinking: A review of the evidence and some suggested directions. In R. W. Pickens & L. L. Heston (Eds.), *Psychiatric factors in drug abuse*. New York: Grune & Stratton.

Parsons, O. A., & Leber, W. R. (1982). Alcohol, cognitive dysfunctions, and brain damage. In *Biomedical processes and consequences of alcohol use* (Alcohol and Health Monograph No. 2). Rockville, MD: National Institute on Alcohol Abuse and Alcoholism.

Pattison, E. M., Sobell, M. B., & Sobell, L. C. (1977). (Authors/Editors). *Emerging concepts of alcohol dependence*. New York: Springer.

Pickens, R. W., & Heston, L. L. (Eds.). (1979). *Psychiatric factors in drug abuse*. New York: Grune & Stratton.

Rachal, J. V., Guess, L. L., Hubbard, R. L., Maisto, S. A., Cavanaugh, E. R., Waddell, R., & Benrud, C. H. (1980, October). *Adolescent drinking behavior. Volume 1: The extent and nature of adolescent alcohol and drug use: The 1974 and 1978 national sample studies.* Final report submitted to the National Institute on Alcohol Abuse and Alcoholism (Contract No. ADM 281-76-0019).

Rachman, S., & Teasdale, J. (1969). *Aversion therapy and behavior disorders.* Coral Gables, FL: University of Miami Press.

Rehm, L. P. (1981). Assessment of depression. In M. Hersen & A. S. Bellack (Eds.), *Behavioral assessment: A practical handbook* (2nd Ed.). New York: Pergamon Press.

Reid, J. B. (1978). The study of drinking in natural settings. In G. A. Marlatt & P. E. Nathan (Eds.), *Behavioral approaches to assessment and treatment of alcoholism.* New Brunswick, NJ: Rutgers Center of Alcohol Studies.

Rimm, D. C., & Masters, J. C. (1979). *Behavior therapy: Techniques and empirical findings* (2nd ed.). New York: Academic Press.

Rosenbluth, J., Nathan, P. E., & Lawson, D. M. (1978). Environmental influences on drinking by college students in a college pub. *Addictive Behaviors, 3,* 117–121.

Rossi, J. J., & Filstead, M. J. (1976). Treating the treatment issues. In M. J. Filstead, J. J. Rossi, & M. Keller (Eds.), *Alcohol and alcohol problems.* New York: Ballinger.

Schaefer, H. H., Sobell, M. B., & Mills, K. C. (1971). Baseline drinking behavior in alcoholics and social drinkers: Kinds of drinks and sip magnitude. *Behavior Research & Therapy, 9,* 23–27.

Schuckit, M. A. (1979). Treatment of alcoholism in office and outpatient settings. In J. H. Mendelson & N. K. Mello (Eds.), *The diagnosis and treatment of alcoholism.* New York: McGraw-Hill.

Sobell, L. C. (1978). Alcohol treatment outcome evaluation: Contributions from behavioral research. In P. E. Nathan, G. A. Marlatt, & T. Loberg (Eds.), *Alcoholism: New directions in behavioral research and treatment.* New York: Plenum Press.

Sobell, L. C., Maisto, S. A., Sobell, M. B., & Cooper, A. M. (1979). Reliability of alcoholics' self-reports of drinking and related behaviors one year prior to treatment in an outpatient treatment program. *Behavior Research and Therapy, 17,* 157–160.

Sobell, L. C., & Sobell, M. B. (1980). Convergent validity: An approach to increasing confidence in treatment outcome conclusions with alcohol and drug abusers. In L. C. Sobell, M. B. Sobell, & E. Ward (Eds.), *Evaluating alcohol and drug abuse treatment effectiveness: Recent advances.* New York: Pergamon Press.

Sobell, L. C., & Sobell, M. B. (1985). *Alcohol abuse education curriculum guide for psychology faculty.* Washington, D.C.: U.S. Department of Health and Human Services.

Sobell, M. B., & Sobell, L. C. (1973). Individualized behavior therapy for alcoholics. *Behavior Therapy, 4,* 49–72.

Sobell, M. B., & Sobell, L. C. (1975). A brief technical report on the Mobat: An inexpensive portable test for determining blood alcohol concentration. *Journal of Applied Behavioral Analysis, 8,* 117–120.

Sobell, M. B., Sobell, L. C., & Sheahan, D. B. (1976). Functional analysis of drinking problems as an aid in developing individual treatment strategies. *Addictive Behaviors, 1,* 127–132.

Sobell, M. B., & Sobell, L. C. (1981). Functional analysis of alcohol problems. In C. K. Prakop & L. A. Bradley (Eds.), *Medical psychology: Contributions to behavioral medicine.* New York: Academic Press.

Sobell, M. B., Sobell, L. C., & VanderSpek, R. (1979). Relationship between clinical judgment, self-report and breath analysis measures of intoxication. *Journal of Consulting and Clinical Psychology, 47,* 204–206.

Stivers, R. Culture and alcoholism. (1976). In R. E. Tarter & A. Sugerman (Eds.), *Alcoholism: Interdisciplinary approaches to an enduring problem.* Reading, MA: Addison-Wesley.

Tarter, R. E., & Schneider, D. U. (1976). Models and theories of alcoholism. In R. E. Tarter & A. Sugerman (Eds.), *Alcoholism: Interdisciplinary approaches to an enduring problem.* Reading, MA: Addison-Wesley.

Victor, M., & Adams, R. D. (1953). Effects of alcohol on the nervous system. In H. H. Merritt & C. C. Hare (Eds.), *Metabolic and toxic diseases of the nervous system.* Baltimore: Williams and Wilkins.

Watson, D. W., Maisto, S. A. & Rosenberg, H. S. (1982). Development of the Alcohol Assertion Inventory. Unpublished manuscript, Vanderbilt University.

Wilson, G. T. (1978). Booze, beliefs and behavior: Cognitive processes in alcohol use and abuse. In P. E. Nathan, G. A. Marlatt, & T. Loberg (Eds.), *Alcoholism: New directions in behavioral research and treatment.* New York: Plenum Press.

Zucker, R. A. (1979). Developmental aspects of drinking through the young adult years. In H. T. Blane & M. E. Chafetz (Eds.), *Youth, alcohol, and social policy.* New York: Plenum Press.

3

CHRONIC HEADACHE

3

The Case of Mr. C.

The patient was a 46-year-old male Caucasian, residing in a moderately sized city in the southeast United States. At the time of the initial interview the patient was unemployed.

The Referral

Mr. C. was referred by a neurologist in private practice. The patient had seen the neurologist for chronic headache. The neurologist could not identify any objective indicant of pathophysiology and diagnosed the patient as having severe tension headache.

Physical Appearance

The patient was rather ordinary looking except for being approximately 30 pounds overweight. He was dressed in casual clothes at the initial interview. There were no outstanding physical appearance features.

Presenting Complaints

The patient described his headache as being present at all times. Mr. C. reported that the pain was present upon awakening and lasted all day long. He indicated that he was aware of the pain even when asleep.

Qualitatively, Mr. C. described the pain as "constant pressure." He reported that the sensations were like that of a "cannon ready to explode." At times, the pain had a "burning" quality, particularly in the center of the head. The patient reported that the pain encompassed his entire head, including his ears.

Mr. C. indicated that just about any task which requires concentration or physical effort seemed to intensify the pain. He stated that "lying down and trying to relax seems to help a little sometimes, but the pain never goes away. Sometimes, watching T.V. helps to keep my mind off it but the pain is still there." The patient reported that he could never predict whether or not these attempts to alleviate the pain would be successful. Similarly, Mr. C. indicated that he could never be sure as to when the headache would intensify. He noted, "The only thing I am sure will make my headache worse is when I have to do something that's an effort." The patient had been unable to work for the past two years.

Mr. C. reported that the headache problem had begun two years ago. The patient was working for a construction company and was involved in an industrial accident. Three weeks prior to the accident, the patient had been promoted to field supervisor by the new owners of the company. Mr. C. stated that he was reluctant to take the position because he did not want all of the responsibility. Nevertheless, he accepted the promotion. He found the position stressful and reported "occasional stomach aches" during this period. Nevertheless, the moderate increase in salary was welcomed.

One day, at one of the construction sites, a wooden plank was accidently dropped by a worker above. The board hit Mr. C. on the top front of the head, knocking him off his feet. Although conscious, the patient felt dizzy, disoriented and in "terrible pain." An ambulance brought Mr. C. to the nearest general hospital. Extensive testing was performed but no apparent physiological damage had occurred. The patient was diagnosed as suffering from a concussion. After four days in the hospital, the medical staff suggested that he be discharged. Since he was still in pain, Mr. C. asked for further testing. The medical staff agreed to "observe" him for three more days. After a week in the hospital, Mr. C. was discharged. Mr. C. reported that his present pain problem originated from this accident at work. The headache had continued without remission since he had been hit on the head.

Following his discharge from the hospital, Mr. C. was referred to a neurologist who could not identify any physiological damage. He referred the patient to a pain clinic.

The pain clinic staff performed psychological tests and diagnosed the patient as "muscle contraction headache." Mr. C. was given extensive training in muscular relaxation. After three months with little relief, the patient was put on an EMG biofeedback training program. At this time, Mrs. C. went to work to support the patient. Biofeedback training was pursued for four months with no appreciable gain. Several standard headache medications were prescribed concurrent with the relaxation and biofeedback training program but seemed to have little effect. After eight months at the pain clinic, Mr. C. terminated his case and consulted a lawyer. A law suit against the construction company was planned.

During the next year and four months Mr. C. saw various physicians and a neurologist, a chiropractor, and hypnotist. Numerous medications were tried but to no avail. Twice it was suggested that he see a psychoanalyst. Mr. C. resisted. His most recent visit to a neurologist resulted in the present referral.

Prior to the accident, Mr. C. reported that he was a very healthy individual. The only physical problem he reported experiencing aside from chronic headache was stomach ache. He reported that as a child he often missed school because of this problem and was once hospitalized for it. No apparent physiological problem was noted.

Currently, Mr. C. is unemployed and spends most of his time at home, reading and watching television. Mrs. C. is employed as a secretary for an appliance company. The patient's lawsuit has yet to come to trial.

Parents and Family

The patient reported that no one in his family suffered from headaches of any kind. Mr. C.'s father was a sanitation department employee and suffered from back problems. His father was operated on twice for problems with his back. The patient's mother was relatively healthy and "took good care of dad." Mr. C.'s older brother was killed in the Korean war.

Interview Behavior

Throughout the discussion of his headache history, Mr. C. was relaxed, pleasant, and verbose. He was very cooperative throughout the interview. Mr. C. explained, "My spirit to go on stems from my wife; she takes great care of me." Finally, he denied that he was experiencing any psychological problems.

Case Formulations of Chronic Headaches

HENRY E. ADAMS

Although Mr. C. appears to be a simple case of "tension" or muscle contraction headache, this case is a good illustration of the complexity of chronic head pain. If one did not look carefully at the situation, the obvious treatment plan would be biofeedback, cognitive therapy, and/or progressive muscular relaxation, which I predict would, and did, end in disaster. Even in the most classic cases of headache, it is always wise to look very carefully before proceeding with intervention.

The approach I use and teach my graduate students is that psychological intervention should be divided into distinct and separate phases: initial interview, assessment tailored for the specific case, case formulation, developing treatment strategies, feedback of case formulation to the patient, and implementation of the treatment plan. Throughout this process it is important to utilize the same procedure in case management as would be used in planning and conducting a research project. This would involve gathering data about the patient (typically through observation), formulating hypotheses, devising tests to rule out less feasible hypotheses, and further testing of more attractive hypotheses. The procedure involves a "hypothesis tree" and continuous feedback which refines or refutes your guesses (Platt, 1966). For example, the initial interview(s) should generate a hypothesis concerning

HENRY E. ADAMS • Department of Psychology, University of Georgia, Athens, Georgia 30602.

the disorder which can be verified, refuted, or replaced during specific assessment. The interview and assessment should result in a case formulation which should indicate how treatment should be conducted. Hypotheses or case formulations may be refuted by further information from the patient or by the fact that the therapeutic intervention does not work. The guiding principle is always to be very skeptical of your hypotheses and ready to refine and replace them if the data do not fit.

In the present case, Mr. C. has been labeled a "muscle contraction" or "tension" headache. Since he has had extensive medical evaluation, it is reasonable to rule out physiological factors. (However, be cautious. Physicians also make mistakes.) In order to do quality clinical work, it is absolutely essential to know the research literature. The first question is, What is known about "tension" headache and how do these facts fit the present case?

ISSUES IN DIAGNOSIS

With headaches, as with any disorder, the initial step is to establish the appropriate diagnosis or classification in this particular case. We can eliminate head pain that is due to traumatic physical injury or disease processes, leaving four major types of head pain associated with psychological disorders, as proposed by the Ad Hoc Committee on Headache over 20 years ago (Friedman, 1962).

1. *Vascular headaches of migraine origin.* Recurrent attacks of headache widely varied in intensity, frequency, and duration. The attacks are commonly unilateral in onset; are usually associated with anorexia and sometimes with nausea and vomiting; occasionally are preceded by or associated with conspicuous sensory, motor, or mood disturbance and are often familial. This disorder is commonly assumed to be due to a cephalic vasomotor disorder.

2. *Muscle-contraction headaches.* Ache, or sensation of tightness, pressure or construction, widely varied in intensity, frequency and duration; sometimes long-lasting; and commonly suboccipital. Associated with sustained contraction of skeletal muscles in the absence of permanent structural change, usually as a part of the individual's reaction to life stress. Notice that a defining characteristic of this disorder is "sustained contraction of skeletal muscles."

3. *Combined headache; vascular and muscle contraction.* Combination of vascular headache of the migraine type and muscle contraction headache, prominently coexisting in any attack. It should be

recognized that the two types of head pain may also occur independently in the same person and on different occasions (Sturgis, Tollison, & Adams, 1978).

4. *Headaches of delusional, conversion, or hypochondriacal states.* Headaches in which the major clinical disorder is a delusion or conversion reaction, and a peripheral pain mechanism is nonexistent. Closely allied are the hypochondriacal reactions in which the peripheral disturbance relevant to the headache is minimal. More recent descriptions of this type of headache have either labeled it as conversion or, more appropriately, as psychogenic head pain. It should be noted that headaches can be a function of other psychiatric disorders such as depression in which the primary disorder should be diagnosed and treated.

In Mr. C.'s case, there are no obvious vascular symptoms or components and therefore there is no further need to discuss migraine headache. On the other hand, it is not so easy to eliminate the possibility of psychogenic head pain if the assessment criteria shown in Table 1 are used. Psychogenic head pain is a topic which has been almost totally ignored in the headache literature; in other pain disorders, such as lower back pain, it is assumed to play a major role in many cases (Adams, Brantley, & Thompson, 1982). It has been my contention that "tension headaches," a term which has been equated with muscle contraction headaches, may be a heterogeneous group of muscle contraction and pyschogenic headaches, as will be suggested by several lines of evidence. The most popular theory and a defining characteristic of the Ad Hoc Committee on Headaches is that muscle contraction headache is due to sustained elevation in muscular activity in the cephalic and neck muscles, although vascular factors may or may not play a role. Presumably, this disorder occurs in individuals whose reponse stereotyping or specificity is in the muscular system and who respond to stress with increased muscle activity. However, in their review of this theory, Haynes, Cuevas, and Gannon (1982) indicated that the data on this issue are not always consistent with the theory. Specifically, they note that some studies have not found a relationship between muscle tension in the affected site and pain or increased muscle tension during the headache state or differences in resting level of EMG activity of normal and muscle contraction headaches individuals. Turkat and Adams (1981), in a particularly puzzling study, found that when normal and muscle contraction individuals were asked to contract their frontalis muscles as long as possible, this procedure produced head pain in both groups but much more rapidly in the muscle contraction group. This indicates that sustained muscle contraction, at least in the frontalis

Table 1. Tripartite Assessment of Head Pain

Headache type	Assessment procedure		
	Subjective	Behavioral	Psychological
Migraine	Usually unilateral onset Prodomes Nausea Pulsating, throbbing pain	Emergency room treatment Bed rest required Avoidance of sound and light Vomiting and other signs of ANS distress	Cephalic vascular lability in headache and nonheadache states Response to vasoconstrictive and potent analgesic or sedative drugs
Muscle-contraction	Dull, aching headband or neck pain Pain attacks less severe; soreness of scalp and neck muscles	Only rarely requires cessation of ongoing activities or bed rest Pain elicited in stressful situations	Elevated muscle tension in facial and neck areas during headache episode and/or non-headache states Often responsive to mild analgesics
Conversion	Pain report typically not fitting pattern of migraine or muscle-contraction Iatrogenic effects	Presence of secondary gain (reinforcement) Presence of an initial precipitating event	Lack of physiological basis for pain (e.g., no elevated EMG or vasomotor disorders)
Combined	Characteristics of both muscle-contraction and migraine, either coexisting in same attack or occurring in separate attacks	Disability a function of type of headache	Physiology may vary as a function of type of pain When both types exist in same attack, physiological changes may involve vascular and musculoskeletal components

area, is a viable mechanism for pain. Turkat also subjected his participants to a Forgione–Barber finger pain stimulator in order to see if those in the muscle contraction population were more sensitive to pain stimuli, as they were. Surprisingly, the majority of muscle contraction participants, over 64%, also developed a headache after this procedure, whereas this happened to only 14% of the normal population. To add to the confusion, the muscle contraction headache subjects did not differ in frontalis EMG from the normal subjects during a non-headache or headache state.

What conclusions can be drawn from these data? If so-called tension headaches do consist of two groups, muscle contraction headaches and psychogenic pain cases, then the confusing results are not surprising. A given experiment will confirm or disconfirm the classic theory of muscle contraction headache depending on the proportion of these two heterogeneous groups included in a particular research sample. The Turkat study apparently had a majority of psychogenic headache subjects in the sample.

In order to evaluate the feasibility of this explanation, Haber, Kuzmiercyzk, and Adams (1985) selected a group of muscle contraction headache subjects, divided them into two groups on the basis of their frontalis EMG level during a headache attack, that is, within normal levels (psychogenic) or elevated (MC) as compared to a normal control sample of subjects. The EMG reactivity of the two groups was then assessed during a non-headache state. The psychogenic headache individuals showed no change in EMG levels, whereas the MC participants (i.e., those with high EMG level) showed a significant decrease during the pain-free state. Normal participants assessed twice in similar time periods with no head pain showed little or no change. The psychogenic group was not significantly different from the normal group, but the MCH groups differed from both of these groups in both states in EMG activity. This experiment was then replicated with a new sample, who were assessed in two pain-free and two headache states to ensure that these differences were consistent and reliable. The same results were obtained with the individuals who had elevated EMG increasing their EMG levels during the pain states and the individuals within the normal range of EMG activity showing little change in headache states. In addition, it was found that the subjects with normal EMG activity in both resting and headache states (labeled as psychogenic headache cases) had more models (parents and relatives) for head pain, were more likely to use head pain to avoid responsibility, and had more atypical developmental patterns of head pain. The atypical pattern of head pains suggests that their pain state may start as quite odd or vague and be gradually shaped to a more classic pattern of muscle contraction headache as a function of iatrogenic effects.

To support this hypothesis further, Figueroa (1981), in a counterbalanced treatment design of EMG biofeedback and progressive muscular relaxation, found that MCH patients (high EMG) responded much better to EMG biofeedback than progressive muscle relaxation. The psychogenic headache group (low EMG) responded equally well to both treatments, but did not show as much reduction in headache activity in the EMG biofeedback condition as the MCH group. These results suggest the possibility that there were both a placebo and a specific effect on the pain mechanism in the muscle contraction group but only a placebo effect in the psychogenic group.

In summary, these data suggest that increased muscle activity may be the pain mechanism in muscle contraction headaches and can be assessed by subjective report, overt behavior, and psychophysiologic indices. On the other hand, the etiology and pain mechanism of psychogenic head pain is not known.

ETIOLOGY OF PSYCHOGENIC HEAD PAIN

If it is assumed that the head pain in the psychogenic disorder is not due to the muscular-skeletal system, what are the factors that are involved in this disorder? Although Fordyce's (1976) model of operant pain is certainly appropriate to this question, I would like to speculate on this issue in more detail. In evaluating any disorder of human behavior, I have found the conceptual developmental model shown in Table 2 to be quite useful as a device to describe or "guess" about the origin

Table 2. Factors in Etiology and Maintenance of Psychological and Medical Disorders

Predisposing	Precipitating	Maintaining	Subsequent elaborations
Biological	Stress	Positive	Emotional
Genetic	Physical trauma	reinforcement	disorders
Prenatal	Somatic illness	Negative	Vocational
Natal		reinforcement	disorders
Trauma			Marital distress
			Social
			relationships
			Financial distress
Environmental			
Reinforcement			
and shaping			
Modeling			
Psychological			
trauma			
	Developmental sequence		
Conception →	Onset →	Course →	Death

of a variety of disorders. As you can see from Table 2 the model evaluates the predisposing, precipitating, maintaining, and subsequent factors along a developmental sequence from birth to death.

PREDISPOSING FACTORS

In general, predisposing factors can be divided into biological factors consisting of genetic, prenatal, and postnatal events which cause changes in anatomical structure or biochemical functioning. Genetic endowment, birth injury, or traumatic event causing physical damage would be examples of this factor. The evidence for such biological influence or lack of influence in psychogenic head pain or other psychogenic disorders has been meager. At this time, there is little reason to believe that such factors including genetic makeup play a significant role in this type of disorder with perhaps one exception.

It is quite possible that individuals are predisposed, because of biological factors, presumably genetic, to respond to stress in terms of specific physiological responses (Lacey, 1967; Malmo & Shagass, 1949). This tendency has been called response stereotyping or specificity. Consequently, people who respond to stress in the cardiovascular system develop cardiovascular disorders; those whose response is in the gastrointestinal tract develop spastic colon, peptic ulcers, and other GI-tract disorders; those who respond in the muscular-skeletal system develop muscular pain disorders. In the case of headaches, response stereotyping may be important in MCH or migraines as suggested by Sturgis (1979) and Thompson and Adams (1984), but the role it plays in psychogenic head pain is questionable since no muscular or other physiological response system dysfunctions have been demonstrated.

Psychological factors appear to play a major role in the development of somatoform and/or psychogenic disorders and may even exaggerate the severity of physical disorders. In general, these effects appear to be due to three factors: (1) direct shaping of illness responses by positive and negative reinforcement, (2) modeling of illness behavior exhibited by family and peers, and (3) a severe psychological trauma that disposes the individual to illness behavior.

The potency of the psychological effect of "sick" behavior can be demonstrated in a number of different ways. For example, many medical patients present illness behavior with no pathophysiological mechanism (Spielberger, Pollans, & Worden, 1983) or display symptoms incompatible with their documented pathophysiology (Wooley, Blackwell, & Winget, 1978). Lipkin and Lamb (1982) claimed that up to 80%

of the substance of general medical practice is determined by psychological or social events. In the specific case of pain, Brena, Chapman, Stegall, and Chyatte (1979) report that 60% of chronic pain patients seeking disability payments have little in the way of identifiable pathophysiology.

The tendency to exhibit pain or other illness behavior in adverse life circumstances probably begins early in life. It is rather obvious in our society that complaints of illness are reinforced by concern by significant others. This tendency is exaggerated in parents who view their children as "sickly" and become overprotective. For example, it has been documented that hypochondriacs come from families of chronic complainers and that male hypochondriacs have overprotective mothers (Baker & Merskey, 1942; Katzenelbogen, 1942). Levy (1980) reports that parents who view their children as "vulnerable to illness" in spite of the fact there is no clinical evidence for this belief utilize medical services significantly more than parents who do not have such beliefs about their children. A very early report by Zborowski (1952) indicated that individuals who were most responsive to pain had mothers who were overprotective of their children's health. Consequently, it is apparent that parents, particularly mothers who are concerned with children's health, may be inadvertently giving them positive reinforcement for illness behavior.

In addition to positive reinforcement for illness or pain behavior, this type of behavior also allows the child to avoid responsible behavior such as attending school, chores, and other unpleasant life events. This is negative reinforcement and verbal complaints are actually avoidance responses, removing the individual from noxious situations.

In addition to these direct influences on behavior, there is little doubt that modeling pain and illness response plays a tremendous role in these disorders. For example, Gentry, Shows, and Thomas (1974) have found that individuals with chronic back pain are more likely to have a parent with a similar disorder. This is also the case with sufferers of abdominal pain (Apley, 1975), dental pain, asthma (Tieramaa, 1979), and other psychosomatic symptoms (Langer & Michael, 1963). Turkat and his colleagues have illustrated this relationship between modeling and illness behavior in a number of studies (Turkat, 1982; Turkat & Noskin, 1983; Turkat & Pettegrew, 1983). Experimentally, Craig (1978) has shown that individuals who view a model receiving aversive stimulus, showing exaggerated pain behavior, and subsequently receiving shock exhibit more pain behavior than subjects who view a tolerant model.

It has also been demonstrated by Hallauer (1972) that verbal positive reinforcement of well statements of medical patients in interviews produces more wellness statements and fewer illness statements than verbal reinforcement of illness statements. In addition, Turkat and his associates (Turkat & Guise, 1983; Turkat, Guise, & Carter, 1983) have shown that experimental subjects who view a model who avoids a work task when exposed to pain show more work avoidance when exposed to pain themselves as compared to subjects who view a non-avoidance model. Turkat, Flasher, Thompson, Hassan, and Mauldin (1983) found that subjects' intensity rating of a standard pain stimulus increased if a high pain rating led to the avoidance of an aversive work task and that intensity ratings to the same pain stimulus decreased when low pain ratings led to the avoidance of an aversive task. In the second study by these investigators, which is more relevant to the headache literature, when a confederate complained of having a severe headache, subjects took on more of the workload than the confederates who asked to be excused from the task but did not complain of head pain. This is an illustration of the potency of complaining and how it may shape an individual's behavior.

There is little doubt that the psychological history of the individual predisposes him to emit verbal complaints of illness and pain more frequently than individuals without such a history. The exact mechanism by which this occurs is not clear, but it may be that chronic complainers have a heightened sensitivity to internal pain stimuli as suggested by Dickinson and Smith (1973). Certainly the reinforcement of pain behavior and the exposure to model for illness behavior could cause an individual constantly to monitor his or her internal state.

PRECIPITATING EVENTS

Precipitating factors involve those events in an individual's life which lead to the appearance of the behavioral and/or somatic symptoms of a psychological, physiological, or psychophysiological disorder. These precipitating events can be broadly divided into stress, physical trauma, and acute or chronic illness.

Stress is a rather nebulous concept which has caused a great deal of controversy and confusion in the psychological and medical literature. It is difficult to define (Selye, 1975). It can be defined in terms of the environmental circumstances that disrupt the normal activity of an

organism (Kagan, 1971) or as a response of the organism either physiologically or psychologically to particular events (Burchfield, 1979;
Selye, 1976). It has also been used as a global label for a field of study
that examines the processes by which organisms adapt to disruptive
events (Averill, 1979). Although all of these definitions have validity,
for our purposes stress will be defined as events which disrupt behavior,
causing negative consequences for the organism. As noted by Leventhal
and Nerenz (1983) in their excellent model of stress, what constitutes
stress is often in the eye of the beholder. Events which would be a
source of pleasure and reinforcement for one individual may be
extremely stressful to another. The interpretation of life events is determined by a number of factors, but certainly the most potent are the
predisposing or life history factors previously discussed. How well
one copes with adversity depends on one's repertoire of coping skills
and how successfully one has implemented them in the past (Janis,
1983).

   With regard to pain behavior, it is fairly obvious that the individual
who is exposed to adverse circumstances and has a history of witnessing
and coping with difficulties by illness behaviors is more likely to exhibit
chronic pain behavior. As noted by Ullmann and Krasner (1975) in
their discussion of conversion reaction, there are two main pertinent
questions. The first is whether the individual is capable of such behavior and the second is under what conditions it will be admitted. A
similar analysis can be used with pain behavior, particularly when there
is no apparent physiological reason for distress. In these circumstances
the previous history of the individual's being exposed to pain models
and/or exhibiting illness behavior under conditions of contingent reinforcement (either positive reinforcement or avoidance conditioning) is
crucial. In cases wherein life stress is not particularly catastrophic but
is consistently present, the acquisition of pain behavior may be gradual
and the exact etiology of pain behavior may be difficult to determine.

   A much more common precipitating factor is an actual illness or
injury: initially there is a physical basis for the pain behavior, but after
the physical difficulty has cleared pain persists. A good example of
such a case was reported by Blanchard and Hersen (1976); an individual
had undergone surgery for a disc fusion and seven years later underwent
additional orthopedic surgery for pain. Five years after the second operation the individual suffered stooping episodes and was unable to walk,
although no physical basis was ever established for the condition. Injuries initially causing back pain or injuries causing head pain when the
physical basis for the pain has been eliminated by medical intervention

but the pain persists are excellent examples of this type of precipitating event.

In summary, chronic pain behavior, including head pain, may be instigated as a maladaptive method of handling life stress or by an accident or physical illness in which the physiological difficulties are remedied but the pain persists.

MAINTAINING FACTORS

A major question in psychogenic pain disorders is why pain continues to occur. This question has usually been addressed in terms of secondary gains, a term introduced by our psychodynamic colleagues, which refers to the fact that the behavior is "paying off" (Packard, 1980). In those cases in which the onset of pain is gradual and there is no apparent physiological illness or injury, the pain behavior may have been gradually shaped to approximate a traditional physical disorder such as muscle contraction head pain by iatrogenic effects. Iatrogenic effects typically occur through repeated examination by physicians whose questions about the person's symptoms inadvertently shape the individual's responses into classic pain syndromes. Unwittingly, a physician may actually be reinforcing or maintaining head pain by his or her concern, which may be verbally conditioning pain statements from the patient. This may also be the reason why Haber et al. (in press) found that head pain changes over the course of illness in psychogenic headaches but not in MCH headaches.

Another major variable is that the pain behavior allows the individual to escape responsibility or avoid unpleasant life circumstances, a major characteristic in identifying psychogenic pain as noted by Haber et al. (1985). Thus, negative reinforcement in the form of avoidance conditioning wherein the pain complaint serves as an avoidance response can be a powerful factor in maintaining complaints of head pain.

Another major factor is positive reinforcement. The majority of individuals who exhibit illness behavior are consistently reinforced for a "sickness" role with attention, sympathy, and concern. Individuals who are prone to use illness behavior as a coping mechanism are most susceptible to the effects of this type of reinforcement. Another kind of positive reinforcement is seen in situations in which there has been an accident or illness causing the disorder resulting in a lawsuit. When this is the case, these disorders have often been labeled as compensation neuroses and are notoriously resistant to therapeutic intervention.

SUBSEQUENT ELABORATIONS

Probably the most devastating effect of psychogenic pain disorders, including head pain, is the severe disruption they often cause in the individual's life. Chronic pain complaints and the behaviors associated with them often initiate a vicious circle which may turn the sufferer into a severely handicapped person. It is important for the clinician to recognize that although these symptoms are byproducts of pain behavior they may be so severe that they require active therapeutic interventions. Chronic pain behavior adversely affects an individual's marital, social, vocational, and emotional adjustment, and this in turn may aggravate the pain disorder.

The impact of pain behavior on a marital relationship is usually quite severe, requiring a major readjustment by the spouse, who often becomes a caretaker required to render assistance on a 24-hour basis. It is not unusual for the very nature of home life of these patients to be greatly altered, with the goals of the family, including the children, to be directed toward providing care to the handicapped individual. This can involve reducing noise level, decreasing social activities, and other remedial techniques which make the home resemble a hospital ward. In addition, the financial resources of the family are usually decimated by medical expenses and job loss or absenteeism. Paradoxically, the more concerned and sympathetic the spouse and family, the greater the likelihood they will aggravate the pain behavior (Fowler, 1975).

The impact of psychogenic head pain on vocational adjustment is even more obvious. A major characteristic of psychogenic pain cases is the inability to cope with responsibility, including mental requirements such as concentration and physical or work requirements which are the basic components of any job. The reduced effort and absenteeism often leave employers with no option but to fire the individual. Pain behavior also interferes with job-seeking activities, and employers are reluctant to offer positions to individuals with a history of illness behavior. Employers may also anticipate absenteeism, which they may perceive as inadequate motivation for performance. Chronic unemployment as well as deterioration of work skills and habits are often the results of this cycle.

The most traumatic effect on the individual, however, is in terms of his or her own emotional adjustment. Needless to say, it is difficult for other people to maintain social relationships with chronic complainers. Although the initial reaction to illness complainers may be

sympathetic, chronic complaints become aversive to other people, particularly in the case of nonterminal illnesses and those in which a
physical illness cannot be readily verified. A common reaction to these
individuals is to avoid the complainer, and on occasion to accuse them
of malingering or of being "weak." Social rejection, combined with
marital discord, vocational disasters, financial distress, and assumption
of the illness role, severly damages the individual's self-confidence and
coping skills.

In the initial stages of pain disorders there is often an almost frantic
attempt to recover from the illness by trying new physicians, new drugs,
or eventually unusual, often ridiculous "cures." The implicit or explicit
accusation of a psychosomatic basis for the illness or even worse, malingering causes many patients to become quite defensive and deny or
react negatively to psychologically based treatments. This is aggravated
by the fact that the public tends to see psychologically based pain
disorders as not being "real." In time, as the individual's attempts to
cope continue to fail, he or she begins to feel helpless, to withdraw, or
to become apathetic. Depression is a prime characteristic of chronic
pain cases—a major reason why antidepressive medication is often used
to treat head pain disorders. However, in the vast majority of these
cases the depression is the consequence and not the cause of the chronic
head pain, a major reason why chemotherapy in these cases often fails.

It is not unusual for people with chronic head pain to become
addicted to pain-alleviating medication, particularly the narcotic and
analgesic drugs. This common by-product of pain causes a whole series
of difficulties, including drug-seeking behavior and other characteristics of addicted individuals. In some cases, the drug craving can actually
serve as an eliciting as well as a reinforcing event for pain behavior.
One of my patients with head pain had become a familiar face in every
hospital emergency room within a 200-mile radius of his home, seeking
Demerol for "migraines." In such cases, the problem of addiction, particularly to narcotics, must be solved before any meaningful progress
can be made with the pain behavior.

COMMENT ON PSYCHOGENIC HEAD PAIN, CONVERSION
REACTIONS, AND MALINGERING

With psychogenic head pain a major question is the relationship
of the disorder to conversion reactions and malingering. Certainly, if
the psychodynamic theorizing surrounding the notion of *conversion*

reaction is ignored, the two disorders are quite common. Both disorders mimic physical illnesses without apparent pathophysiology. In both disorders previous bona fide physical illnesses serve as instigators and models for specific illness disorders (Levy & Jankovic, 1983). Suggestibility or susceptibility to modeling illness behavior is present in both conditions. There are always serious questions about the possibility of malingering and the authenticity of the disorders in both conditions. I would argue that psychogenic head pains (and perhaps other types of psychological pain) are specific subtypes of what has been called *conversion disorders*. Although the symptoms may be different, the etiology, the development, and the course of the disorders are quite similar.

Another major problem is the question of malingering. This is a particularly relevant topic since in many of these cases there are secondary gains, often involving a lawsuit. Malingering implies that the individual purposely planned and enacted a psychological or medical condition for personal gain. Although secondary gains are always a consideration in these disorders, I do not believe that these patients purposely plan such behavior or, more to the point, even understand it. Awareness or consciousness implies that the individual cognitively comprehends and can verbally report the basis of his or her behavior. As Levy and Jankovic (1983) have demonstrated in their case with hysterical seizures, events which control an individual's behavior may not be available to the individual's consciousness or awareness. As a matter of fact, those states that we call *awareness* or *consciousness*, contrary to the belief of some cognitive behavior therapists, may be more controlled conditions than controlling conditions as Levy and Jankovic point out. Learning can occur without consciousness or an awareness of the contingency of reinforcement by the individual. The belief that our attitudes and beliefs control all aspects of our behavior, including pain, or that changing attitude and belief is necessary for the control of all types of behavior is a rather ludicrous proposition in view of the evidence.

THE CASE OF MR. C.

Mr. C. is an excellent example of the usefulness of the research literature as a method for understanding clinical cases, since he has many signs of the psychogenic headache disorder. In terms of predisposing factors, his father suffered from back pain which required surgery twice, and he apparently received a great deal of attention and sympathy from his wife for this handicap. The father thus served as an excellent model for illness behavior for the son. The fact that Mr. C. was imitating his father's sick role is well illustrated by the report of the chronic stomachaches he suffered as a child with no apparent physical basis, which allowed him to escape an onerous task, that is, going to school. His stomachaches continued to occur as a reaction to stress, such as the negative reaction he experienced caused by his job promotion. In addition, Mr. C.'s employment was apparently distasteful to him because of the additional responsibility placed on him by recent promotion before the accident.

In terms of the precipitating event, there was a bona fide physical disorder which served as the model for the specific pain behavior. He was hit on the head and did suffer from a concussion. When the physical effect of the concussion cleared, the pain persisted, not surprisingly in view of this individual's past history. Why does the pain continue to persist if in fact there was no physical basis? Pain behavior has, in many ways, served a very useful purpose for Mr. C. He has escaped a job that he despised. He is a man of leisure, spending most of his time at home reading and watching television. The secondary gain associated with a possible lucrative settlement of his lawsuit is all too obvious.

What about Mr. C.'s behavior would suggest that his pain was psychogenic rather than muscle contraction? In the first place, his description of his head pain is not typical of muscle contraction headaches. Rather, he notes a "burning" sensation in the center of the head and says that the pain encompasses his entire head including his ears. Neither the "hatband" nor the neck distribution of pain observed in muscle contraction headache is present. As is sometimes typical in these cases, he has a dramatic, exaggerated description of his pain, "a cannon ready to explode." The reinforcing nature of this type of pain behavior is obvious since any effort makes the headache worse, yet he is able to read and watch television—activities that typically aggravate other types of headache.

How do we verify that this is in fact a psychogenic headache rather than a muscle contraction headache disorder? As I have noted before, one should be continuously skeptical of one's diagnosis and case formulation and must continuously evaluate the validity of one's guesses. In this particular case, it is obvious that the next move is to assess the individual in terms of his muscle activities in the cephalic areas during pain-free and headache states. If there is no increase in EMG activity from pain-free to pain state, then we are on the right track. If there is, then the conceptualization is probably wrong.

If our conceptualization is right, the next question is which treatment strategy would be most useful with this particular case. Quite frankly, in my experience, I doubt that any treatment procedure will be effective until the most potent reinforcer is eliminated, that is, until his court case is settled. However, since I doubt very seriously that this individual is malingering, a settlement of his court case is not likely to eliminate the head pain since there are many other reinforcers for this behavior. In this particular case, the treatment program which is designed to eliminate the reinforcement for illness behavior and enhance the possibility of reinforcement for well behavior has the greatest chance of success. I refer specifically to an operant approach as described by Fowler (1975). In such a treatment program, the wife and other individuals in Mr. C.'s environment would have to be instructed to be neutral to his pain behavior, encourage increased activity and effort on his part through contingent, positive reinforcement, and generally shape him into a functioning, coping individual. The basic strategy would be to extinguish pain complaints and reinforce active, healthy behavior. Needless to say, this type of approach would require gathering a great deal more information about Mr. C. and soliciting the cooperation of the people in his environment.

In summary, head pain without a physical basis cannot be divided simply into muscle contraction or tension headaches and migraine-type disorders. A major difficulty, both in clinical work and research with these disorders, has been the fact that the psychogenic basis for many individuals with head pain complaints has been consistently ignored because of the tendency to match symptoms with treatment techniques. In other words, if the individual had a muscle contraction (tension) headache, the treatment of choice was either EMG biofeedback or cognitive therapy. In the case of migraines, the treatment of choice was temperature biofeedback or, in some cases, cognitive-type therapy. Because of the fact that these approaches ignore the reinforcement contingencies for psychogenic headaches, their effectiveness with these disorders is often minimal and transient. The most successful treatment intervention for headache disorders (and other types of psychological disorders as well) is one which is based on an understanding of an individual and a treatment plan which is devised for the characteristics of that particular patient.

REFERENCES

Adams, H. E., Brantley, P. J., & Thompson, K. (1982). Biofeedback and headache: Methodological issues. In L. White & B. Tursky (Eds.), *Clinical biofeedback: Efficacy and mechanisms.* New York: Guilford Press.

Apley, J. (1975). *The child with abdominal pains.* Oxford: Blackwell Scientific Publications.

Averill, J. R. (1979). A selective review of cognitive and behavioral factors involved in the regulation of stress. In R. A. Depue (Ed.), *The psychobiology of the depressive disorders: Implications for the effects of stress.* New York: Academic Press.

Baker, B. & Mersky, H. (1982). Parental representations of hypochondriachical patients from a psychiatric hospital. *British Jouranl of Psychiatry, 141,* 233–238.

Blanchard, E. B., & Hersen, M. (1976). Behavior treatment of hysterical neurosis: Symptom substitution and symptom return reconsidered. *Psychiatry, 39,* 118–129.

Brena, S. S., Chapman, S. L., Stegall, P. G., & Chyatte, S. B. (1979). Chronic pain studies: Their relationship to impairment and disability. *Archives of Physical and Medical Rehabilitation, 60,* 387–389.

Burchfield, S. R. (1979). The stress response: A new perspective. *Psychosomatic Medicine, 41,* 661–672.

Craig, K. (1978). Social modeling influences on pain. In R. A. Sternbach (Ed.), *The psychology of pain.* New York: Raven Press.

Dickinson, J. R., Jr., & Smith, B. D. (1973). Nonspecific activity and habituation of tonic and phasic skin conductance in somatic complainers and controls as a function of auditory stimulus intensity. *Journal of Abnormal Psychology, 82,* 404–412.

Figueroa, J. L. (1981). The relationship between frontalis EMG level and response to treatment with EMG biofeedback and relaxation training in headache. Unpublished doctoral dissertation, University of Georgia.

Fordyce, W. (1976). *Behavioral methods for chronic pain and illness.* St. Louis: C. V. Mosby.

Fowler, R. S., Jr. (1975). Operant therapy for headaches. *Headaches, 15,* 63–68.

Friedman, A. P. (1962). Ad hoc committee on classification of headaches. *Journal of American Medical Association, 179,* 747–748.

Gentry, W. D., Shows, W. D., & Thomas, N. (1974). Chronic low back pain: A psychological profile. *Psychosomatics, 15,* 174–177.

Haber, J., Kuzmiercyzk, A. R., & Adams, H. E. (1985). Tension headache: Muscle overactivity or psychogenic pain? *Headache, 25,* 23–29.

Hallauer, D. (1972). Illness behavior: An experimental investigation. *Journal of Chronic Disease, 25,* 599–610.

Haynes, S. N. Cuevas, J., & Gannon, L. R. (1982). The psychophysiological characterlstics of muscle-contraction headaches. *Headache, 22,* 122–132.

Janis, I. L. (1983). Stress inoculation in health care: Theory and research. In D. Meichenbaum & M. E. Jarenko (Eds.), *Stress reduction and prevention.* New York: Plenum Press.

Kagan, A. (1971). Epidemiology and society, stress and disease. In L. Levi (Ed.), *Society, stress and disease* (Vol. 1). London: Oxford University Press.

Katzenelbogen, S. (1942). Hypochondriacal complaints with special reference to personality and environment. *American Journal of Psychiatry, 98, 815–822.*

Lacey, J. T. (1967). Somatic response patterning and stress: Some revisions of activation theory. In M. H. Appley & R. Turnbull (Eds.), *Psychological Stress: Issues in Research.* New York: Appleton-Century-Crofts.

Langer, T. S., & Michael, S. T. (1963). *Life, stress and mental health: The mid-town Manhattan study* (Vol. 2). London: Free Press of Glencoe.

Leventhal, H., & Nerenz, D. R. (1983). A model for stress research with some implications for the control of stress disorders. In D. Meichenbaum & M. E. Jarenko (Eds.), *Stress reduction and prevention.* New York: Plenum Press.

Levy, J. C. (1980). Vulnerable children: Parents' perspectives and the use of medical care. *Pediatrics, 65,* 956–963.

Levy, R. S., & Jankovic, J. (1983). Placebo-induced conversion reactions: A neurobehavioral and EEG study of hysterical aphasia, seizure, and coma. *Journal of Abnormal Psychology, 92,* 243–249.

Lipkin, N., & Lamb, G. S. (1982). The couvade syndrome: An epidemiologic study. *Annals of Internal Medicine, 96,* 509–511.

Malmo, R. B., & Shagass, C. (1949). Physiologic study of symptom mechanisms in psychiatric patients under stress. *Psychosomatic Medicine, 11,* 25–29.

Packard, R. C. (1980). Conversion headache. *Headache, 20,* 266–268.

Platt, J. R. (1966). Strong inference. *Science, 146,* 347–353.

Selye, H. (1975). Confusion and controversy in the stress field. *Journal of Human Stress, 1,* 37–44.

Selye, H. (1976). *Stress in health and disease.* London: Butterworth.

Spielberger, C. D. Pollans, C. H., & Worden, T. J. (1983). Anxiety disorders. In S. M. Turner & M. Hersen (Eds.), *Adult psychopathology: A behavioral perspective.* New York: Wiley.

Sturgis, E. T. (1979). Liability and reactivity in the headache response. Unpublished doctoral dissertation, University of Georgia.

Sturgis, E. T., Tollison, C. D., & Adams, H. E. (1978). Modification of combined muscle contraction-migraine headaches. *Journal of Applied Behavior Analysis, 11,* 215–233.

Thompson, J. K., & Adams, H. E. (1984). Psychophysiologic characteristics of headache patients. *Pain, 18,* 41–52.

Tieramaa, E. (1979). Psychic factors and the inception of asthma. *Journal of Psychosomatic Research, 23,* 253–262.

Turkat, I. D. (1982). An investigation of parental modeling in the etiology of diabetic illness behavior. *Behaviour Research and Therapy, 20,* 547–552.

Turkat, I. D., & Adams, H. E. (1981). An investigation of muscle contraction head pain: Psychophysiologic pain mechanisms and classification issues. Paper presented at the 15th annual meeting of the Association of Behavior Therapy, Toronto, November, 1981.

Turkat, I. D., Flasher, L. V., Thompson, T. D., Hasson, S. & Mauldin, M. (1983). Negative reinforcement in the development of illness behavior: Two analogue experiments. Unpublished manuscript.

Turkat, I. D., & Guise, B. J. (1983). The effects of vicarious experience and stimulus intensity on pain termination and work avoidance. *Behaviour Research and Therapy, 21,* 241–245.

Turkat, I. D., & Noskin, D. E. (1983). Vicarious and operant experiences in the etiology of illness behavior: A replication with healthy individuals. *Behaviour Research and Therapy, 21,* 169–172.

Turkat, I. D., & Pettegrew, L. L. (1983). Development and validation of the Illness Behavior Inventory. *Journal of Behavioral Assessment, 5,* 35–47.

Turkat, I. D., Guise, B. J., & Carter, K. N. (1983). The effects of vicarious experience on pain termination and work avoidance: A replication. *Behaviour Research and Therapy, 21,* 491–493.

Ullmann, L. P., & Krasner, L. (1975). *A psychological approach to abnormal behavior* (2nd ed.). Englewood Cliffs, NJ: Prentice-Hall.

Wooley, S., Blackwell, B., & Winget, T. (1978). The learning theory model of chronic illness behavior: Theory, treatment, and research. *Psychosomatic Medicine, 40,* 379–401.

Zborowski, M. (1952). Cultural components in responses to pain. *Journal of Social Issues, 8,* 16–30.

4

ANTISOCIAL PERSONALITY DISORDER

4

The Case of Mr. V.

Sociopathy is one of the most fascinating types of psychopathology, yet it raises considerable controversy and often appears to be misunderstood. Accordingly, the authors of Chapter 4 felt that it might be to the reader's advantage if the case presentation was to follow a discussion of the sociopathy literature and that such a case should be an ongoing one from the authors' clinical practice. The editor wholeheartedly agreed. Thus, the case of Mr. V. is presented within the following chapter.

4

Antisocial Personality Disorder
Assessment and Case Formulation

PATRICIA B. SUTKER and ALAN R. KING

Habitual rule breaking and chronic disregard for sociolegal restraints are behavioral characteristics attributed to individuals labeled *antisocial personality*. Authors of the DSM-III (American Psychiatric Association, 1980) deemphasized underlying traits and negative intentions and enumerated specific types of behavior seen as definitive of antisocial personality disorder. Diagnosis of pathologically nonconforming individuals was predicated firmly on documentation of a history of continuous and chronic antisocial involvements. Not too many years ago, however, primary attention had been given to cataloguing unwholesome personality traits to describe individuals labeled *sociopath* and *psychopath*. It was assumed that socially deviant behaviors were energized by such personality substrates as selfishness, impulsivity, and callousness. Historically, these notions replaced even more uncomplimentary terms which described antisocial persons as "morally deranged," "psychopathically inferior," and "morally insane." Even today, to observe a constellation of antisocial characteristics may be

PATRICIA B. SUTKER • Psychology Service, Veterans Administration Medical Center, Department of Psychiatry and Neurology, Tulane University School of Medicine, New Orleans, Louisiana 70146.   **ALAN R. KING** • Department of Psychology, Southern University, New Orleans, Louisiana 70118.

tantamount to inferring the presence of negative personality traits or person deficits.

The literature on abnormal behavior is testimony to clinical fascination with individuals whose social deviance has become exaggerated. Antisocial personality disorders comprise the major focus for most didactic presentations of the range of personality disorders. Accounts of their etiologies vary from attributions of intellectual deficiencies to abnormalities in central nervous system functioning. Contemporary writers focus predominantly on genetic, constitutional, and learning contributions to antisocial behaviors. Despite disagreements among theorists about the possible causes of chronic deviance, clinical observers are likely to converge in their assessment of associated personality features and in their views that individuals so characterized represent a challenge to therapeutic intervention. For example, studies have shown surprising agreement regarding the essential features of the antisocial personality (Albert, Brigante, & Chase, 1959; Gray & Hutchinson, 1964). As Robins (1978) observed, if the notion of the antisocial personality is a myth, it is one told over and over among different groups of people in different places at varying times—yet with amazing similarity.

Negative descriptions of antisocial individuals and their potential for change are common in the psychiatric and psychological literature. Cleckley (1955; 1976) provided the most comprehensive characterization of psychopathy. Among its descriptors, he called attention to such features as superficial charm, good intelligence, absence of delusions, seemingly rational thinking, unreliability, untruthfulness, insincerity, lack of remorse, poor judgement, failure to learn from experience, pathological egocentricity, incapacity to love, and general affective poverty. The clinical features listed as diagnostic of antisocial personality in the DSM-II (American Psychiatric Association, 1968) also included references to selfishness, impulsiveness, irresponsibility, callousness, and guiltlessness. Concentrating primarily on the socialization process, Gough (1948) proposed that psychopaths are pathologically deficient in role-playing ability and hence unable to view their actions from the perspective of another or to judge personal behaviors against group standards.

Recent descriptions of antisocial personality disorder tend to perpetuate negative assumptions regarding individuals characterized as psychopaths. This trend continues largely without regard for an accumulating literature deemphasizing negative person constructs and pointing to situations in which psychopathic behaviors may be seen as similar to those of so-called normals. For example, Adams (1981) wrote of psychopaths:

> Such individuals are incapable of significant loyalty to other individuals, groups, or social values. They are grossly selfish, callous, irresponsible, impulsive, and unable to experience guilt or to learn from experience or punishment. Their frustration tolerance is low, and they tend to blame others or rationalize their behavior. (pp. 253–254)

Heilbrun (1982) noted that conceptualizations of psychopathy are based on postulated deficient socialization processes in which loyalty, guilt, and frustration tolerance are poorly developed and a selfish, callous, impulsive, and irresponsible life-style is maintained as a consequence. Hence, psychopaths are seen as unable to profit from experience, rarely distressed by their behaviors or the suffering of others, and concerned primarily with the present and the circumstances of immediate gratification. It is not surprising, then, that pessimism reigns as to their potential for constructive behavior change (Suedfeld & Landon, 1978).

Equating the concepts of sociopathy and habitual criminality, Halleck (1981) expressed the view that chronically antisocial behavior is amenable to positive change through psychotherapy. Vaillant (1975) reasoned that many of the negative conceptualizations of sociopathy constitute construction of a mythical beast, and he pointed to the human dynamics associated with the disorder and to its potential treatability. Ray and Ray (1982) called attention to the more desirable personality characteristics associated with psychopathy, and other researchers have identified areas in which psychopathic functioning is neither deficient nor maladaptive (Sutker, Archer, & Kilpatrick, 1981). To illustrate some of the negative and positive characteristics which may be encountered in association with antisocial behavior among patients labeled *psychopathic*, a brief outline of recent research findings is presented. For greater detail, readers are referred to comprehensive reviews of the literature offered by Hare and Schalling (1978) and Brantley and Sutker (1984).

CORRELATES OF ANTISOCIAL PSYCHOPATHOLOGY

Antisocial Behavior

DSM-III (1980) descriptions of the antisocial personality reflect current trends to operationalize definitions of the disorder by referring to observable behaviors and documented historical facts. Evidence must be obtained of a history of continuous and chronic antisocial behavior in which it appears that the rights of others have been violated repeatedly. Such behaviors must be shown to have had origins in childhood or adolescence and to have persisted over time and across several types of situations. Based in part on the research findings of Spitzer, Endicott, and Robins (1975), criteria for diagnosis of antisocial personality make reference to such problems as erratic work performance, parental irresponsibility, failure to accept social norms, and illegal activities. The clinician is encouraged to determine whether aggressive or sexual behavior occurred in the early years and whether there were signs of emerging antisocial symptoms during adolescence, for example, evidence of lying, stealing, fighting, truancy, running away from home, and/or resisting authority. Use of drugs and alcohol should be carefully documented for critical life periods.

As Heilbrun (1982) noted, the pattern of personality characteristics associated with psychopathy may suggest greater risk for violent behaviors. Nevertheless, there is no consistent evidence of a relationship between violence and psychopathic personality, although violent behaviors occur among psychopaths as they do among other psychiatrically defined groups of individuals. Adams (1981) characterized psychopaths as irrationally violent and cited Charles Manson as prototypic. However, if one considers the behavioral definition of the antisocial personality disorder as outlined in the DSM-III, the stereotype of a deranged killer hardly seems applicable. The syndrome presented is one of antisocial adults characterized by adolescent unruliness and delinquency and continuing adult nonconformity. The picture is one of individuals who have engaged in repeated, antisocial behaviors over time, and it is assumed that such behaviors are directed purposively toward need satisfaction or survival. Although the needs of antisocial persons may be assumed to be exaggerated or more demanding of immediate fulfillment, they are not necessarily thought to reflect bizarre mentation or the derangement associated with unusual or seemingly senseless killings.

When people are classified psychiatrically by a tally of their antisocial activities, especially those judged deviant by the greater societal whole, it can be assumed that a heterogeneous group may be represented. In many cases, it is likely that the group is too heterogeneous and may include individuals who have engaged in heinous crimes prompted by cognitive disorganization or distortions. Such individuals might best be evaluated carefully to determine whether the characteristics common to the schizophrenias are applicable. Further, common behaviors may not be assumed to imply shared etiological factors or even similar facilitating stimuli as precursors. Nevertheless, there is ample evidence that the category of antisocial personality does include individuals of low intelligence who appear irresponsible, violent, disloyal, and selfish at one extreme as well as those who are more clever. Complex sociopaths, as Arieti (1967) indicated, often bring themselves into conflict with authority, but they tend to experience the more negative possible consequences of their actions with less frequency.

In any event, the most critical element for diagnosing antisocial personality is evidence of early nonconformity which has extended into adulthood and become maladaptive in consequences. Antisocial behaviors must be shown to be persistent and to encompass several areas of functioning such as work and social involvements. Other diagnoses, for example, borderline personality disorder, are more appropriate to individuals seen as irrational or psychotic on a temporary basis. Violent behaviors are not necessarily assumed to be diagnostic. One must explore the extent to which negative affect is present or has prompted socially deviant acts. Rather than look to the irrationally violent as prototypic, it is more appropriate from a clinical standpoint to cite examples of drug-addicted men and women, subsets of alcoholics, and substantial portions of men and women incarcerated for crimes against property (Sutker & Archer, 1984).

Learning and Performance Behavior

Eysenck (1964) characterized psychopaths as slow learners who tend to extinguish slowly, and Cleckley (1955; 1976) has commented over the years that psychopaths seem unable to profit from experience, especially that involving punishment. Consistent with these notions, studies have shown psychopaths inferior in verbal conditioning (Johns & Quay, 1962; Quay & Hunt, 1965; Stewart, 1972), passive avoidance learning (Lykken, 1957), and classical conditioning and generalization of autonomic responses (Hare, 1965; Hare & Quinn, 1971). More recently, Gorenstein (1982) showed that psychopathic psychiatric patients performed less well than did nonpsychopathic psychiatric patients on tasks requiring cognitive flexibility and control, and he speculated that psychopaths' difficulties in modifying ongoing response sets were similar to those exhibited by patients with frontal lobe lesions.

Other investigators, however, have found the performance of psychopaths to equal that of control subjects on tasks involving social learning (Fairweather, 1954; Kadlub, 1956), learning sets (McCullough & Adams, 1970), verbal conditioning using social reinforcement (Bryan & Kapche, 1967), probability learning in a card game in which punishment was a near certainty (Siegel, 1978), and paired-associate learning without delay in feedback information (Gullick, Sutker, & Adams, 1976; Sutker, Gil, & Sutker, 1971). In addition, studies have shown that psychopaths are not necessarily deficient in avoidance conditioning (Gendreau & Suboski, 1971; Persons & Bruning, 1966; Schmauk, 1970) or on tasks requiring planning and foresight (Sutker, Moan, & Swanson, 1972) and modification of dominant cognitive response sets and cognitive flexibility (Sutker, Moan, & Allain, 1983).

Apparent contradictions in research findings suggest the need to identify the factors which may have contributed to a pattern of results emphasizing deficits as opposed to those which have not. These factors may be important to consider in assessing possible areas of deficiencies among psychopaths and in planning strategies to improve upon demonstrated weaknesses. In addition, findings may shed light on areas of potential strength for exploitation in therapeutic intervention efforts. To summarize, it has been observed that the following variables affect learning and performance among psychopaths: (1) probability and type of reinforcement, (2) timing of reinforcement, (3) preference for reward or reinforcing stimuli, and (4) perceptions of task and surrounding conditions. That is, psychopaths have been shown to perform better under conditions of uncertain but positive possible rewards which are delivered as close to the behaviors as possible. Their efforts are also enhanced when they have positive perceptions of the task and/or person administering the task and when they are interested in what they are doing.

It is evident, then, that psychopaths are not necessarily deficient in acquiring learned responses or in performing tasks under structured conditions. There is consensus that they may behave idiosyncratically or differently than do most so-called normals in learning situations, and the quality of their efforts appears to be more influenced by salient and perhaps subtle differences in learning contexts. Psychopaths may also be predicted to exhibit sophisticated problem solving in one context juxtaposed with marked deficits in another. Whereas the effects of important variables affecting human learning and performance in normal subject groups have been relatively well elucidated, the influence of these factors may be paradoxical among psychopaths. As Lykken (1978) warned, we should not restrict ourselves to obvious situational variables but should attempt to assess the extent to which the "game" of our contrived context strikes the fancy of the psychopathic subjects. In any case, we must not assume that learning performance is deficient or that psychopathic behaviors are inflexible and unamenable to modification. Using multimethod assessment, it is our task to design a treatment package which exploits individual preferences and strengths, modifies and minimizes personal weaknesses, and offers maximum likelihood for individual gains.

Problem-solving Sophistication

Arieti (1967) classified psychopaths into simple and complex types and pointed to level of intelligence as an important determinant of the extent and type of antisocial behaviors. He characterized the complex psychopath as one who, having average to superior intelligence, exhibits sufficient judgment to achieve self-determined goals while disregarding social morality. Heilbrun (1979, 1982) also pointed to intelligence level as a person factor influencing expression of violent behaviors among psychopaths. Supporting these notions, Sutker, Moan, and Allain (1983) found that highly intelligent psychopaths were less likely to exhibit cognitive inflexibility, perseveration, and impulsivity in a structured problem-solving situation than were those characterized by average intelligence. Such findings suggest that higher intelligence may mitigate against the expression of inflexible, impulsive behaviors among psychopathic patients. It is critical, then, to assess levels of intelligence as related to impulse control and cognitive mechanisms for coping. High intelligence may represent a mediator of adaptive behavior among psychopathic patients and as such may be considered in treatment planning as a factor to be used toward attenuation of behavior disinhibition.

Interpersonal Behavior

Among the characteristic interpersonal behavior patterns attributed to adult psychopaths are irritability and aggressiveness, sexual promiscuity or infidelity, irresponsibility in parenthood or to dependents, and manipulation of others for personal profit. Such behaviors are thought to be related to deficiencies in social development and functioning. For example, Gough (1948) saw psychopaths as having failed to reach appropriate adult standards of socialization. Over the years, Cleckley (1955; 1976) has argued that psychopaths are apathetic to suffering in others and insensitive in social situations. More recently, Rime, Bouvy, Leborgne, and Rouillon (1978) concluded that psychopaths exhibited increased nonverbal activity during interview interactions, representing highly intrusive and troublesome behaviors and lack of social awareness or skill. Gorenstein and Newman (1980) also pointed to social disregard as a prominent psychopathic feature and indicated that underlying their social behaviors were efforts to gratify transient desires as immediately as possible.

Many of these more extreme claims, especially those suggesting lack of social awareness and interpersonal deficits, are offered in the face of accumulating contradictory evidence on interpersonal postures and interactions attributed to psychopaths. Sociopaths, for example, have been shown to be as sensitive to social cues and affective stimuli as control subjects in a vicarious conditioning paradigm (Sutker, 1970), and socially relevant stimuli were more easily acquired in a verbal learning task than were socially nonrelevant stimuli among sociopaths (Sutker, Gil, & Sutker, 1971). Sociopaths have also been shown to score better than normals on measures requiring observation for detail in the tangible and social environments (Sutker, Moan, & Allain, 1974). In an impressive series of studies (Widom, 1976; 1977) found that psychopaths did not behave more selfishly or egocentrically, show more concern with personal gain, or act less responsibly than normal subjects.

Despite claims that psychopaths are socially insensitive and callous, as well as selfish and nonaccommodating, observers of their behavior have noted apparent social skillfulness and successful interpersonal manipulations as characteristic (Maher, 1965; Ullman & Krasner, 1975). The literature suggests that psychopaths are as capable as others of monitoring social interactions with propriety in novel assessment or initial interpersonal situations. However, over time and across situations, the effects of their more deviant interpersonal behaviors become additive, if not synergistic, and sequences of behavior including negative interpersonal interactions and unhappy feelings are initiated and maintained. It is not surprising, then, that those who know them best are most likely to complain about their repeated antisocial behaviors and the seemingly unending string of troublesome situations which complicate their lives. Problems with sexual indiscretion, lawlessness, substance abuse, low frustration tolerance, and exaggerated sensation seeking obviously put psychopaths at risk for failure in maintaining enduring attachments to sexual partners, and even friends.

Data collected in research studies over the past 10 years suggest that psychopaths tend to be keen observers of social behavior and capable of responding with appropriate emotions evidenced by verbal and nonverbal enthusiasm. Psychopaths find themselves stimulated by socially relevant cues, and they have been shown to participate in various types of game situations with regard for the rules of cooperation. Support has been found for Gough's (1948) speculation of deficiencies in role taking, however, and these seem to be attributed to difficulties in understanding what others are thinking and feeling because of their own peculiar or idiosyncratic thought constructs. For the most part, psychopaths may compensate for these cognitive peculiarities in that they demonstrate at least adequate superficial social skills—especially in structured interpersonal situations. Smith (1978) has, in fact, characterized psychopaths as survivors in American society, and personal impressions suggest that psychopathic prisoners adjust to the interpersonal demands of incarceration with the least distress and greatest effectiveness.

Cognitive Activity

Clinical investigators have focused increasingly on the role of cognition in the etiology, expression, and treatment of various types of psychopathology with emphasis on depressive symptoms (Bandura, 1977; Beck, 1976). Writers of the DSM-III (1980), however, minimized the importance of identifying cognitive content and processes characteristic of psychopaths. As yet, there have been no systematic attempts to catalogue cognitive statements, clusters of self-statements, or possible cognitive distortions which might be associated with antisocial behavior expression. An exception is the work of Widom (1976), who used the repertory grid technique to explore the interpersonal and personal construct systems of primary and secondary psychopaths and control subjects. Widom found that psychopaths showed misperceptions about people in general and specific misperceptions along a construct dimension labeled *dull–exciting*. Her work suggested that psychopaths have difficulties in acknowledging that people construe events differently than they do, that such perceptions are persistent, and that psychopaths fail to modify their construct systems accordingly.

If it can be assumed that psychopathy may be represented by characteristic cognitive processes or clusters of self-statements, it is important to attempt to understand cognitions associated with antisocial behaviors. Given traditional descriptions of psychopaths, at least five areas come to mind which could be targeted for research study among groups of psychopaths or using single-case design. These areas are: (1) egocentric thoughts or thoughts about self; (2) goal-directed persistency messages; (3) views about authority figures and rules; (4) self-statements focusing on depression or boredom states; and (5) fantasy behaviors, themes, and content. For example, it has been hypothesized that psychopaths think about themselves and their plans inordinately. References to self and personal plans could be identified and recorded for frequency in certain situations and compared with those of normal subjects in the same contexts.

The extent to which psychopaths admit thinking about the immediacy of obtaining important goals and the lengths to which they will go to achieve satisfaction could be studied using a cognitive framework. Psychopaths are credited with blatantly resisting authority and risking censure, but the conditions under which they exhibit these behaviors are not understood. It is suggested here that psychopaths tend to disregard sociolegal restraints when at least one of two conditions are met: (1) anticipated rewards/gains are greatly desired; and (2) negative consequences are judged to be minimal or easily avoided. It is also suggested that fantasy behaviors are indulged minimally among psychopaths when behavioral options are feasible given their system of constructs. Recently, Sutker and Allain (1983) found a strong association between conceptualizing behavior options and acting upon them in individuals characterized by sociopathic features as opposed to subjects considered normal who were more likely to think about deviant actions but avoid their expression.

Classification of the cognitive messages precursory to impulsiveness could prove helpful as an adjunct to understanding seemingly erratic behaviors, working to achieve modification in maladaptive behavior and emotional patterns, and encouraging prosocial involvements. One might identify the thoughts or cognitive content which communicate a state of boredom or intolerance for sameness as well as the cognitive processes which precede and accompany efforts to remedy the perceived need—both in psychopaths and normal subjects. Covert self-statements urging action should be determined as well as those which check, modify, or order the direction of given activities. Such inventories could prove useful to therapists working with individual patients and are needed to describe commonalities in thinking among psychopaths compared to normals and psychiatrically defined groups. As yet, virtually no data exist describing the cognitive content or processes, including fantasy behaviors, common to psychopaths or underlying their antisocial as well as prosocial activities. In addition, self-statements indicating lack of self-worth and feelings of depression should be a focus for measurement.

Emotional Activity

Using a content analysis of approximately 70 publications on the psychopathic personality, Albert, Brigante, and Chase (1959) reported that clinicians reached consensus that psychopaths were characterized by absence of conflict, anxiety, and guilt. In addition, many researchers and practicing clinicians have accepted Cleckley's (1955; 1976) notions that psychopaths exhibit poverty in major affective reactions and are unlikely to be driven to suicidal acts. Taking another view, Thorne (1959) wrote,

> The sociopath leaves a swath of disillusioned, hurt, and seriously damaged people in his wake [and] . . . does not emerge unscathed from his irregularities. At heart, he knows what he is, and this causes an increasing burden of self-hate, however well disguised or repressed. In the beginning, the sociopath can escape from anxiety by simply leaving the site of failure and securing ego inflation from the spurious security of new sexual conquests. But gradually it becomes necessary to consume increasing amounts of alcohol or drugs to anesthetize anxiety. . . . Also, the sociopath is getting older, less physically attractive, and outwardly ravaged by the wages of sin. . . . [He] gravitates socially downward until finally ending in the slums, broken financially, in and out of delirium tremens, shunted from prison to hospital, and finally expiring in the poor house or mental hospital. (p. 325)

In the same vein, Vaillant (1975) saw the antisocial behaviors of sociopaths as immature expression of negative affect states and discontent. In this sense, psychopaths were seen as more adolescent than ineducable.

Writers of the DSM-III (1980) suggested that psychopathic patients frequently present, or are found, with signs of personal distress. Complaints of depression, dissatisfaction, and anger are common, and data generated by research efforts show that indices of depression are elevated in subsets of groups which are largely antisocial. Weissman and her colleagues (Weissman, Pottenger, Kleber, Ruben, Williams, & Thompson, 1977) found secondary depressive symptoms in alcoholics and opiate addicts, and objective test measures have reflected depression in hospitalized alcoholics (Overall, 1973; Sutker, Archer, Brantley, & Kilpatrick, 1979) and addicts in treatment (Gilbert & Lombardi, 1967; Sutker, 1971). In many instances, depression and anxiety are associated with stressing life circumstances related to antisocial behaviors and abate with time and environmental stabilization (Sutker, Allain, & Cohen, 1974). In any case, the relationships between depression and acting-out behaviors are complex. Regardless of which came first, depression and antisocial psychopathology are inextricably linked in large numbers of patients called psychopaths.

Even this cursory review of extant literature suggests that simplistic conceptualizations of psychopathy are outdated and that antisocial behaviors are multidetermined. Documentation of a wide variety of nonconforming activities over time does not necessarily rule out the possibility of more serious psychopathology such as schizophrenia, and it is the task of the clinician to recognize the psychological heterogeneity among individuals who present with a constellation of antisocial behaviors. Studies have shown that psychopaths can become moderately to severely depressed and/or anxious, whereas others may evidence minimal neurotic symptomatology. There are psychopaths who are bright and adaptive in most settings and circumstances, and there are those who are less intelligent and facile in coping with stress. The question of whether violence is a component of the constellation of behavioral features characteristic of psychopathy is yet unanswered, and there are probably gender differences in the expression of antisocial inclinations. Individuals may also be identified who share emotional and behavioral characteristics with psychopaths but maintain their behaviors within the bounds of legal propriety. The extent to which such individuals permeate defined occupational or social groups is a question for research.

For purposes of this text, it is assumed that psychopath, sociopath, and antisocial personality disorder labels can be used interchangeably. Psychopathy is defined simply in terms of repetitious, chronic pathological nonconformity which has taken on maladaptive, inflexible expression. It is assumed that psychopaths, though perhaps distressed by their behaviors, persist in antisocial activities which are maintained by yet unidentified mechanisms of anticipated rewards. It is also assumed that psychopaths experience a range of emotional states—many of which are negative—and that depression is within their emotional repertoire. Psychopaths are not likely to appear in the all-or-none variety, and patients with psychopathic features present themselves with varying types of antisocial behaviors, differing in duration and frequency. Similarly, they differ in presenting mood states, problem-solving sophistication, physical problems, and degree to which their behaviors have become maladaptive, fixed, and troublesome to themselves and others. These differences suggested the need for individually focused assessment and treatment efforts, including identification of person strengths and weaknesses, evaluation of events or situations in the past environment and family background, and appraisal of the ongoing context of behavior–behavior sequences. A systematic approach to assessment and treatment necessitates careful identification of the presenting symptoms, long-standing target problems, and situational and behavioral factors which have impinged on the person over time.

ASSESSMENT AND CASE FORMULATION

Individual assessment and case formulation for purposes of psychological diagnosis and treatment may be conceptualized in terms of problem identification, response measurement, developmental analysis, and case formulation. More important than assigning individuals to categories is understanding the clusters of symptoms of disordered behaviors, cognitions, and emotions which characterize them. To point out that the diagnosis of antisocial personality may have negative consequences seems unnecessary. Yet, there have been cases in which individuals assigned this label have suffered harsh dispositions, because persons with decision-making powers focused on deficit-prone explanations and disregarded the possibilities of positive behavior change. Emphasis must be given to assessment of individual performance characteristics and specific targeting of behaviors, thoughts, and emotions for therapeutic change, for example, facilitation or discouragement

The assessment techniques used most frequently to specify problems common among psychopaths have been described at length by Brantley and Sutker (1984) and will not be reviewed here. Adequate assessment encompasses the use of clinical interviews, self-report inventories, behavior observations and checklists, and the option of psychophysiological monitoring over time. Choices of strategies vary among clinicians as do the content of their selected instruments; however, each approach may be seen to have its merits. A composite of strategies is recommended for individual case assessment, and those which are most appropriate to the case presented in this chapter will be elaborated.

Referral Circumstances

The mechanism of patient referral was telephone contact to the clinical psychologist by a family practice physician who provided clinical services within the confines of a family practice department in a large medical university complex. The patient, known as Mr. V., was a 28-year-old white man who had scheduled appointments at the family practice clinic regularly over the past four months. His initial visit was prompted by referral from an orthopedic surgeon whom he contacted regarding back pain subsequent to an automobile injury. His visits to the clinic had been characterized by complaints of lower back pain and requests for pain medication. Mr. V. had voiced feelings of depression and requested assistance in processing claims for disability insurance and other compensation related to automobile injury. The clinical psychologist was requested to "assess the contribution of psychological factors to complaints of pain and evaluate the extent of depression in the context of describing Mr. V. as a person." At the time of referral, the physician had been unable to identify specific organic referents for the pain and had noted patient requests for different and additional types of narcotic drugs.

Problem Identification

In this case, problem identification was seen to require at least three steps: (1) initial clinical interview with patient, (2) review of medical charts, and (3) interview contact with significant others in the patient's life, for instance, his wife. Meyer and Turkat (1979) described the effective clinician as the "supreme theoretician and detective," and this is an appropriate role for the psychologist in the assessment process. It might be noted parenthetically that the limits of the referral request are not mandated on the psychologist. Rather, assessment is viewed as a comprehensive process which may extend beyond the initial suggestion of the referring party. Mr. V. was scheduled for an initial interview, and the clinician used this opportunity to develop an outline of the problems which Mr. V. was experiencing from his perspective. The psychologist attempted to construct a rudimentary picture of the patient's childhood, adolescence, and adjustment to work and social involvements as an adult. Questions regarding depression, anxiety, back pain, and plans for the future comprised another aspect of the interview. Permission was obtained to telephone the patient's wife to obtain her view of the situation, and an appointment was made for the patient to return for more comprehensive evaluation.

During the initial interview, Mr. V. behaved in a manner which could be described as verbally facile, emotionally responsive, and relatively uninhibited. The patient talked freely about his past and presented himself as a person who was confused about directions for the future, worried about the stability of his marriage and "minor" legal difficulties, and concerned that he might have injured his back substantially in the recent automobile accident. Although he admitted to antisocial behaviors in adolescence such as occasional fighting, truancy, and shoplifting, he attempted to present himself as having "grown out of this" and as minimally interested in drugs or alcohol, except by prescription. He was eager to describe his pain symptoms and to indicate that he required more powerful drugs to cope with back pain which accompanied strenuous exercise or work. Mr. V. was cooperative with the examiner throughout the session, and he agreed to complete the assessment process, including a two-week period of self-monitoring.

Summarizing results from the initial interview, the psychologist compiled a statement of target problem areas which were conceptualized as the patient presented and ordered them in terms of emphasis. As can be seen in Table 1, the problems were back pain and resulting physical disability and depression. Marital discord and legal difficulties were relegated to secondary focus, and any emphasis they might have

Table 1. Patient-Identified Problem Targets: Data from Initial Assessment

Back pain	Depression	Marital discord	Legal difficulties
Manifestations			
Pain complaints	Unhappiness	Arguments, fights	DUI arrest
Medication	complaints	with wife	Speeding tickets
requests	Boredom talk	Sexual infidelities	Injury litigation
Facial grimaces	Loss of interest	Reduced affection	
Reduced activity	Reduced activity	to and from wife	
Slowed	Sleep disturbances	Wife left the home	
movements	Indecisiveness	Wife threatened	
	Antisocial	divorce	
	behaviors		
	Drug and alcohol		
	intoxication		
Situational factors			
Constant across	Increased at night,	Increased by	Increased by
situations	in early morning	unemployment	alcohol and
Increased by	Increased by idle	Increased by drugs	drugs
activity	time	and alcohol	Increased by acting
Increased at	Increased by stress	Increased by	out
night, in early	Decreased initially	infidelity	Increased by idle
morning	by alcohol and	Increased by legal	time
Decreased by	drugs	pressures	
alcohol and	Increased over	Increased by back	
drugs	time by alcohol	pain	
Aggravated by	and drugs	Decreased by	
perceived	Increased by work	prosocial	
stress	failures,	activities (e.g.,	
	unemployment	sports)	

been given may have been prompted by interviewer questions. Manifestations of target problems were identified as well as the situations in which discomfort became exaggerated or attenuated. The exercise of listing problems as the patient saw them was selected to obtain his input in compiling a more exhaustive list of target problems, formulating a conceptualization of his case, and outlining avenues for treatment recourse.

The second step in assessment constituted efforts to secure information from medical records and significant others. In this case, there was no medical documentation for physical disability contributing to ongoing pain complaints. The patient's wife supported her husband's claims of back pain, but discussions with her pointed to excessive alcohol use, long-term abuse of prescription drugs, chronic marital conflicts, and repeated sexual infidelity on his part. She in turn did not use drugs, engage in extramarital affairs, or drink alcohol to excess, except when under stress. Mrs. V. noted that her husband typically showed diminished concern with his back when he was having a "good time" with friends. She said he tended to change jobs frequently and without advance warning, and she was troubled by fears that their marriage was irreparably jeopardized. She indicated that although they had been happy during the early months of marriage, they had become increasingly unhappy. Several years back, her husband had joined the Marine Corps, and he had seemed more interested in the marriage at that time. However, when he completed service requirements, he returned to old habits which necessitated her frequent initiation of marital separations. She indicated that she took responsibility for paying the bills most of the time and that without her intervention they would have found themselves in grave financial crisis. She concluded the interview by affirming that she loved her husband no matter what and that she wanted him desperately to settle down with her and find work which he liked.

Response Measurement

Once this background was obtained, the patient was rescheduled for comprehensive assessment. Instruments to be administered were selected on the basis of information gathered, such that initial hypotheses could be tested by more direct means. For example, data obtained from the patient and his wife suggested that substance abuse and other antisocial activities were problematic, as well as significantly related to the patient's pain complaints. Therefore, one hypothesis to be explored was that the patient deliberately exaggerated pain reports to obtain narcotics from a legitimate source. The extent of antisocial activities during adolescence and adulthood was documented in this regard. Essential to answering the consultation request was an assessment of the severity, duration, and nature of depressive symptoms and an identification of determinants of perceptions of being physically disabled and needing drugs. Intelligence levels, problem-solving strengths and weaknesses, and characteristic approaches to stress were targets for evaluation. Response measurement included assessment of common attitudes about self, others, and life, emotional states and enduring moods, possibility of psychotic complications, and signs of character disorder symptomatology other than those suggesting psychopathy. In addition, data contributing to the formulation of a typology of important situations in childhood, adolescence, and adulthood life stages were obtained.

Data were obtained by self-reports, reports from others, direct observations and ratings, and individually administered standardized tests. Mood state changes were measured over a two-week monitoring period, as were alcohol and drug consumption, pain complaints, and important activities or events, including those which were antisocial and prosocial. As an example, depression was measured at the time of assessment using the Minnesota Multiphasic Personality Inventory (MMPI) Scale Depression (D), the Beck Depression Inventory (BDI), the Multiple Affect Adjective Checklist (MAACL), and clinician ratings of depression using the Brief Psychiatric Rating Scale (BPRS). The MAACL was used to assess depression, anger, and anxiety over the two-week monitoring period as well. Propensities for antisocial involvements and sensation seeking were evaluated by scores on the MMPI Scale Psychopathic Deviate (Pd), Gough's (1960) California Personality Inventory (CPI) Socialization Scale (So), Zuckerman's (1979) measure of sensation seeking (SSS), and a listing of antisocial activities reported during adolescence or before age 15 years, during adulthood, and over the two-week period of monitoring. Given this patient's complaints of back injury, records of pain and medications were required, and the extent to which he was inclined to somatize problems in the past was explored.

State-of-the-art assessment strategy assumes that in addition to person characteristics, behaviors and environmental or situational factors operate in interaction with reciprocal influence to determine given sets of behaviors, to initiate or modulate feelings, thoughts, and other person factors, and to contribute to situations in which the person has been found. It is important, then, to measure variables from the three systems, to obtain data by several methods, to employ a time-sampling approach, and to determine relationships among variables as much as possible. A summary of the data obtained in initial assessment and derived from administration of the battery of test instruments is presented in Table 2. Such information was used to generate a list of hypotheses about behaviors and situations to be explored further in clinical interview or by other assessment procedures. The clinical interview in this case was scheduled for a time at the close of the two-week monitoring period, such that all materials were available for constructing a profile of target problems. This profile was used to suggest relationships between target problems and the environment, logical and experienced consequences of problems, varied manifestations of symptoms, and contributions of person, situation, and behavior factors as reciprocal agents. Assessment of the patient's repertoire of coping strategies was also seen as important. An exhaustive list of hypotheses cannot be presented, but several are discussed for purposes of illustration.

Table 2. Summary of Data Derived from Traditional Assessment Instruments

Cognitive characteristics		Personality characteristics	
Intellectual resources		Depression	
WAIS-R full-scale score	122	BDI total score	21
WAIS-R verbal score	124	MMPI scale D (T-score)	77
WAIS-R performance score	112	MAACL depression score	23
Flexibility and control		Anxiety	
WCST categories completed	6	MMPI scale Pt (T-score)	60
WCST total errors	11	MMPI Scale A (T-score)	67
WCST perseverative errors	3	MAACL Anxiety Score	13
WCST nonperseverative errors	8	Anger	
Forethought and impulse control		MMPI scale Pa (T-score)	62
Porteus test quotient	132	MAACL anger score	9
Porteus qualitative score	8	Social nonconformity	
SSS total score	29	MMPI scale Pd (T-score)	81
MMPI scale Ma (T-score)	73	CPI scale So (standard score)	31

Developmental Analysis

Developmental analysis may be conceptualized as an attempt to compile a list of common behaviors by type and frequency and situations common to the patient over time using all test and interview data. Looking at the findings presented in Table 2, it is obvious that Mr. V. is an intelligent, verbally facile man with more than adequate abilities for observation. He demonstrated capabilities for planning, changing response sets as needed, and exercising cognitive control in structured situations. It is assumed that the capacity for forethought is related to one's facility for enhancing, attenuating, or nullifying the effects of personal or others' behaviors. Mr. V.'s performances across the Wechsler Adult Intelligence Scale—Revised (WAIS-R) subtests were qualitatively inconsistent, and it was hypothesized that he typically became impulsive, inattentive, and distracted when required to persist in routine tasks or to execute nonpreferred assignments. Mr. V. was thought to be a chronic underachiever and a person who had failed to maximize his cognitive strengths. It was thought likely that he was inconsistent in work situations as well as sporadically productive, depending upon perceived incentives and other circumstances. Given this constellation of cognitive strengths and weaknesses, it was hypothesized that Mr. V. was bored frequently with most of the situations in which he found himself. Further, he seemed unable to find employment which offered intellectual challenge, satisfactory financial remuneration, and the element of excitement.

To address questions regarding medication requests, the problems of pain complaints, depressed affect and mentation, and extent and frequency of antisocial behaviors were examined. It was predicted that Mr. V. was a socially nonconforming, sensation-seeking man who had been living on the verge of trouble, evidenced by involvement in a series of "sticky" situations, juvenile acting-out, and adult indiscretions. The patient was questioned about truancy, school suspensions, fighting, substance abuse, law-breaking, and sexual promiscuity as defined by the DSM-III (1980). The question of whether Mr. V.'s back pain was related to organic factors was left to the physician; however, it was seen as critical to determine the possible role of psychological variables in contributing to pain complaints and behavior. It was also necessary to gain perspective on the reasons for requesting medications and the extent to which drug use was superimposed on already existing patterns of alcohol and illicit drug use. It was possible that the patient had maintained feelings of depression coupled with lack of fulfillment and poor self-esteem and that the accident had triggered a reason to visit the doctor, seek solace in drugs of a different type, and gain therapeutic attention. It was also possible that the patient was looking for drugs and physician validation of his disability and that he was not the least interested in changing life-style patterns or enhancing his moods other than through chemicals.

The clinical interview was conducted with these and other notions in mind; however, it was recognized from the outset that there are no simple answers to any of the questions posed and that most of the hypotheses generated were neither mutually exclusive nor capable of conclusive affirmation or disconfirmation. During the interview, the clinician attempted to build a picture of the patient's behavior in childhood and adolescence, including a view of situations in which he found himself during various life stages, his adjustment to school and home demands, his strategies for managing unhappiness or stress, and his most characteristic interpersonal styles. He was asked about the sources of enjoyment in his life and his aspirations for career development, both when he was a youth and as he grew older. A list of the types of antisocial and prosocial behaviors was generated (see Table 3), and the events surrounding his seeking medical assistance were explored.

Data from the comprehensive interview showed that Mr. V. was the oldest of three children and raised in an environment in which parental supervision was largely lacking. His father was a merchant seaman while Mr. V. was a young child but later worked as a construction foreman. His mother built a career teaching in middle school. His father and mother engaged in frequent domestic fights which centered

Table 3. Summary of Data Derived from Behavioral Assessment

Observed behaviors

Presenting symptoms
  BPRS thinking disturbance   0   BPRS hostile/suspiciousness   4
  BPRS withdrawal/retardation   0   BPRS anxious/depression   8

Self-reported past behaviors

Antisocial behaviors before age 15 years
  Truancy more than 5 days/school year
  Suspended from school on at least 2 occasions
  Repeated sexual intercourse in casual relationships
  Repeated drunkenness and substance abuse
  School grades markedly below expectations

Antisocial behavior since age 18 years
  Inconsistent work involvement and behaviors
  Frequent job changes and unemployment
  Problems with sustaining enduring attachment to sexual partner
  Two or more marital separations
  Flagrant sexual promiscuity
  Financial irresponsibility
  Disrespect for sociolegal norms, DUI, and speeding arrests
  Use of illegal drugs

Prosocial behaviors before age 15 years
  Childhood paper route and other odd jobs
  Sporadically good grades in elementary school
  Regular participation in sports activities in school
  Organization of games and sports in neighborhood
  No suspensions or failures in elementary school
  High frequency of social contacts
  Social successes with peers

Prosocial behaviors since age 18 years
  Active participation in neighborhood sports
  Satisfactory or excellent adjustment in military service
  Dedication to program of physical fitness on sporadic basis
  Numerous social contacts other than substance-abuse related
  Social successes with peers

Self-reported ongoing behaviors[a]

Alcohol and drug use
  Alcohol or drugs used on 90% of days
  Average daily consumption of 2.12 oz. absolute alcohol
  Daily use of marijuana, pain medications

Impulsive, nonconforming behaviors
  Sexual infidelity on 3–4 occasions each week
  Fights with wife on 6 occasions each week
  Seeking new sources of drugs for use

Prosocial, positive behaviors
  Resumption of regular exercise routine, 3–4 times each week
  Maintained behavior, mood, and event logs as requested

[a]Examples of data collected over two-week monitoring period

around the father's drinking, staying out late, and becoming involved with other women. Mr. V.'s father was described as physically strong, fun-loving, and hardworking, and his mother was seen as hardworking, overly critical, and controlling. When Mr. V. reached the age of 11 years, his parents were in the process of divorce. From that time, Mrs. V. worked even harder and ultimately became principal of a middle school. She maintained high expectations for all her children but rarely spent time with them except in maintenance or instruction kinds of functions. Mr. V. was the only son among the three children, and Mrs. V. was particularly critical of him. She was said by him to comment frequently, "He is just like his father."

Mr. V. described few periods of unhappiness in his early life, except that he did not enjoy school (except sports and recess) and that he was deeply hurt by his father's leaving the home. He was annoyed by his mother's criticisms, but since she was not home much of the time he was able to do as he pleased. He saw himself as "well-liked" by his classmates, despite occasional fights. He was inclined to gain attention by showing off, and he experimented with drugs and sex at an early age. At the age of 8 years, he began smoking cigarettes, and by the time he was 13 he was using marijuana regularly. First sexual intercourse was reported at the age of 14 years, and the impetus to this encounter was said to be the encouragement of an older girl, 17 years. During his high school years, he was truant with friends, and he indulged in occasional thefts and burglaries with them. For the most part, he attempted to avoid serious legal offenses. He did not excel academically, and he was bored in school. Usually he was liked by his teachers, and he was able to avoid punishment for wrongdoing by using his quick wit. An attractive physical appearance and endurance, clever verbalizations, and sporadic good school performances worked to his advantage. Mr. V. acknowledged that he was "intellectually superior" but that he found few things which really interested him over time, excepting physical types of activities.

Mr. V. maintained an active, visible, and popular life-style as an adolescent. He enjoyed sexual promiscuity, participated minimally in school, and engaged in minor though reportedly exciting criminal acts. During his senior year, however, he burglarized a drugstore and was almost apprehended. By this time, he was also drinking more alcohol and engaging in more frequent drug use. In retrospect, Mr. V. reported having been discontent at this time in his life, uncertain about the future, and bitter about his father having left home. He hoped to extricate himself from this negative state of affairs by attending college and becoming a lawyer. Nevertheless, he performed poorly during his last high school year, and his academic problems were compounded by the unexpected pregnancy of one of the girls whom he had been dating. He married this woman and sought employment immediately following graduation. The first two years of married life were said to be more settled than those in school, and Mr. V. remained home much of the time when not working. He drank less alcohol and maintained steady employment. He admitted, though, that his wife tended to be demanding and controlling, as well as less affectionate with the coming of the baby. He said that he felt trapped and bored in this marriage and noted that he saw his wife as intellectually unsophisticated and easy prey to his manipulations and fabrications. He returned to old habits and in fact expanded his antisocial behavior by frequent drinking and drug use to intoxication, staying out late or not coming home, and initiating a series of love affairs.

Prompted by unhappiness, Mr. V. enlisted in the Marine Corps for two years of active duty. He found initial training at Paris Island rigorous, but he enjoyed the challenge of physical exertion and the camaraderie of man-to-man situations. He was stationed in the Philippines for most of his service commitment, and he did not see active combat. During his tour of duty, he found a ready supply of drugs, cultural approval for sexual promiscuity, and new interests in opiates and potent marijuana. Upon discharge, he felt mild withdrawal symptoms, but he remained abstinent from opiates for several months after returning to the United States. His situation with his wife was improved upon his return for a few months, but in time their relationship deteriorated. In fact, Mr. V. began a series of indiscreet extramarital affairs, heavy substance abuse, and frequent work changes. By the age of 27, he reported that he felt he was "losing control" over his life. He was using marijuana, amphetamines and cocaine, and opiate derivatives heavily. In addition, he was drinking to intoxication periodically. About 10 months prior to his appearance at the Family Practice Clinic he was arrested for Driving under the influence (DUI), and this followed two previous arrests for speeding.

The DUI offense was described by Mr. V. as the "straw that broke the camel's back." His wife complained bitterly about his lack of responsibility and his not caring for her and the child, and she left him, threatening to file for divorce. She had left him before, but this time she contacted a lawyer who filed papers on Mr. V. for official separation. Mr. V. reported that he felt greater depression, loneliness, and emptiness than he had ever known. He said that it seemed to him that the more he had tried to relieve the boredom and to have a good time, the more unhappy he became. He also struck upon the notion that alcohol and drugs exerted a "depressing" effect on him, but he thought that physician-prescribed drugs might have the opposite effect. He insisted that his back was painful to him and that he was worried about the physical repercussions of the accident. In any event, Mr. V. used the accident and injury to lure his wife home so that she could "take care of him." Nevertheless, he said that their relationship was tenuous and that if he did not improve his behavior he would surely lose her and the little girl. In addition, he would sustain financial losses because his wife was paying most of the bills. Contact with Mrs. V. confirmed these reports, but Mrs. V. revealed that she was "hopelessly in love" with Mr. V. She was certain that if she waited sufficiently long, she could influence him to become the man she had always wanted.

Case Formulation

Paramount in formulating Mr. V.'s case was deriving an understanding of the ongoing behaviors, emotions, and situations which characterized his life. The intricacies of person, behavior, and situation factors in influencing each other have been discussed by Bandura (1983). For purposes of this text, behaviors, situations, and person factors are seen to act reciprocally to influence ongoing behaviors, situations, and person variables. For instance, involvement in negative, acting-out activities is associated with other types of antisocial activities over time and the experience of negative outcomes. Unfortunate consequences lead to depression, and depression may provoke acting out, more negative situations, and greater depression. Looking at the evidence, Mr. V. can be described as a nonconforming, socially facile, and often charming man with strengths in cognitive functioning, physical appearance and energy, and productive behaviors when in structured environments or with supervision, for example, the Marine Corps. It is clear that his home environment during the formative years was characterized by situations which have been shown to be associated with adolescent drug use, antisocial behavior, and underachievement. A sampling of situations occurring over time in Mr. V.'s life is presented in Table 4. Examples of distal factors which have been found associated with drug use and delinquency are minimal parental supervision, absence of paternal influence, poor communication between and with parents, unreasonable parental standards, peer encouragement of deviance and drug-taking, and parental tolerance of deviance in general (Sutker, 1982).

During adolescence, few negative consequences resulted from Mr. V.'s antisocial involvements, and he continued to pursue his desires

Table 4. Summary of Situations and Events Characteristic over Time

Distal situations	Proximal situations
Parental fighting	Marital conflicts
Father absent from home	Troubles with employers
Minimal parental supervision	Work terminations
Adequate finances	Speeding tickets
Unreasonable maternal standards	Automobile accident
Peer encouragement of drugs, crime	Back injury
Drug and alcohol availability	DUI arrest
Few early illnesses	Chronic drug and alcohol intoxication
No hospitalizations	Conflicts with female lovers
No psychiatric treatment	Male encouragement of drug use
Two school suspensions	Minimal exercise
Stealing with peers	Poor physical fitness, tiredness
Unwanted pregnancy	Repeated sexual indiscretions
Forced marriage	Wife pressure for work, fidelity, time,
Career plans cancelled	attention, money
Forced employment	Idle time and nothing to do
Wife pressure for time, attention	No contacts with parents
Marine Corps basic training and duty	
Chronic drug and alcohol intoxication	
Regular exercise	

of the moment. As he became older, he realized that steps were necessary to encourage certain changes, and he attempted to settle down with his wife. When that failed, he tried the military to find the discipline which he thought important for him. Although he found himself happier in the Marines than ever before, social pressure for drug use, ready availability of drugs, and the stresses of the military system influenced him. He found that he could manage emotional problems, disappointments, and frustration by using potent drugs. As a boy, he had already learned that acting out relieved his energies and provided other satisfactions as well. By the time he reached the twenties, however, these strategies were well practiced but unsatisfactory in contributing to a sense of personal happiness over time. Mr. V. reported that he did not know how to extricate himself from the miserable situation in which he found himself. When questioned about possible self-generated solutions, Mr. V. recited reliance on a few censure statements which were derived from his mother's or wife's views of his behaviors, but he voiced no statements or cautions originating in his own system or related to self-established goals and values.

It was the judgment of the clinician that marital separation, financial and legal difficulties, lingering depression, and an automobile accident culminating in back injury and some degree of pain prompted

Mr. V.'s recognition of requiring assistance. He certainly did intend to exploit physician visits for all the narcotic drugs he could obtain, but he was ambivalent about this and in part desperately sought relief for his drug-related discontent and cavalier life-style. Mr. V. was seen as bored with his life, his wife, and himself. He was also frustrated by back pain which was believed by the clinician to be experienced genuinely but exaggerated for effects. Given these assumptions, a typology of target problems was constructed as seen in Table 5. The three target manifestations which required the most immediate attention were excessive alcohol use, drug dependence, and depressed thoughts and behaviors. The assessor was also mandated to propose ways in which the more global constellation of self-defeating antisocial behaviors could be reduced and appropriate prosocial activities encouraged and substituted. This would include outlining plans for Mr. V. to accomplish the following: (1) maintain a relatively alcohol and drug-free existence; (2) identify exciting alternatives to drug-induced states and sexual promiscuity, if married; (3) acquire and practice strategies for managing high levels of tension, anger, and depression; (4) add a dimension of behavioral self-discipline to his life; (5) improve his relationship with

Table 5. Clinician Identified Problem Targets

Problem area	Target manifestation
Antisocial psychopathology	Abuse, dependence on alcohol
	Abuse, dependence on drugs
	Repeated, flagrant sexual promiscuity
	Work, financial irresponsibility
	Reckless driving, driving under influence
Depression, negative affect	Complaints of unhappiness, boredom
	Reduced prosocial activities (e.g., work)
	Fighting with wife, others
	Thoughts of hopelessness, no direction
	Thoughts of needing drugs, fun, pleasure
	No program of physical exercise
	Exaggerated perceptions of pain
Cognitive and behavior dyscontrol	Poor judgment, little impulse control
	No plans for future, work, social life
	Meager self-discipline even in exercise
	No resources established for leisure time
	Meager resources for delay of gratification
Social immaturity and dependence	High demandingness of significant others
	Minimal investments in relationships
	No satisfaction with personal relationships
	Childish behavior around family members

his wife or facilitate its dissolution; and (6) define occupational and schooling options for the present and future.

The aggregate of assessment findings shows that Mr. V. met the criteria for the DSM-III (1980) diagnosis of antisocial personality disorder. As illustrated in Figure 1, he also produced the prototypic MMPI profile of the psychopath. Unlike many of his antisocial counterparts, he was raised in a middle-class home, was not associated with hardcore criminality, and did not vent himself to full-fledged juvenile delinquency or practice antisocial behaviors to the extreme. In addition, he was smarter perhaps than what one might call the average psychopath, and he was bright, engaging, and clever in avoiding harsh negative consequences of his behaviors. It was only as he became older that his boyish charms began to wear thin, and he himself became unhappy with meager career, marriage, and other personal goal achievements. Mr. V. also exhibited signs of dysthymic disorder as defined by DSM-III (1980), and it was hypothesized that his depression had contributed chronically to his patterns of drug use, as his drug use and antisocial activities contributed to his negative affect. Looking at the sequence of life events, it is difficult to ascertain whether depression or antisocial involvement came first chronologically. Most probably, Mr. V. was basically antisocial, but it was likely that most people minimized Mr. V.'s depression as he did himself. For the most part, people focused on the constellation of nonconforming and sometimes outrageous behaviors which Mr. V. expressed and failed to notice his negative mood states and their relationships to his nonconformity.

Mr. V., then, was seen as a bright psychopath whose antisocial behavior had begun to yield sufficiently negative consequences that he was willing to consider the possibility of life-style changes, if only to give himself a "breather." Evidence showed that he realized his exaggerated tendencies to have his way and to indulge himself. Given the literature on psychopathy which has been reviewed, one could assume that Mr. V. would sustain few lasting changes unless he himself decided that these were inescapable or offered greater possibility for personal gratification. That is, situational pressures converged with the anticipation of alternative rewards to pique Mr. V.'s potential motivation for change. One could assume also that antisocial activities would not be relinquished unless satisfactory substitutes were found and anticipation of important, tangible rewards were viewed as attainable.

Mr. V. had to be able to look forward to working in a situation which was viewed as exciting, meaningful, or challenging in some manner. If he were to be happy interpersonally, he would have to decide whether he wished to remain with his wife or to set his course alone

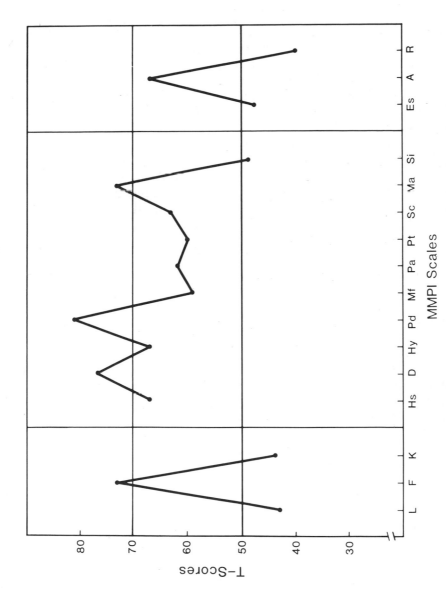

Figure 1. T-score elevations on MMPI validity, clinical, and selected special scales.

for a time. These choices were, of course, left to the patient, but the therapist acknowledged that it was unlikely to achieve therapeutic gains without establishing plans for a satisfactory work situation, hopes for a meaningful career, and at least partial resolution of marital discord. Mr. V. would have to be encouraged to reduce use of alcohol and drugs immediately and to begin to engage in behavior and thinking which he could perceive as positive or rewarding so as to counteract his depression and offer substitutes for excessive alcohol and drug use. Whether Mr. V. enjoyed sky diving, mountain climbing, or expanded sports participation, he would have to be prompted to identify these interests and indulge himself in such prosocial types of energy discharge. Further, if he could obtain release from his physician, he would be encouraged to begin a regular program of exercise similar to that he had maintained to keep in shape in the Marines. Indeed, he might well be exhorted to reconsider career alternatives in this branch of the service.

Among his most critical problems were impulsiveness, ambivalence and anger in close interpersonal relationships (especially with women), poor capacity for dealing with stress, social immaturity manifested in such features as high demandingness and difficulties in delaying gratification, and meager appreciation (fear) of the consequences of antisocial acts. On the positive side, his strengths included intellectual sophistication, facility with words, potential cognitive and behavioral control, adequate resources for forethought, willingness to work diligently at something he enjoyed, and ease in relating to others. He was also a physically attractive man who in the past had profited from the supervision, structure, and camaraderie of the military. There was evidence of guilt feelings and remorse over things having gone awry. Given these strengths and weaknesses, the psychologist was faced with the task of outlining possible mechanisms for impacting on defined problem targets. Before suggesting therapeutic strategies which might be important for psychopathic patients, we must examine several more common assumptions regarding antisocial behavior and the potential treatability of nonconforming persons.

TREATMENT DESIGN AND IMPLEMENTATION

First and foremost, the clinician should be convinced that treatment efforts are not necessarily doomed at the outset. It is assumed by the writers of this text that antisocial and related behaviors are determined or influenced by the ongoing reciprocal interplay of person, situation, and behavior factors. It is posited that antisocial individuals can learn to relinquish negative activities and adapt to life conditions with greater maturity and responsibility. It is unlikely, however, that treatment could succeed without genuine patient interest in modifying living patterns beyond the period of immediate discomfort and for clearly defined personal reasons. Should Mr. V. continue alcohol and drug abuse, it would be naive to anticipate his achieving lasting improvements in mood states, changes in employment habits, or more satisfying interpersonal interactions. Even if he did avoid the more blatant forms of antisocial expression, such gains would be threatened if he were unable to resolve many of his marital conflicts, develop positive alternatives to antisocial activities, and secure an employment situation which satisfied his needs.

Because Mr. V. was a bright man who was hypothesized to be motivated for behavioral change by unhappiness and frustration, he was seen as a reasonable candidate for treatment. That he was at the time of assessment actively seeking drug supplies, preoccupied by concerns about his back injury, and feeling unhappy with his home situation were negative points. The assumption behind his treatment was that a working therapeutic relationship could be used as a context in which behavior and emotional changes could be initiated, reinforced, practiced, and generalized through the processes of consistent structuring, shaping, and monitoring. Successes could be achieved only, however, if the bonds between patient and therapist were developed strongly over time and if the therapist became an important reinforcer per se. Under these conditions, Mr. V. could be influenced by the therapist toward positive changes, and his vulnerability for acceptance, approval, and adventure could be used to two advantages: facilitation of prosocial activities and discouragement of antisocial expression and associated consequences. That is, once Mr. V. had begun to maintain regular contacts with the therapist, to sense ongoing approval and acceptance, and to grasp the need for greater behavior control, it would be possible to discourage self-defeating activities in favor of more adaptive pleasure-seeking pursuits, both for the present and for the future. All of this would be impossible to achieve if the patient perceived feelings of repugnance or judgment in the therapist. That is, the therapist who sees himself or herself as removed from the vulgarity of antisocial behavior might best focus on other therapy candidates.

An important hypothesis related to management of antisocial patients is that they are reluctant to rid themselves of potent sources of pleasure without anticipation or realization of specific positive events. Ideally, pleasurable pursuits must be incompatible with maintaining antisocial expression. For example, heroin addicts have been known to turn their backs on narcotics because they have found work or love situations which offered them at least as much, and perhaps more, personal satisfaction than did drugs. Therefore, the therapist should develop in conjunction with the patient a treatment plan focusing directly on behaviors, situations, and person factors such as attitudes or moods which serve to initiate or maintain substance abuse. A period of hospitalization or residential treatment may be required to manage drug dependence, and if so this is the first step in treatment. Gains realized in the residential modality may then be maximized in an enduring aftercare relationship. Although there are data to suggest that most substance abusers profit from periods of hospitalization (Sutker, Allain, & Cohen, 1974; Zuckerman, Sola, Masterson, & Angelone, 1975), significant relapse problems occur because aftercare supervision is perfunctory or entirely lacking.

Clinicians generally inform patients of their assessment conclusions, and Mr. V. was given a down-to-earth explanation of his target problems, suggested mechanisms for their resolution, and possible options for behavior and emotional change. It is suggested that antisocial individuals will modify their behaviors only if they so wish and decide to do so and that intentions and desires are necessary but insufficient to maintain changes, even once begun. Therefore, the clinician would present the case findings in a straightforward, compelling manner with an elaboration of patient strengths and weaknesses. Lion (1978) indicated that therapists working with psychopaths must be "continually vigilant" to possible distortions and fabrications. This is not necessarily true across situations or antisocial patients, but the therapist must learn to determine when exaggerations are being offered or distortions implemented for effect. In any event, it is critical to secure patient endorsement of the needs for treatment and to enlist patient input for developing a treatment plan, guidelines for progress measurement, and realistic goals for achievement. Goals must be established with appreciation for patient strengths and weaknesses, and setbacks in goal attainment must be anticipated. It is also important to avoid advancing goals which are impossible to achieve or unrealistically phrased.

It is important to address the issue of behavioral-emotional setbacks when considering management and treatment of antisocial patients. Regression to self-defeating, antisocial acts is to be expected from time to time and must be managed in a calm, well-structured manner without the negative affect or judgmental censure associated with such behaviors in the patient's life (excluding, of course, heinous violent acts or person offenses). The antisocial patient is seen to be in therapy with an objective individual who behaves differently, and perhaps even unpredictably, in conditions through which antisocial behaviors are admitted or discovered. Relapse does not signal failure unless relapses are repeated and inexplicable. As Marlatt (1982) has said of alcoholics and smokers, antisocial individuals must learn to manage relapse constructively and to develop a new repertoire of coping strategies to achieve progress in overcoming behavioral slips. Hence, the therapist does not assume the role of judgmental parent or spouse but offers consistent acceptance of the person and discourages antisocial (or adolescent) behaviors which emerge over the course of time. These are the symptoms which constitute psychopathic psychopathology, and the patient should not be rejected for the very problem behaviors which necessitated treatment. As an illustration of the censure-punish-banish model, the delinquent youth is expelled from school to fend alone and unsupervised on the streets. It is no surprise that freedom begets antisocial expression and antisocial behaviors lead to greater deviance.

Essential to treatment is encouragement of whatever positive characteristics were identified during assessment, for example, social facility, personal creativity, physical prowess, sense of humor. Favorable patient features and situations must be exploited to facilitate acquisition of adult coping strategies and better management of high-risk situations which prompt antisocial acts. To whatever extent possible, the environmental stimuli associated with past antisocial expression should be minimized. For example, Sutker (1974) found that stimuli in the environmental context may exert powerful influences on behaviors among heroin addicts attempting to remain drug-abstinent. Thus, the ideal treatment situation is designed to enhance self-esteem, feelings of mastery, and personal confidence over the environment and life circumstances as they may arise and signal antisocial involvements. As feelings of mastery are improved and accomplishments realized, more productive and prosocial behaviors may be anticipated. Such behaviors are typically seen as their own rewards, but they provide a good focus for therapeutic reinforcement. One of the critical points in treatment of antisocial individuals occurs in conjunction with early successes or relief of negative moods, strengthening of confidence, and emerging perceptions of self-sufficiency. These changes may lead the patient to conclude that treatment has accomplished its purpose and may be discontinued. In most cases, premature interruption of treatment will result in returns to antisocial expression, although there are exceptions.

One of the problems encountered in treatment of antisocial individuals is the therapist's reluctance to attend to or believe patient statements reflecting unhappiness, depression, loneliness, and anxiety. As in the case of health professionals who reason that alcoholics, for example, have created their own sickness and deserve to suffer, so some clinicians assume that negative affect states, if they exist at all among psychopaths, constitute their "just desserts." It is not necessary to belabor the point that such attitudes are not helpful in the therapeutic process. Rather, it is important to highlight the necessity of monitoring a range of positive and negative thoughts and feelings toward the goal of lifting depression and encouraging more positive affect. Numerous studies have shown a highly complex, entangled relationship between negative moods and self-defeating behaviors such as antisocial expression, for example, abuse of illicit substances, repeated DUI arrests, and other forms of criminality. It is incumbent upon the therapist and patient to work out a depression, or perhaps boredom, management program which includes self-monitoring, self-reporting, and collecting traditional assessment data. As the patient learns to enhance strategies for identifying and dealing with unhappy moods (exclusive of marked antisocial expression), chances for success are multiplied.

Research data have shown psychopaths to be minimally deterred by threats of punishment or censure and favorably influenced by social rewards such as praise, especially that which is immediate. Psychopaths have been found to be cooperative with others when working jointly to solve problems, but there is also evidence of competitiveness, especially within paired members of the same gender. The therapist, of course, does not wish to become involved in a power struggle with the antisocial patient. Psychopaths tend to be sensitive to "games" which the therapist might attempt and to resent obvious superficiality and obvious information feedback delays. One must also work to sustain therapeutic contact with the antisocial patient. It is hypothesized that efforts to maintain patient behavioral controls and continue patient cooperation with the demands of therapy over time improve the chances for success. That is, early goals are to keep the patient in treatment. Usually, the fact that psychopathic patients appear regularly for treatment represents a positive gain in and of itself. As with adolescents, it is true that the longer the antisocial expressions may be postponed or their severity and frequency lessened, the better the chances to continue delay of antisocial behaviors and the negative consequences which accompany them. In their place, one may hope to substitute positive health-engendering options for obtaining pleasure.

As yet, there is scant evidence that therapeutic efforts are effective among psychopathic patients. In part, limitations in our fund of research knowledge and methods of treatment assessment account for this. In addition, however, psychopaths are found most frequently in drug and alcohol treatment programs, in prisons, or in other settings to which their antisocial behaviors have brought them. Such persons may represent the "worst" component of the antisocial expression cluster, so to speak, whereas those who may have profited in treatment in less dramatic precipitating circumstances tend to go unnoticed. Regardless of these issues, antisocial behaviors are seen as relatively constant over time with slim possibilities for "burn out" in the middle years (Maddocks, 1970; Robins, Gentry, Munoz, & Marten, 1977). Review of the evidence suggests that antisocial behaviors, ranging from mildly idiosyncratic to highly maladaptive, are subject to prescribed principles of acquisition and modification as are any sets of behaviors described categorically. Although constitutional explanations for behavioral aberrance have been advanced (Fowles, 1984; Gorenstein, 1982) and the contingencies for controlling antisocial expression may not be immediately apparent, we are not led to the conclusion that antisocial problems are intractable. In this sense, it is critical that certain events not be reasoned *a priori* to be punishing or rewarding for individuals classified as antisocial but that the characteristics of classes of punishing and rewarding stimuli be identified and tested among antisocial groups and for individual patients.

We have urged an objective look at individuals characterized as antisocial personality disorder—a view which for the most part excludes overtones of repugnance, distaste, and disdain. Despite numerous descriptions of antisocial patterns and the generalizations offered in this text, psychopaths should not be seen as a homogeneously extreme and irrationally violent conglomerate of individuals who share proclivities to behave similarly and predictably over time and across situations. As an example, there are psychopaths who are significantly less intelligent and more impulsive than others, and some psychopaths are bright and adaptive in almost any setting. The possible existence of behavioral or cognitive differences between the sexes in expression of antisocial psychopathology is also open for exploration. We have also found that there are individuals who share characteristics with those called antisocial and yet maintain behaviors largely within the bounds of societal propriety. Hence, there should be emphasis in assessment, treatment, and research efforts on determining the strengths of individuals labeled antisocial or deviance-prone.

If we may offer some generalizations, psychopaths as a group appear to be robust, socially facile, ingenious, and capable of forethought. As we have noted previously (Brantley & Sutker, 1984), among their ranks are daring, adventuresome, resourceful persons who may have been disposed by situations, person traits or constitutional factors, or behavioral sequences toward repeated ill-advised activities. Certainly, it is time for us to turn our assessment and research efforts toward understanding some of the strengths these individuals may have to offer. By this means, we may encourage their prosocial behavior expression as well as minimize their social deviance—the ultimate goals for behavioral intervention among psychopaths or sociopaths. Additionally, we may come to understand some of the mechanisms by which psychopaths manage fears, delay worry about behavior consequences, cope with impending stressors, and achieve successful interpersonal manipulations. Such knowledge could have application to their treatment as well as to that of individuals in other diagnostic categories whose psychopathology appears to represent in many ways the converse of that exhibited in psychopathy.

As for closure on Mr. V., he showed strengths during assessment as described and might be imagined to achieve improvements in target behaviors, including substance abuse and interpersonal conflicts. If he should secure an ideal therapeutic relationship for him, one in which he finds himself genuinely motivated to maintain treatment contacts over time and inclined to continue to work toward personal changes, there is a favorable probability for success. Identification of appropriate career goals and interesting social involvements are essential to treatment progress, and in straightforward terms Mr. V. must learn to differentiate those impulses he may be allowed to indulge from urges inevitably associated with self-defeat. Given structure, support, and consistency in the treatment approach and Mr. V.'s continued interest in treatment efforts, the prognosis is good. Nevertheless, the therapist must be prepared to deal constructively with relapse behaviors and to maintain an interpersonal stance with Mr. V. which does not mimic that of significant others in his life. Continual evaluation of treatment progress, monitoring of Mr. V.'s behaviors, moods, and mentation over time, and reevaluation of patient goals as he makes progress are essential.

We are now at a point in time which allows an objective look at the epidemiological, longitudinal course of antisocial psychopathology from childhood to the adult years. Follow-up of antisocial children has not been markedly useful in predicting adult recovery or amelioration of adult antisocial expression (Robins, 1981). Nevertheless, it has been shown that childhood antisocial expression is more predictive of serious adult deviance than any other factor identified to date. Severe economic hardships and other situational factors of negative impact, models of antisocial behavior or criminality in one or both parental figures, lack of parental supervision, and outright physical and/or sexual abuse do increase the risk of adult carry-over of antisocial behaviors

(Sutker, 1982). Further, antisocial behaviors perpetuate themselves. Obviously, to break the chain of ongoing social deviance is the goal we have in mind—a feat which is assumed to be more difficult among adult patients than in children or adolescents.

Regardless of one's point of view on the controversial topics related to antisocial behaviors, it must be conceded that the concept of psychopathy incorporates multidimensional phenomena which taken together are of great cost to American society. Antisocial behaviors are seen to be remarkably stable and enduring over time and may coexist with neurotic symptomatology such as depression and anxiety. We have learned that antisocial psychopathology does not necessarily imply violent behavior and that there are often positive person features associated with a constellation of blatantly nonconforming behaviors. Because antisocial behaviors do not respond favorably to "insight-oriented" psychotherapy, a different tact has been proposed in the chapter. This approach emphasizes recognition of person strengths, facilitation of adult strategies for coping with stress, disappointment, tension, and frustration, enhancement of prosocial behaviors as potential substitutes for negative forms of self-gratification, and discouragement of self-defeating, nonconforming behaviors. Positive mechanisms to encourage behavior change, for example, therapist approval and social rewards, are discussed in contrast to management models based on strategies of censure, punishment, and banishment.

ACKNOWLEDGMENTS

Appreciation is expressed to Dr. Irving Kauffman for his critical evaluation of this manuscript and to Albert N. Allain, Jr., for his editorial assistance.

REFERENCES

Adams, H. E. (1981). *Abnormal behavior.* Dubuque, IA: Wm. C. Brown.
Albert, R. S, Brigante, T. R., & Chase, N. (1969). The psychopathic personality: A content analysis of the concept. *Journal of General Psychology, 60,* 17–28.
American Psychiatric Association (1968). *DSM-II: Diagnostic and statistical manual of mental disorders* (2nd ed.). Washington, DC: Author.
American Psychiatric Association. (1980). *DSM-III: Diagnostic and statistical manual of mental disorders* (3rd ed.). Washington, DC: Author.
Arieti, S. (1967). *The intrapsychic self.* New York: Basic Books.
Bandura, A. (1977). *Social learning theory.* Englewood Cliffs, NJ: Prentice-Hall.
Bandura, A. (1983). Temporal dynamics and decomposition of reciprocal determinism: A reply to Phillips and Orton. *Psychological Review, 90,* 166–170.

Beck, A. T. (1976). Cognitive therapy and the emotional disorders. New York: International Universities Press.

Brantley, P. J., & Sutker, P. B. (1984). Antisocial behavior disorders. In H. E. Adams & P. B. Sutker (Eds.), Comprehensive handbook of psychopathology. New York: Plenum Press.

Bryan, J. H., & Kapche, R. (1967). Psychopathy and verbal conditioning. Journal of Abnormal Psychology, 72, 71–73.

Cleckley, H. (1955). The mask of sanity (3rd ed.). St. Louis: Mosby.

Cleckley, H. (1976). The mask of sanity (5th ed.). St. Louis: Mosby.

Eysenck, H. J. (1964). Crime and personality. London: Methuen.

Fairweather, G. W. (1954). The effects of selected incentive conditions on the performance of psychopathic, neurotic and normal criminals in a serial rote learning situation. (Doctoral dissertation, University of Illinois, 1953). Dissertation Abstracts International, 14, 393–394 (University Microfilms No. 6940).

Fowles, D. C. (1984). Biological variables in psychopathology: A psychobiological perspective. In H. E. Adams & P. B. Sutker (Eds.), Comprehensive handbook of psychopathology. New York: Plenum Press.

Gendreau, P., & Suboski, M. D. (1971). Classical discrimination eyelid conditioning in primary psychopaths. Journal of Abnormal Psychology, 77, 241–246.

Gilbert, J. G., & Lombardi, D. N. (1967). Personality characteristics of young male narcotic addicts. Journal of Consulting Psychology, 31, 536–538.

Gorenstein, E. E. (1982). Frontal lobe functioning in psychopaths. Journal of Abnormal Psychology, 91, 368–379.

Gorenstein, E. E., & Newman J. P. (1982). Disinhibitory psychopathology: A new perspective and a model for research. Psychological Review, 87, 301–315.

Gough, H. G. (1948). A sociological theory of psychopathology. American Journal of Sociology, 53, 359–366.

Gough, H. G. (1960). Theory and measurement of socialization. Journal of Consulting Psychology, 24, 23–30.

Gray, K. G., & Hutchinson, H. C. (1964). The psychopathic personality: A survey of Canadian psychiatrists' opinions. Canadian Psychiatric Association Journal, 9, 452–461.

Gullick, E. L., Sutker, P. B., & Adams, H. E. (1976). Delay of information in paired-associate learning among incarcerated groups of sociopaths and heroin addicts. Psychological Reports, 38, 143–151.

Halleck, S. L. (1981). Sociopathy: Ethical aspects of diagnosis and treatment. In J. H. Masserman (Ed.), Current psychiatric therapies, (Vol. 20). New York: Grune & Stratton.

Hare, R. D. (1965). Acquisition and generalization of a conditioned-fear response in psychopathic and nonpsychopathic criminals. Journal of Psychology, 59, 367–370.

Hare, R. D., & Quinn, M. J. (1971). Psychopathy and autonomic conditioning. Journal of Abnormal Psychology, 77, 223–235.

Hare, R. D., & Schalling, D. (Eds.). (1978). Psychopathic behaviour: Approaches to research. New York: Wiley.

Heilbrun, A. B. (1979). Psychopathy and violent crime. Journal of Consulting and Clinical Psychology, 47, 509–516.

Heilbrun, A. B. (1982). Cognitive models of criminal violence based upon intelligence and psychopathy levels. Journal of Consulting and Clinical Psychology, 50, 546–557.

Johns, J. H., & Quay, H. C. (1962). The effect of social reward on verbal conditioning in psychopathic and neurotic military offenders. *Journal of Consulting Psychology,* *26,* 217–220.

Kadlub, J. J. (1956). The effects of two types of reinforcements on the performance of psychopathic and normal criminals. Unpublished doctoral dissertation, University of Illinois.

Lion, J. R. (1978). Outpatient treatment of psychopaths. In W. H. Reid (Ed.), *The psychopath: A comprehensive study of antisocial disorders and behaviors.* New York: Brunner/Mazel.

Lykken, D. T. (1957). A study of anxiety in the sociopathic personality. *Journal of Abnormal and Social Psychology, 55,* 6–10.

Lykken, D. T. (1978). The psychopath and the lie detector. *Psychophysiology, 15,* 137–142.

Maddocks, P. D. (1970). A five-year follow-up of untreated psychopaths. *British Journal of Psychiatry, 116,* 511–515.

Maher, B. A. (1965). *Principles of psychopathology.* New York: McGraw-Hill.

Marlatt, A. (1982). Relapse prevention: A self-control program for the treatment of addictive behaviors. In R. B. Stuart (Ed.), *Adherence, compliance and generalization in behavioral medicine.* New York: Brunner/Mazel.

McCullough, J. P., & Adams, H. E. (1970). Anxiety, learning sets, and sociopathy. *Psychological Reports, 27,* 47–52.

Meyer, V., & Turkat, J. D. (1979). Behavioral analysis of clinical cases. *Journal of Behavioral Assessment, 1,* 259–270.

Overall, J. E. (1973). MMPI personality patterns of alcoholics and narcotic addicts. *Quarterly Journal of Studies on Alcohol, 34,* 104–111.

Persons, R. W., & Bruning, J. L. (1966). Instrumental learning with sociopaths: A test of clinical theory. *Journal of Abnormal Psychology, 71,* 165–168.

Quay, H. C., & Hunt, W. A. (1965). Psychopathy, neuroticism, and verbal conditioning: A replication and extension. *Journal of Consulting Psychology, 29,* 283.

Ray, J. J., & Ray, J. A. B. (1982). Some apparent advantages of subclinical psychopathy. *Journal of Social Psychology, 117,* 135–142.

Rime, B., Bouvy, H., Leborgne, B., & Rouillon, F. (1978). Psychopathy and nonverbal behavior in an interpersonal situation. *Journal of Abnormal Psychology, 87,* 636–643.

Robins, E., Gentry, K. A., Munoz, R. A., & Marten, S. (1977). A contrast of the three more common illnesses with the ten less common in a study and 18-month follow-up of 314 psychiatric emergency room patients. II. Characteristics of patients with the three more common illnesses. *Archives of General Psychiatry, 34,* 269–281.

Robins, L. N. (1978). Sturdy childhood predictors of adult antisocial behaviour: Replications from longitudinal studies. *Psychological Medicine, 8,* 611–622.

Robins, L. N. (1981). Epidemiological approaches to natural history research: Antisocial disorders in children. *Journal of the American Academy of Child Psychiatry, 20,* 566–580.

Schmauk, F. J. (1970). Punishment, arousal and avoidance learning in sociopaths. *Journal of Abnormal Psychology, 76,* 325–335.

Siegel, R. A. (1978). Probability of punishment and suppression of behavior in psychopathic and nonpsychopathic offenders. *Journal of Abnormal Psychology, 87,* 514–522.

Smith, R. J. (1978). The psychopath in society. In D. T. Lykken (Ed.), *Personality and psychopathology* (Vol. 19). New York: Academic Press.

Spitzer, R. L., Endicott, J., & Robins, E. (1975). *Research diagnostic criteria.* New York: Biometrics Research, New York State Department of Mental Health.

Stewart, D. J. (1972). Effects of social reinforcement on dependency and aggressive responses of psychopathic, neurotic, and subculture delinquents. Journal of Abnormal Psychology, 29, 76–83.

Suedfeld, P., & Landon, P. B. (1978). Approaches to treatment. In R. D. Hare & D. Schalling (Eds.), Psychopathic behaviour: Approaches to research. New York: Wiley.

Sutker, P. B. (1970). Vicarious conditioning and sociopathy. Journal of Abnormal Psychology, 76, 380–386.

Sutker, P. B. (1971). Personality differences and sociopathy in heroin addicts and non-addict prisoners. Journal of Abnormal Psychology, 78, 247–251.

Sutker, P. B. (1974). Field observations of a heroin addict: A case study. American Journal of Community Psychology, 2, 35–42.

Sutker, P. B. (1982). Adolescent drug and alcohol behaviors. In T. Field, A. Huston, H. Quay, L. Troll, & G. Finley (Eds.), Review of human development. New York: Wiley.

Sutker, P. B., & Allain, A. N. (1983). Behavior and personality assessment in men labelled adaptive sociopaths. Journal of Behavioral Assessment, 5, 65–79.

Sutker, P. B., Allain, A. N., & Cohen, G. H. (1974). MMPI indices of personality change following short- and long-term hospitalization in heroin addicts. Psychological Reports, 34, 495–500.

Sutker, P. B., & Archer, R. P. (1983). Drug abuse and dependence disorders: Psychopathology and deviance. In H. E. Adams & P. B. Sutker (Eds.), Comprehensive handbook of psychopathology. New York: Plenum Press.

Sutker, P. B., Archer, R. P., Brantley, P. J., & Kilpatrick, D. G. (1979). Alcoholics and opiate addicts: Comparison of personality characteristics. Journal of Studies on Alcohol, 40, 635–644.

Sutker, P. B., Archer, R. P., & Kilpatrick, D. G. (1981). Sociopathy and antisocial behavior: Theory and treatment. In S. M. Turner, K. S. Calhoun, & H. E. Adams (Eds.), Handbook of clinical behavior therapy. New York: Wiley.

Sutker, P. B., Gil, S. H., & Sutker, L. W. (1971). Sociopathy and serial learning of CVC combinations with high and low social-content ratings. Journal of Personality and Social Psychology, 17, 158–162.

Sutker, P. B., Moan, C. E., & Allain, A. N. (1974). WAIS performance in unincarcerated groups of MMPI-defined sociopaths and normal controls. Journal of Consulting and Clinical Psychology, 42, 307–308.

Sutker, P. B., Moan, C. G., & Allain, A. N. (1983). Assessment of cognitive control in psychopathic and normal prisoners. Journal of Behavioral Assessment, 5, 275–287.

Sutker, P. B., Moan, C. E., & Swanson, W. C. (1972). Porteus Maze Test and qualitative performance in pure sociopaths, prison normals, and antisocial psychotics. Journal of Clinical Psychology, 28, 349–353.

Thorne, F. C. (1959). The etiology of sociopathic reactions. American Journal of Psychotherapy, 13, 319–330.

Ullmann, L. P., & Krasner, L. (1975). A psychological approach to abnormal behavior (2nd ed.). Englewood Cliffs, NJ: Prentice-Hall.

Vaillant, G. E. (1975). Sociopathy as a human process: A viewpoint. Archives of General Psychiatry, 32, 178–183.

Weissman, M. M, Pottenger, M., Kleber, H., Ruben, H. L., Williams, D., & Thompson, W. D. (1977). Symptom patterns in primary and secondary depression. Archives of General Psychiatry, 34, 854–862.

Widom, C. S. (1976). Interpersonal and personal construct systems in psychopaths. *Journal of Consulting and Clinical Psychology, 44,* 614–623.

Widom, C. S. (1977). A methodology for studying noninstitutionalized psychopaths. *Journal of Consulting and Clinical Psychology, 45,* 674–683.

Zuckerman, M. (1979). *Sensation seeking: Beyond the optimal level of arousal.* Hillsdale, NJ: Lawrence Erlbaum.

Zuckerman, M., Sola, S., Masterson, J., & Angelone, J. V. (1975). MMPI patterns in drug abusers before and after treatment in therapeutic communities. *Journal of Consulting and Clinical Psychology, 43,* 286–296.

5

PARANOID PERSONALITY DISORDER

5

The Case of Mr. P.

Mr. P. was a 26-year-old Caucasian. He resided in a small college town in the southeast United States and worked as a clerk in city government. Prior to this job, he had spent a brief period of time as a policeman.

The Referral

The patient was self-referred. He had sought the help of a professional because he wanted to learn assertive skills. He reported having read a considerable number of self-help books on assertiveness but worried that he was not following these correctly. Accordingly, he was hoping to receive systematic training in assertiveness.

Physical Appearance

The patient was average in height but a bit chubby for his size. His dress was neat but very conservative. His hair was short and brown. He wore thick-lensed and black rimmed eyeglasses.

Presenting Complaints

The patient believed that he was being treated unfairly and picked on by numerous individuals. Because of this, he sought assertiveness training, so that he "could stand up for his rights." He reported feelings of being treated unfairly in interactions at his job, at church functions, and in normal everyday encounters with strangers.

Mr. P. indicated that he was socially isolated. He reported having no friends and spending the majority of his time either at work, at church functions, or by himself. He argued that the reason he did not have any friends was his very busy schedule at work and at church. Nevertheless, he wished that he did have some friends.

The patient reported a fear that he was going to be murdered. Although he could not specify the particular person who was after him, he gave numerous illustrations of this fear. For instance, coming home from work, he was fearful of leaving his house because he was afraid he might be attacked, perhaps by a Doberman Pinscher. Further, he would not go into bars because he was afraid that someone might kill him. At other times he felt that some type of personal injury might come to him, although he did not necessarily have an idea what that might be. Finally, he indicated that at certain times he felt as if Satan was trying to kill him.

The patient indicated that he had had no sexual experiences with other individuals. He was a virgin and had never kissed a woman. He reported having considerable difficulty in interacting with women and had numerous explanations as to why he would not want to become involved with one. As an example, he reported that at times when he felt sexual attraction to a woman, hours later he would feel pain through his penis. Further, he argued that he did not want to become involved with a girl because that might lead to her family's breaking up because of him.

The patient experienced considerable depression from time to time and occasionally experienced suicidal thoughts. These mostly related to the theme of being lonely and to the idea that Satan was trying to kill him.

History

Mr. P. reported being the youngest of four children all of whom, he said, "were intelligent, but never lived up to their potential." He mentioned the fact that his "brother was a scientology freak who lived in California, who had recently had a nervous breakdown and that one of his sisters had married a rapist who was now in jail."

As a child, the patient indicated that he had frequent anxiety attacks and terrible nightmares about bad things happening to him. He recalled vividly being scolded for telling family-related information to a friend at an early age. This included such information as "dad's pimples on his buttocks" and that "granddad drank beer."

As a child, Mr. P. always felt that people were watching him and were interested in him. He described himself as a loner when a child, fearful of becoming an adult. He reported that his teachers talked about him and that they were out to get him. He never seemed to develop any close relationships with anyone outside his family. Mr. P. was a devout Catholic and spent much of his time involved in church functions. He reported that as a child he felt that some serious injury would come to him because he was a Catholic. He also reported that his parents frequently criticized him for being so fearful and he developed a fear that his parents would blame him for tragedies that he could not help.

Parents

The patient described his father as "deaf, paranoid, neurotic, sometimes terrible" and feared being like him. Mr. P. described his mother: "She tried to possess me, baby me, she exploited me all my life and didn't respect my manhood." He said that his parents were extremely concerned about what other people thought of them. Accordingly, it was a close-knit family that avoided social interaction. He recalled numerous instances of his parents' concern about putting on a good front to others. Further, he described his background as an overcritical environment which "turned me into a perfectionist." He reported numerous instances of intense criticism from his parents which made him feel unworthy, unintelligent, and always fearful of doing the wrong thing.

Interview Behavior

At the beginning of the interview, it was explained to the patient that the session would be videotaped since this was a teaching clinic. The patient seemed extremely uncomfortable about the idea of being videotaped and asked numerous questions about the purpose of it and who would be seeing it. After considerable discussion about the utility and purposes of videotaping the session, the patient agreed to sign the appropriate consent form.

Throughout the interview, Mr. P. appeared interested in pleasing the therapist but often spoke in detail about things unrelated to the question posed to him. He also seemed to spend considerable time thinking about his replies before giving them. Nevertheless, Mr. P. appeared highly motivated to participate in a treatment.

5

Formulation of Paranoid Personality Disorder

IRA DANIEL TURKAT

> At Basel I founded the Jewish State. If I were to say this
> today, I would be met by universal laughter. In five years
> perhaps, and certainly in fifty, everyone will say it.
> Theodor Herzl (1897)

The above extract from Herzl's diary (Silverberg, 1972) seems well suited to serve as an introduction to a chapter on paranoid behavior. Individuals who hold beliefs of grandeur ("I founded the Jewish State") in the face of contradictory data (the State of Israel did not exist in 1897) and who anticipate immediate ridicule for these beliefs ("I would be met by universal laughter") but future admiration ("everyone will say it") are viewed as paranoid. The fact that in 1948 Herzl's prediction became reality would not have reduced the temptation by some in 1897 to label Herzl as a paranoid.[1]

Does the above example suggest that paranoid beliefs are always correct? Hardly so. However, as well shall see later on, the case of Herzl highlights some important aspects of paranoid phenomena.

The present chapter has several objectives. First, the history of the construct *paranoia* will be traced. Second, the currently accepted

[1]To diagnose anyone on such limited information would certainly be inappropriate. The present author is an admirer of Herzl and in no way means to imply that this great figure was paranoid.

IRA DANIEL TURKAT • Department of Psychology, University of North Carolina at Greensboro, Greensboro, North Carolina 27412.

161

classification of paranoid phenomena will be examined and prevalence estimates for its categories will be provided. Third, theories of paranoid pathology will be discussed. Fourth, a new approach to paranoid personality disorder will be outlined. Finally, tactics in formulating clinical cases of paranoid personality disorder will be illustrated.

HISTORICAL PERSPECTIVE

Paranoia has enjoyed a long and lively history. Millon (1981) pointed out that observations of paranoid phenomena were noted over 2,000 years ago. Excellent reviews of the history of the term are available (Kendler & Tsuang, 1981; Lorr, Klett, & McNair, 1963; Manschrek, 1979; Millon, 1981; Millon & Millon, 1974; Swanson, Bonhert, & Smith, 1970), and these serve as the primary sources for the chronological account below.

Hippocrates (460–377 B.C.) is credited with introducing the term *paranoia* (Swanson, *et al.*, 1970). It derives from the Greek *paranoia* "besides oneself" (Millon & Millon, 1974). Interestingly, the term was used in a general sense to indicate the presence of disorganized, delirious thinking or insanity. Although the term paranoia was not widely used in early writings, constructs related to it were noted. Plato, over 2,500 years ago referred to "religious madness." Asclepiades (A.D. 90) outlined distinctions between delusions, hallucinations, and illusions. Aretaeus (A.D. 100) discussed "divine mania" and Caelius Aurelianus (A.D. 400) described traits such as animosity and suspiciousness.

Most writers on the subject note that the term *paranoia* was not used again until sometime in the eighteenth century, although during the Renaissance Schenck and Zacchias discussed pathological "fanaticism," "prophesying," and "religious exaltation." In the 1700s Arnold, Kant, and others referred to delusions of grandeur and persecution. Finally, in 1772, Vogel explicitly used the term *paranoia* in a manner somewhat consistent with current practice (see Swanson *et al.*, 1970), although Heinroth is often credited with the term's revival (e.g., Millon & Millon, 1974). By the mid-1800s, the construct was generally accepted and attempts to distinguish subcategories began, particularly among prominent psychiatrists (Lorr *et al.*, 1963).

In the late 1800s, the psychiatrist Emil Kraepelin introduced the first comprehensive nosology of psychiatric disorders (Adams, 1981). As noted by Lorr *et al.* (1963), Kraepelin attempted to organize the newly emerging and proliferating contributions in the area. Not only did Kraepelin's work on nosology have a major impact on the diagnostic schemes of today; he also formalized attempts to subclassify paranoid phenomena (Kendler & Tsuang, 1981). In the course of eight editions of his textbook, the stage was set for controversy over proper classification of paranoid phenomena as well as the relationship between paranoia and other disorders.

The early 1900s witnessed considerable debate about the classification of paranoid phenomena. Eugen Bleuler objected to Kraepelin's classification of paranoid psychoses and argued that these were actually schizophrenic disorders, a position which was opposed by Kretschmer and a variety of other European psychiatrists. In America, the debate continued, as evidenced by the changing categorizations and criteria in the various nosologies proposed by the American Psychiatric Association over the past 50 years. Today, some of the aforementioned issues remain with us (cf. Kendler & Tsuang, 1981; Magaro, 1981; Meissner, 1981).

In short, although the concept of paranoia has been around for thousands of years and is widely accepted as valid today, how to classify it, subclassify it, understand it, and treat it remains highly controversial.

CLASSIFICATION

The most widely utilized classification system today is the third edition of the American Psychiatric Association's (1980) *Diagnostic and Statistical Manual of Mental Disorders* (DSM-III). According to the DSM-III, paranoid phenomena are classified into three major categories: (a) paranoid disorder, (b) paranoid schizophrenia, and (c) paranoid personality disorder.

Paranoid Disorder

The defining characteristic of paranoid disorder is the presence of persistent persecutory delusions or delusional jealousy not due to some other disorder such as schizophrenia. A delusion is a false belief that does not change in the face of obvious contradictory data. The individual suffering from paranoid disorder behaves in line with the delusion that he or she experiences. Thus, for example, a man who believes that his wife is unfaithful to him, despite convincing evidence to the contrary, will justify his belief by pointing to changes in his wife's work schedule, spots on the bedroom sheets, and so on.

DSM-III specifies three types of paranoid disorder: (1) paranoia, (2) shared paranoid disorder, and (3) acute paranoid disorder. Paranoia is defined as a chronic persecutory delusional system of at least six months' duration. Although the delusional system is unshakable, the individual's thinking style is clear and well organized. Shared paranoid disorder involves two or more people. Here, one person meets the criteria for paranoia and, as a result of a close relationship, a second person shares the delusion(s). Acute paranoid disorder is defined as paranoia of less than six months' duration.

Paranoid Schizophrenia

This nosologic category involves meeting the criteria for schizophrenia (i.e., presence of hallucinations, loose associations, incoherence, or bizarre delusions such as "my appendix was replaced with a radio transmitter") and the presence of persecutory or grandiose delusions or hallucinations. The major distinction between this disorder and paranoid disorder is the presence or absence of schizophrenic symptoms.

Paranoid Personality Disorder

The primary characteristics of paranoid personality disorder are generalized suspiciousness and mistrust, hypersensitivity to slights and threats, and restricted affect. These traits are stable, inflexible, and maladaptive and cause significant impairment and/or distress. By definition, the individual diagnosed as having paranoid personality disorder does not have a well-systemized delusion or schizophrenic symptoms.

Discussion

The relationship between paranoid disorder, paranoid schizophrenia, and paranoid personality disorder is unclear, according to DSM-III. The issue has been debated for decades and continues to be today (e.g., Kendler & Tsuang, 1982; Magaro, 1980; 1981; Meissner, 1981). Interestingly, there is little if any disagreement about the validity of the construct of paranoia; arguments develop mostly from differing views on how to subclassify paranoid phenomena. Whereas DSM-III lists paranoid personality disorder, paranoid disorder, and paranoid schizophrenia as distinct psychopathological entities, many view these disorders as representative of the same construct, differing only in their location on a continuum (e.g., Magaro, 1981; Swanson et al., 1970).

Others (Kendler, 1982; Meissner, 1981) are more concerned with viewing paranoid schizophrenia as a type of paranoid disorder and less concerned with paranoid personality disorder.

The nosologic debate on paranoid phenomena appears to be facilitated by at least two factors. First, the term *paranoid* has been used loosely in the literature (Munro, 1982), promoting confusion as to which disorder (e.g., paranoid disorder versus paranoid schizophrenia) is being investigated. This is similar to the problems noted in use of the term *compulsive* (Turkat & Levin, 1984): does it mean presence of obsessions, ruminations, motor rituals, cognitive rituals, or a personality style? Second, there is a paucity of research on the classification of DSM-III's three major disorders of paranoid phenomena. One cannot determine the relationship between paranoid personality disorder, paranoid schizophrenia, and paranoid disorder if these are not separated a priori in research. Thus, classification of paranoid pathology remains an empirical question which requires rigid adherence to current classification criteria, proper use of diagnostic labels, and evidence for reliable diagnosis before one can examine the similarity or dissimilarity of these disorders on variables such as etiology and treatment.

EPIDEMIOLOGY OF PARANOID PATHOLOGY

Torrey (1981) notes that epidemiological research in this area is notably poor in terms of data quality, methodology, and classification practice. Accordingly, estimates of prevalence and incidence which are detailed below should be viewed with caution.

Paranoid Disorder

Kendler (1982) reviewed hospital admissions and epidemiological data from various countries for paranoid disorder. His extensive review led him to conclude the following: (1) paranoid disorder represents 1–4% of all psychiatric admissions; (2) 2–7% of all psychotics admitted to psychiatric hospitals are classifed under paranoid disorder; (3) each year, 1–3 individuals per 100,000 are admitted for the first time to a psychiatric hospital for paranoid disorder; and (4) in the general population, paranoid disorder is present in 24–30 individuals per 100,000. These data led Kendler to conclude that paranoid disorder is neither rare nor common in comparison to other psychopathological conditions.

Paranoid Schizophrenia

The prevalence and incidence of schizophrenia is considered to be substantially higher than such rates for paranoid disorder. It is estimated that 6% of the general population are schizophrenics and that approximately one-half of all psychiatric in-patients are schizophrenics (Adams, 1981).

Torrey (1981) reviewed studies from various countries on the prevalence of paranoid schizophrenia among all schizophrenics. This review indicated a considerable range in prevalence estimates. For example, in Indonesia (Pfeiffer, 1962, 1963) paranoid schizophrenics represented 4% of all schizophrenics, whereas in China (Cerney, 1965) 46% of schizophrenics were classified as being of the paranoid type. Of the nine prevalence estimates reported by Torrey (1981), I have calculated the medium prevalence estimate of paranoid schizophrenics among all schizophrenics to be 24%.

Paranoid Personality Disorder

Hardly any prevalence data exist for paranoid personality disorder although some believe the disorder to be quite common (e.g., Manschreck, 1979). However, a recent report by Kass, Spitzer, and Williams

Table 1. Epidemiological Data on Paranoid Personality Disorder[a]

DSM-III field trials (phase two)		Vanderbilt Clinic (Columbia-Presbyterian)
Total number of patients	2,712	531
Total number of personality disorder cases	1,120	272
Total number of female personality disorder cases	599	168
Total number of male personality disorder cases	521	104
Number of female paranoid personality disorder cases	19	4
Number of male paranoid personality disorder cases	26	10
Total number of paranoid personality disorder cases	45	14
Percentage of paranoid personality disorder cases among personality disorders	4.0	5.2
Percentage of paranoid personality disorder cases among all psychiatric cases	1.7	2.6

[a]Derived from Kass et al. (1983).

(1983) on sex ratios in diagnoses based on DSM-III sheds some light on the issue. These authors provide data on the distribution of personality disorder diagnoses in two settings: (1) phase two of the DSM-III field trials for adult patients and (2) the Vanderbilt Psychiatric Clinic of Columbia Presbyterian Medical Center in New York. Data from the former indicate that paranoid personality disorder represents 4% of all personality disorders and 1.7% of all psychiatric cases. The Vanderbilt Clinic data revealed similar results: 5.2% of all personality disorder cases were paranoid personality disorders and 2.6% of all cases were paranoid personality disorders. Table 1 summarizes relevant statistics which I have gleaned from the Kass *et al.* (1983) study.

THEORETICAL APPROACHES

Several theories have been proposed to account for paranoid pathology. The majority of these theories attempt to explain paranoid pathology in general but for the most part are aimed at paranoid disorder (i.e., delusion present). A smaller set of theories are specifically restricted to paranoid personality disorder. For organizational purposes, this distinction is maintained.

Theories of Paranoid Pathology

Seven major theories of paranoid pathology can be gleaned from the literature: (1) homosexuality, (2) hostility, (3) homeostasis, (4) shame–humiliation, (5) operant, (6) exclusion, and (7) pseudocommunity. The most prominent explanation of paranoia was contributed by Freud (Chalus, 1977), with which the discussion below begins.

Homosexuality. According to Freud, paranoia originates with a homosexual desire. Because such a desire is anxiety-provoking, it is defended against by an unconscious reaction formation. Here, the original thought of homosexual desire is transformed into a hostile one, as follows (for a male):

"I love him"→Anxiety→Reaction Formation→"I hate him"

Unfortunately, the thought "I hate him" is also anxiety-generating and requires an additional transformation. Thus, anxiety is reduced by the unconscious use of projection:

"I hate him"→Anxiety→Projection→"He hates me"

This unconscious transformation serves to crystallize three simultaneous functions. First, the unacceptable homosexual wish is repressed. Second, a resolution of anxiety is achieved. Third, the view that "he hates me" now justifies "I hate him." Thus, paranoia is viewed as a delusional system ("he hates me") stemming from an unacceptable homosexual desire.

Does homosexuality theory account for paranoid pathology? Several points appear to vitiate the theory's viability (cf. Adams, 1981; Chalus, 1977; Colby, 1975). First, although homosexuality is a concern of many paranoids, it is not a concern for many others. Second, although homosexuality is *correlated* with paranoia to a certain degree, it has never been shown to be *causative*. Third, the correlation between paranoid and homosexual tendencies apparently exists for males but not for females. Finally, the Freudian view of paranoia seems capable of making two contradictory predictions simultaneously. For example, if homosexual tendencies are present, this supports the theory; however, if homosexual tendencies are not present, this can still support the theory because such tendencies are unconscious.

Hostility Theory. In his review of the evidence pertinent to Freud's homosexuality theory of paranoia, Chalus (1977) concluded that Freud was partially correct. Basically, Chalus agreed with Freud that unconscious hostility which is projected unto others can account for paranoid pathology but he argued that homosexual desire is not necessarily the precipitant of paranoid projection. According to Chalus, paranoia originates with cruel and sadistic parental behavior toward the child.

The hostility theory of paranoia postulates the following developmental sequence: A child who is treated sadistically by his or her parents will develop hostile impulses toward them. Since expression of such hostility toward one's parents is anxiety-provoking, the hostility is repressed. Under sufficient stress, the unconscious hostility becomes intolerable and must be discharged. Here, the hostility is projected unto others. Given the strong tension-reducing properties associated with such a defense mechanism, the projection process is intensified, leading to a paranoid psychosis. Thus, the hostility theory of paranoia seems similar to homosexuality theory in all respects except one: the origin of the paranoid projection process.

What are the advantages of the hostility theory of paranoia compared to the homosexuality viewpoint? First, hostility theory specifies particular parental behaviors as the origin of paranoia. This hypothesis is directly testable. Second, the theory postulates one less unconscious transformation than the homosexuality view. Finally, hostility theory can account for homosexuality as a precipitant of paranoia if it is viewed as a stressor, provided the patient has had cruel or sadistic parents.

Hostility theory does have its problems. For example, the "stress" needed to trigger a paranoid psychosis is ambiguously defined:

> Presumably, the paranoid psychosis will then be precipitated when, *for whatever reason* (italics added) . . . the adult paranoid's hostile impulses become overwhelmingly intolerable, thereby "triggering" an excessive discharge of the aversive hostility through its projection onto others. (Chalus, 1977, p. 185)

Further, the theory appears somewhat circular. For example, in paranoid personality disorder, hostility is a defining symptom (e.g., hypervigilance, hypersensitivity, readiness to counterattack at any perceived threat). This leads the theory to the discomforting position of using part of a disorder's definition to "explain" the disorder. Finally, although hostility theory postulates one less unconscious transformation than does homosexuality theory, it still relies on unconscious mechanisms which remain difficult to study scientifically.

Homeostasis Theory. In their excellent text on paranoia, Swanson *et al.* (1970) discuss the homeostasis view of paranoid behavior. Here, it is assumed that all individuals pursue equilibrium, both biologically and psychologically. Any factor which produces disequilibrium is reacted to by attempts to restore homeostasis.

The homeostatis view of paranoia postulates that any factor (e.g., joblessness) which produces psychological disequilibrium (e.g., feelings of inadequacy) activates attempts to restore the balance. Such restorative attempts involve the "paranoid mode" (e.g., "I lost my job because I'm too clever for this company"). As noted by others (Adams, 1981; Colby, 1977), the homeostasis view of paranoia is too general to be considered a useful proposition.

Shame–Humiliation Theory. In his widely quoted review article, Colby (1977) argues that (what he considers to be) the three major psychological theories of paranoid phenomena (i.e., homosexuality, hostility, and homeostatic) are inferior in explanatory power to his theory, termed "shame–humiliation." In fact, Colby views the homosexuality, hostility, and homeostatic positions as special cases which can be accounted for by the shame–humiliation theory. Colby's theory has led him to develop a computer model of paranoid thinking, resulting in considerable discussion in the literature (Abelson, 1981; Agassi, 1981; Colby, 1975; 1976; 1977; 1981; 1983; Colby, Fraught, & Parkison, 1979; Colby, Hilf, Weber, & Kramer, 1972; Gunderson, 1981; Izard & Masterson, 1981; Lindsay, 1981; Magaro & Shulman, 1981; Maher, 1981; Manschreck, 1983; Reid & Reidler, 1981; Swanson, 1981).

The shame–humiliation theory is primarily an information-processing view of paranoia. Here, paranoia is seen as a thinking mode or style which attempts to prevent feelings of shame or humiliation. More specifically, any stimulus which signals to the paranoid that he or she is inadequate, the unpleasant effect of shame or humiliation, is prevented by projecting blame unto others. To illustrate the paranoid mode (i.e., shame–humiliation avoidance thinking), Colby devised a computer simulation and attempted to show its relevance to paranoid patients (cf. Colby, 1981).

How useful is the shame–humiliation theory? On the one hand, it has allowed Colby to develop an ingenious use of computer technology for studying paranoid thinking. Further, it is postulated that such thinking is activated by any signals of inadequacy in the paranoid. On the other hand, Colby's theory has numerous problems. First, it does not address how paranoia develops. Rather, it focuses only on thinking strategy in an active paranoid. Second, the computer model has been questioned regarding its validity as an analogue of clinical paranoia. Finally, shame–humiliation theory seems quite similar to other theories, (e.g., hostility theory) in that it takes projection to be the sin qua non of paranoid thinking. In many respects, the differences among theories seem semantic in nature.

Operant Explanation. An operant view of paranoid behavior has been proposed by Ullman and Krasner (1975). The basic premise of this viewpoint is that paranoid behavior is a result of environmental contingencies. More specifically, the person who has become paranoid is one whose life experiences have shaped him or her to attend to information selectively. Given fragmentary information on which to base his actions, the paranoid behaves in line with the narrow stimuli perceived. This behavior is viewed by others as strange, and this view establishes interpersonal contingencies which perpetuate paranoid behavior. Thus, the operant view details paranoid behavior as appropriate to one's learning history and argues that the paranoid's learning experiences differ from those of people who do not become paranoid.

The operant account of paranoia has several attractive features. First, it views paranoid behavior as a learned phenomenon. This hypotheses is testable. Second, the operant view argues that normal and paranoid behavior are both acquired through the same process: learning. What differentiates the paranoid and the normal individual is the content of the developmental history. Finally, the operant explanation does not utilize unconscious mechanisms to account for paranoid behavior. Rather, the factors which promote paranoia are considered to be observable.

The major difficulty with the operant account is that it fails to specify the precise environmental circumstances which are postulated to generate paranoid behavior.

Exclusion Theory. Lemert (1962), a well-known sociologist, has offered an intriguing account of paranoia. Called the exclusion theory, it greatly influenced Ullman and Krasner (1975) in their development of the operant view of paranoia.

According to Lemert (1962), psychopathology can only be understood in terms of the individual and his or her interaction with other members of society. An individual who has consistent interpersonal difficulties is viewed as a threat to the normal rules of a group and according to Lemert this is the originating point of paranoid development.

When a normal individual behaves atypically, others usually tolerate such behavior. For example, when a person complains excessively about receiving a speeding ticket unjustly, most individuals still accept the individual (e.g., "Oh, Henry is just having a bad day"). However, the individual who persists in such behavior and chronically exhibits interpersonal difficulties will be viewed negatively by others. Eventually, those around the individual will view him or her as a stimulus for intense interaction. Accordingly, attempts will be made to avoid this person. If one cannot avoid the troublemaker, then one humors or patronizes him. Lemert labeled this process *informal exclusion.*

Once the informal exclusion process develops, the troublemaker begins to pick up subtle cues that people seem to be against him. If he persists in behaving out of line, the cues will no longer be subtle (e.g., he is thrown out of a club or demoted in his job) and the process of *formal exclusion* has begun. The individual is now isolated and views others as really against him. If he persists in threatening the rules of the group (e.g., complaining to authorities), the process of exclusion solidifies. Persistent threatening behavior (e.g., a law suit) unites the entire community (e.g., justice department, occupational setting) against the individual. Thus, the exclusion theory of paranoia postulates that people really are against the individual labeled as paranoid.

Lemert's view of paranoia contributes some intriguing hypotheses. In many respects, the paranoid is viewed as one who behaves in ways which generate a hostile reactions by others. Thus, the paranoid individual and his or her social network both contribute to the development of what we call paranoid behavior. Clearly, it raises an important question about paranoid beliefs: is it appropriate to label the paranoid as delusional if others really are against him?

The exclusion theory offers useful hypotheses about paranoid behavior and would be strengthened with greater specification of the behaviors and conditions in which exclusion promotes paranoia.

Pseudocommunity Theory. One of the most comprehensive accounts of paranoid pathology has been proposed by Cameron (1963). Almost all introductory abnormal psychology textbooks discuss Cameron's postulated *pseudocommunity*, but hardly any cover the detailed observations and inferences about paranoid pathology that he provides.

Cameron believes that individuals who develop paranoid disorder (i.e., delusions of persecution or jealousy) have much in common with normals. Specifically, all individuals develop inferences based on incomplete information and act upon these inferences. For example, when we drive to work we assume that we still have a job. When we arrive at work and the secretary says hello with a smile, we assume that she is in a good mood. In both instances we assume a lot but neither assumption is always correct. Cameron argues that most of our daily attitudes and activities are based upon hypothesized probabilities derived from small bits of information.

The way we feel at a particular time may alter the inferences we make about fragmented information. For example, if one is feeling anxious and insecure while driving to work, one may wonder if one's job is on the line. When the secretary smiles, one might feel that "something is up." However, on a day when we are feeling good, such inferences may never come to us. These two notions, that all of us behave in accord with inferences made from limited information and that our feelings affect our inferences, are central to Cameron's view of paranoid reactions. According to Cameron, a delusion is an inference that becomes fixed, is inflexible, and is unaffected by contradictory evidence. The goal of a delusion is to reduce anxiety and tension.

Cameron argues that all individuals experience delusional thinking in ordinary life but only certain individuals are likely to develop well-systematized delusions. These individuals, called paranoids, experience a unique developmental history.

Paranoid disorder is viewed by Cameron as the consequence of two primary events: (1) early training in distrust and (2) certain triggering situations. He believes that an underlying personality of suspiciousness and distrust is a prerequisite for the development of systematized delusions. According to Cameron, individuals who cannot trust others, who are unable to tolerate suspense, and are deficient in viewing events from various perspectives when under stress are likely to develop delusions when particular events occur. Thus, Cameron believes that paranoid disorder develops when a paranoid personality faces certain environmental circumstances. In fact, he hypothesizes seven precipitating factors specific to paranoid reactions.

These may be summarized as any events which: (1) increase feelings of envy, jealousy, hatred, resentment, and/or inferiority; (2) isolate the individual socially; (3) permit the paranoid personality to ruminate while isolated from others, even for short time periods; and (4) increase feelings of suspicion and distrust.

Once the paranoid personality experiences intolerable frustration from any of the above precipitating events, he or she seeks to resolve this psychological disequilibrium. All alone and feeling under attack, the paranoid becomes selectively hypersensitive. Hypotheses become intensely focused but especially narrow. Inferences are viewed as facts. Accordingly, Cameron speculates that unconscious conflicts propel intolerable frustration, pressures, and tension; to reduce this uncomfortable state, individuals reconstruct reality by regressing to early life. Here, the expectations of sadistic treatment that they experienced as children are projected unto others and they search for a target or focus for the hostility feelings. This is the beginning of the paranoid pseudocommunity. As Cameron (1963) notes:

> The paranoid pseudocommunity is a reconstruction of reality. It organizes the observed and the inferred behavior of real and imagined persons into a conspiracy, with the patient as its focus. This organization of a hostile pseudocommunity does not comfort or reassure a paranoid person, but it does satisfy his overwhelming need for closure. He "finds out what it is all about." He . . . now has some idea of what to expect . . . whom he must watch and why. The fright is no longer a nameless, formless terror. It is now organized and has a focus. (p. 487)

Once the pseudocommunity has developed, it serves many useful purposes which perpetuate the reconstruction of reality. According to Cameron, the pseudocommunity allows discharge of destructive psychic energy. Hostile impulses are focused unto others. Guilt is denied—the patient feels an innocent victim. Comfort is provided by the "logical" explanation. Interactions with others can now occur, for the person now knows "what to look for and how to deal with it."

Discussion. The seven theories described above must be viewed as potential viable accounts of paranoid pathology until they are tested sufficiently in research. However, examination of the range of explanations each theory offers can serve to highlight certain advantages of one account over another.

To begin, homeostatic theory appears much too general to be considered a useful account of paranoia. It offers few if any specific predictions. The operant view also appears too general, although it does offer some testable predictions (e.g., paranoids are shaped by their experiences, they develop selective attention, their actions are appropriate to their inferences). I consider Cameron's theory to be the most comprehensive and in most respects to account for the predictions of the other theories. This conclusion can be best understood by examining the proposed etiological accounts in terms of predisposing, precipitating, and maintaining factors.

Three of the seven theories propose factors which render an individual vulnerable to develop paranoid delusions, given appropriate precipitants. Hostility theory specifies sadistic parents, exclusion theory postulates interpersonal difficulties, and pseudocommunity theory views paranoid personality as a predisposition. The latter hypothesis is discussed in greater detail later on, but for present purposes it should be recognized that Cameron's view of the paranoid personality is an individual who is distrustful and has difficulty relating to others (e.g., inability to take others' perspectives). Thus, Cameron's postulation subsumes the predisposing factors specified by both Chalus and Lemert. Further, not only does Cameron specifically hypothesize the types of interpersonal problems involved (which Lemert does not), he specifically referred to sadistic or brutal parental behavior in paranoid development long before Chalus.

In regard to those hypothesized variables which can trigger a paranoid delusion in a predisposed individual, Cameron is the only theorist to propose specific precipitating factors. These can be summarized as events which produce intense negative emotion and/or social isolation. The hypothesized precipitants of the other theories are covered by Cameron's speculation, be they anxiety related to homosexual desire (Freud), stress (Chalus), psychic disequilibrium (Swanson *et al.*), inadequacy feelings (Colby), or exclusion (Lemert).

Finally, Cameron speculates that the paranoid delusion has many useful functions which serve to maintain it. The pseudocommunity allows the discharge of psychic energy and anxiety and gives the individual the *feeling* that he or she now knows how to interact with the hostile community (even if such behavior does elicit negative reactions). Thus, paranoid delusions are maintained because they are useful, whether to discharge psychic energy or anxiety (homosexuality and hostility theory), restore equilibrium (homeostatic theory), avoid negative affect about self (shame–humiliation theory), or obtain certain consequences (operant and exclusion theories).

In short, Cameron views the delusional paranoid as one who was first a paranoid personality (i.e., distrustful, socially difficult) and later experienced certain precipitants (e.g., social isolation, intense negative affect). Clearly, his formulation appears to be the most comprehensive among its competitors. However, it raises the question as to what causes paranoid personality disorder.

Theories of Paranoid Personality Disorder

Two theorists have provided formulations specific to paranoid personality disorder. These theorists are Millon and Cameron.

Millon. The personality disorder section of the DSM-III was greatly influenced by Theodore Millon (1981, 1983), who has published extensively on personality and clinical psychology issues (Millon, 1969; Millon & Millon, 1974). In particular, his *biosocial-learning theory* led him to construct and coordinate a set of personality syndromes which are reflected in the DSM-III personality disorder sections. For Millon, personality development is determined by the interplay of numerous factors such as heredity, neuropsychological states, maturation, and learning variables.

Millon believes that paranoid personality covaries with other personality types and that a "pure" case is hard to come by. Not only is there "no universal attribute" of the paranoid personality, but, he believes, there is "no unique" developmental sequence. In his 1981 text, Millon outlines five major subtypes of paranoid personality disorder and speculates on potential etiological factors for each.

1. *Paranoid-narcissistic personality.* Such individuals are characterized by Millon as haughty, pretentious, ungenerous, naively self-confident, exploitative, expansive, presumptuous, and arrogant. Millon believes that such individuals were unrestrained, overvalued and over-indulged by their parents and that this treatment aided the development of deficits in interpersonal responsibility, cooperativeness, and empathy as well as a self-perception of excessive importance. Accordingly, once such individuals leave the shelter of their home setting they are faced with objective reality. Rather than face their shortcomings, they retreat into fantasies of omnipotence.

2. *Paranoid-antisocial (aggressive) personality.* Millon describes the paranoid-antisocial person as one who is belligerent, intimidating, power-oriented, ruthless, cunning, and brutal. The development of such a syndrome is seen as being affected by biogenic factors. As Millon notes:

> Many of these patients appear to come from families with a disproportion-
> ately high number of members who display vigorous energy and an irascible
> temperment. As children, these patients are likely to have been active and
> intrusive; they exhibited frequent temper outbursts and were considered to

be difficult to manage and found to precipitate difficulties. Aspects of their
thick-skinned and aggressive temperament may be traced to constitutionally
low thresholds of reactivity in the limbic and reticular systems. (Millon,
1981, p. 393)

Millon speculates that such individuals as children received harrass-
ment and antagonism from their parents. Thus, they learned to view
the world as harsh, a view which led to rebellious, manipulative, and
hostile behavior. They are therefore rejected by others, become isolated,
and eventually delusional (persecution).

3. *Paranoid-compulsive personality.* Millon characterizes the
paranoid-compulsive person as rigidly conforming, nonspontaneous,
perfectionistic, humorless, tense, inflexible, small-minded, and self-
righteous. Such people desperately seek independence by aiming to be
perfect and faultless. Millon believes that the parents of these individuals were overcontrolling (i.e., generating numerous rules to be enforced
with contingent punishment). Accordingly, as children, paranoid-
compulsive persons seek to avoid making errors so as to prevent parental punishment. By following parental rules stringently, such individuals become quite like their parents: overcontrolling, rule-following,
perfectionistic. Such training promotes a lack of spontaneity, fear of
the unknown, and intolerance of suspense. As adults they withdraw.
Since they are all alone and aware of their isolation, self-criticism runs
high. This hostility toward the self is then projected unto others.

4. *Paranoid-passive aggressive personality.* Millon (1981) describes
the paranoid-passive aggressive person as discontent, stubborn, pessimistic, aggressively fault-finding, obstructive, and resentful. Vacillation is frequent. Such behavior prevents the development of good
social relationships, which perpetuates negativistic behavior. Millon
believes that the paranoid-passive aggressive personality emerges from
"irregular infantile patterns and an uneven course of maturation"
(p. 394), affected by low neurophysiological thresholds or responsive-
ness. This in turn leads to inconsistent parental reactions, promoting
an irritable, negativistic child, unable to develop stable relations. Isolation promotes delusion jealousy.

5. *Decompensated paranoid personality.* The paranoid personality who becomes easily strained by life stress is highly vulnerable to
psychotic episodes and such is the case with Millon's description of
the decompensated paranoid personality. This personality is viewed
in some respects by Millon as the bridge between paranoid personality
and paranoid disorder or paranoid schizophrenia.

Cameron. Perhaps the most useful account of the paranoid
personality to date can be found in Cameron's writings (1963, 1974).

Interestingly, almost all abnormal psychology textbooks discuss Cameron's pseudocommunity, which is a description of the structure and function of a paranoid delusion. Hardly any texts discuss Cameron's view of the paranoid personality. This is particularly surprising given Cameron's view that a paranoid delusion can develop only in a paranoid personality; the merits of his analysis deserve full consideration.

According to Cameron, paranoid personality originates from a basic lack of trust. As infants, these people have not been protected from excessive tension and anxiety. Many have been treated sadistically or brutally by their parents and many have been denied consistent parental love. This early training in distrust leads the individual always to be on guard for possible attack. Because of this fearfulness and suspicion, the individual cannot tolerate suspense and is unable to perceive things from others' (e.g., nonbelligerent) points of view. Thus, Cameron believes that early sadistic parental treatment leads to three primary problems in the offspring:

1. An inability to trust others
2. An inability to tolerate suspense
3. An inability to shift role perspectives

All three of these problems lead the individual to act inappropriately under stress.

Cameron points out that the normal person under stress puts faith in others when frightened, can hold off from premature action until he has reasoned things through, and can momentarily detach himself from the stressful situation and view it from various perspectives. Because the paranoid individual lacks these abilities, he or she acts in a hypersensitive, narrow-minded, impulsive manner and is likely to jump to conclusions. Expecting sadistic treatment from others, the paranoid individual becomes especially tense under stress and withdraws.

According to Cameron, four additional problems seem to characterize the paranoid personality. First, the paranoid personality is *exquisitely sensitive to the unconscious attitudes of others*. As Cameron (1963) notes:

> All of us harbor minute traces of hostility even in some of our most favorable attitudes toward others. Most of us at times feel indifferent toward everyone, especially when preoccuppied. . . . A passing resentment toward a good friend, a temporary annoyance with someone whom we love . . . nearly all of us manage to get along, without suffering serious disturbance, in a social atmosphere that . . . has its negative moments in its overall friendliness. Not so the paranoid personality. He detects our contradictory traces clearly and consciously, even when we are unaware of them. . . . They disturb him because he experiences them as though they were conscious, dominant and

intentional . . . he greatly magnifies what he perceives. He may make a
molehill of momentary dislike into a mountain of external hatred. . . . Even
hostility that is aimed at someone else is apt to be picked up by the paranoid
person and misinterpreted as hostility aimed at him. (p. 478)

Although the paranoid personality is supersensitive to unconscious hostility in others, Cameron (1963) points out a second major
problem, *insensitivity to his or her own attitudes:*

Along with this exquisite sensitivity . . . goes an equally striking unawareness of the hostile, contemptuous, critical and accusing attitudes the paranoid person has himself. This unawareness is unfeigned. One trouble with
these unrecognized attitudes is that they stimulate avoidance and dislike
in others; and this seems to the paranoid person objective evidence that his
expectation of being discriminated against was justified. (p. 479)

In addition to their extreme sensitivity to others' hostility and
hyposensitivity to their own hostile attitudes, Cameron points out that
paranoid personalities *lack self-esteem* and *secretly feel inferior sexually.* Both problems are viewed as consequences of a basic lack of
trust.

Discussion. Both Millon and Cameron provide intriguing and useful accounts of paranoid personality. Neither has been the subject of
systematic research. This of course should not detract from their potential usefulness since there is no research on paranoid personality disorder at all. Accordingly, the theories proposed by Cameron and Millon
provide a good background from which to approach paranoid personality scientifically. In the next section, I outline an approach to paranoid
personality disorder which has similarities to and differences with the
previously reviewed theories.

PARANOID PERSONALITY DISORDER: A NEW APPROACH

Given the considerable speculation about paranoid personality
disorder (PPD) and the absence of research data on it, how should we
proceed in attempting to understand this disorder scientifically? It would
seem most efficient to begin at the single-case level (Adams & Calhoun,
1974; Shapiro, 1957, 1961, 1970, 1975). Once systematic study of the
single case has yielded important findings, efforts toward further understanding should proceed using experimental designs (e.g., controlled
group) appropriate to the more sophisticated questions being asked.
Such an approach seems applicable to PPD in particular (Turkat, Maisto,
Burish, & Rock, in press), the personality disorders as a class (Turkat

& Alpher, 1982), and poorly understood psychopathologies in general (Carey, Flasher, Maisto, & Turkat, 1984).

PPD: An Initial Course of Inquiry

Turkat and Maisto, 1985, recently reported on their attempt to study systematically a clinical series of personality disorder cases (N = 35), with particular emphasis on their formulation. Their study of eight PPD cases, including a laboratory experiment with one particular case, led them to develop a general formulation of PPD. This formulation has guided the present author to a program of research on PPD.

Pathogenesis of PPD. In our work with numerous cases of PPD (including the eight cases reported by Turkat & Maisto, 1985, and numerous others before and thereafter) we have noticed a common etiological sequence, which we have come to call the *evaluative-uniqueness theory.* Although descriptive in nature, it remains a theory (see Shapiro, 1979, for discussion of the observation-inference distinction in clinical work) of PPD pathogenesis.

In our view, PPD appears to unfold in five stages as follows:

1. *Parental training.* The individual destined to develop PPD seems to come from parents who emphasize two major themes to their child: "You must be careful about making mistakes" and "You are different from others." These messages teach the child to view himself or herself as being special and to be on guard for others' evaluations. Hence, the interaction of these parental training themes have led to the term *evaluative–uniqueness.*

All PPD cases we have seen clinically report retrospectively that at least one of the parents was a perfectionist who demanded an error-less way of life. Constant concern was expressed in the home that mistakes should be avoided, be they social (e.g., presentation to others outside of the home) or nonsocial (e.g., house chores). Accordingly, the child developed early to be anxious about making errors, especially social ones.

In addition to perfectionist training, PPD cases report that early on they were labeled by others (i.e., parents) as being different or unique. Messages along this theme have included "You are much brighter than your peers," "You are more attractive than others," "You are closer to God than your (nonreligious) friends," and so on. *Critical here is the presence of a distinguishing attribute that is identified and exaggerated in its importance by others.*

Given these early messages, the child is taught that he or she is unique and that others' evaluations are very important. Thus, PPD cases often report being warned by their parents to watch out for others' teasing, attacks, and jealousy. Coupled with this training is family closeness, secretiveness, and a clear concern about the distinction between family and nonfamily.

2. *Acting different.* Given evaluative–uniqueness training, it is natural to see relevant behavior outside the home at an early age. It is not uncommon for such a child to be said to be "genius quality" by a teacher, a "bookworm" by classmates, or a "bore" by neighborhood children. The child trained in this mode appears socially anxious and hence guarded and awkward. Critical here is the fact that the child appears different to others *outside the home*, which strengthens early parental training.

As the child progresses through school, social anxieties and "different" social behavior increase. Often, derogatory nicknames are applied (e.g., "computerhead," "Harvey Q. Asshole"), reflecting peer rejection. Such experiences not only reinforce early parental training but further set the individual apart from others. Naturally, guardedness and suspiciousness increase, inviting further criticism for such social behavior; this of course prevents the individual from learning more appropriate social skills.

During teenage school years, such experiences can intensify greatly. Developmentally, most people go through increased social awareness and concern during this period and much cruelty can occur. Often, a group of "cool" or "in" classmates will unite to ostracize the individual in a public manner. Jokes are played. Humiliating pranks are employed. Accusations fly. Bearing the brunt of these attacks, the individual withdraws.

3. *Social isolation.* At this point, the individual is alone. Ostracism is deeply felt. Others cannot be trusted. All of the person's social fears are confirmed. Insecurity permeates and intensifies.

How can the person trained in this pattern of evaluation and uniqueness resolve the anxiety from social isolation? Attempts to be accepted by the group are not an option; the person does not have the skills to carry it off successfully and is too fearful of further rebuke. Thus, the person remains alone, insecure, and anxious. At this point, the individual is highly motivated to reduce the intense anxiety about being isolated but cannot do it through social means. Only one recourse is available: rumination about the predicament.

4. *Explanations.* Spending hours alone, day after day, ruminating about being socially isolated, is a very uncomfortable dilemma to find oneself in. Naturally, the individual seeks to find a rational explanation for his or her social isolation (Maher & Ross, 1984). In attempting to

understand the question, "why am I isolated from others?" the most appropriate answer is one of *persecution:* "Others are against me, something is wrong with me." Clearly, the individual has sufficient data to make such a conclusion. Further, such an explanation is consistent with evaluative–uniqueness training (i.e., "Others have evaluated me negatively and I am different from others"). Unfortunately, although such a conclusion does indeed seem to explain the data (i.e., isolation, peer ostracism), it is quite anxiety-generating. At this point, the only option available to reduce the intolerable affect catalyzed by persecutory thinking is to create a more comfort-generating explanation for "why people are against me." This new explanation must: (1) explain why people are against him, (2) logically fit the data, and (3) be anxiety-reducing. Accordingly, the individual utilizes prior evaluative–uniqueness training and develops an explanation of *grandeur:* "The reason people are against me is that they are jealous of my special skills." Now when others torment or tease or ignore the individual, the anxiety associated with it ("see, they are against me") can be alleviated ("because I'm superior"). The chain of such thinking is diagrammed below:

"Others are against me."
↓
ANXIETY ELEVATED
↓
"There is something wrong with me."
↓
ANXIETY ELEVATED
↓
"There is something wrong with me;
it's that I'm better than others."
↓
ANXIETY REDUCED

Once the explanatory system of the paranoid personality has developed, the social interaction style becomes more understandable. When others reject the person, it makes good sense (e.g., "See, they are against me because I'm special"), even though rejection still causes anxiety. However, if others try to become close to (or accept) the individual, this is especially threatening. First, suspiciousness exacerbates (e.g., "They've screwed me before, they're setting me up again"). Second, *if another person attempts to accept the paranoid personality, then the explanatory system is threatened* (e.g., "maybe I'm not so different after all"). Thus, any signs of evaluation (positive or negative) by others engender anxiety in the paranoid personality.

5. *Cycle perpetuation.* Given the hypothesized etiological sequence described above, the DSM-III specified traits for paranoid personality disorder become quite understandable. If one is *hypersensitive* to others' possible threats, then one must be suspicious around others and guarded in one's interactions (*restricted affect*). Further, such behavior only serves to repel others thereby perpetuating a vicious cycle. This not only helps to prevent the individual's learning more appropriate social skills but also solidifes his existing social skills problems.

In understanding the social behavior of the paranoid personality disorder case, we have found Adams' model of social skills (cf. Turkat & Maisto, in press) to be quite helpful. Here, social skills are compartmentalized into four major categories: attention, information processing, response emission, and feedback.

In terms of *attention*, the paranoid personality often misses important social cues and/or selectively attends to inappropriate ones. Further, the person often *processes information* in an idiosyncratic way (e.g., "She didn't ask for my opinion because she thought I would make her look foolish, even though I wouldn't have"). In addition, the person often *emits responses* which turn other people off (e.g., awkward, guarded, humorless behavior). Finally, such individuals, do not seem to profit well from *feedback* (e.g., a criticism is seen as an attack, never as constructive). These behaviors serve only to perpetuate a vicious cycle which maintains social isolation.

In sum, the etiological theory advocated here is that paranoid personality disorder stems from early parental training in evaluative-uniqueness, acting different from others, becoming isolated socially, explaining isolation in terms of persecution and grandeur, and perpetuation of a vicious cycle.

Research. There is virtually no published research on paranoid personality disorder (Turkat *et al.*, in press). However, we have begun to test some of our hypotheses and a portion of our preliminary (unpublished) data is described below.[2]

First, to identify a cohort of paranoid personalities, several points had to be considered: (1) an accepted protocol to identify PPD cases was not available in the literature; (2) by definition, such cases are guarded and thus may avoid being studied scientifically; (3) use of DSM-III criteria would be essential. With these points in mind, we decided to begin with a college student population (since they were

[2] I am indebted to my students, particularly David Banks, for their help in the development and execution of this research program.

required by their course in general psychology to participate in research projects).

A search through the literature yielded three psychometrically sound instruments which seemed to match the major PPD traits specified by DSM-III: (1) SCL-90, paranoid ideation subscale (Derogatis, 1978) to measure suspiciousness; (2) Fear of Negative Evaluation scale (Watson & Friend, 1969) to measure hypersensitivity; and (3) Superego subscale of the Lazare–Klerman–Armor Inventory (1970) to measure restricted affect. These instruments were applied to several hundred students, and those individuals scoring 1.5 standard deviations or greater above the mean on the measures were labeled as paranoid personalities (as opposed to paranoid personality *disorder*). Three studies (including a replication) revealed the following:

1. Paranoid personality (PP) subjects reported experiencing significantly more paranoid thoughts (e.g., "I am a genius," I am God") compared to normals.
2. PP subjects reported experiencing significantly more paranoid thoughts during high school and junior high school compared to controls.
3. PP subjects had participated in fewer research projects than their non-PP counterparts and were more reluctant to participate in a study of social interaction which included being videotaped.
4. PP subjects and controls could be successfully discriminated by their reactions to personal history questions reflecting evaluative–uniqueness training (e.g., "Was your father especially concerned about social evaluation?").

Current investigations include testing aspects of Adams' model of social skills as applied to PP, the relationship between college student PP and clinically diagnosed PPD, and other related questions.

FORMULATION OF THE CASE OF MR. P.

With the previous review of theory, clinical experiences, and research, we now turn to the case of Mr. P. which precedes this chapter. It should be noted that I encountered the presented case several years preceding this writing. Therefore, it will be used as a starting point for clinical issues to be discussed. A more extensive PPD case illustration can be found in Turkat and Maisto (1985).

At this point it is probably to the reader's advantage to return to the case description before moving on to the sections below.

The Initial Clue

By definition, the paranoid personality is cautious, guarded, suspicious, and hypersensitive. Accordingly, one would expect such a case to act in this manner during a good deal of the initial interview. In this respect, perhaps the earliest clue that Mr. P. might be a paranoid personality was his reaction to being videotaped.

Almost all teaching clinics require their clients to sign a consent form which indicates that sessions may be audiotaped, videotaped, discussed with supervisors, presented in staff meetings, and/or used in other forms (confidentially) for teaching purposes. Many individuals will sign such a consent form without discussion. Others will ask a few questions to clarify their understanding. Only rarely will a person spend considerable time discussing it. Further, although many people will feel a bit uncomfortable about being videotaped, few become especially concerned. It has been my experience that atypical concern about videotaping (and other teaching tools involving others besides the attending clinician) often is a strong clue that one is dealing with a paranoid personality.

In dealing with the person who is highly suspicious and thus especially inquisitive about videotaping and so forth, it is important for the clinician to be reassuring but matter-of-fact. A defensive posture will only arouse further suspicions and impede progress.

Although the paranoid personality may show excessive concern about the consent form and the activities it may lead to in the future, I have never known a patient to refuse to sign the consent form or to leave the clinic before treatment had begun.

Some other initial clues for identifying possible paranoid personalities include the following:

- The patient may scan the clinic, its lobby, and/or the therapy room more intensely and frequently than is usual.
- The patient may seem very anxious and tense compared to typical cases.
- The patient may fill out a pretherapy screening questionnaire (e.g., presenting problems, history, demographics) in a perfectionistic and guarded manner.
- The patient may ask the therapist to outline and defend his or her credentials.

The Referral

Mr. P.'s reason for self-referral was that he wanted professional guidance in developing assertiveness skills.[3] He reported that his attempt to develop these skills through self-help books generated concern that he was not performing the skills appropriately.[4] In our experience, it is critical to understand *why* individuals want to learn a particular skill such as assertiveness whether they are paranoid or not, but even more so if one is dealing with a PP. Mr. P. seems to be assuming that his problem will be resolved if he is assertive. If this assumption is false, then assertiveness training is contraindicated. Thus, understanding why Mr. P. wants assertiveness training would allow the clinician to test the viability of Mr. P.'s assumption as well as shed light on Mr. P.'s more central problems if indeed his assumption is false.

Mr. P. indicated that he felt that others were picking on him and thus he needed to "stand up for his rights." Critical here is the question, "Why does Mr. P. feel that others are picking on him?" In a general sense, if his feeling is inappropriate (i.e., others are *not* picking on him), Mr. P. clearly has a serious problem. On the other hand, if his feeling is appropriate (i.e., others are picking on him) then one must determine why others are picking on him. If we assume that Mr. P. is correct (i.e., his problem is purely a lack of assertiveness), then we are forced to assume further that almost all unassertive people are picked on by many people in their environment; this is a difficult position to defend. Nevertheless if he is doing something to elicit being picked on (e.g., acting weird) this would be a critical target for treatment. Finally, given the data that Mr. P. feels picked on by co-workers, church participants, and even strangers, it would seem reasonable (to me) to conclude that Mr. P. probably acts in ways which elicit being picked on by some and that he also inappropriately interprets innocuous behavior by some as persecutory. The facts that Mr. P. at age 26 had no friends (because of a

---

[3]It is unfortunate that the behavior therapy literature has been obsessed with assertiveness training for years. Equally if not more disturbing is that many behavior therapists seem to think that assertiveness training is a synonym for social skills training. I believe that assertiveness is a small aspect of social skills in general and is contraindicated in many cases presenting social skills problems.

[4]I have been and continue to be quite concerned about the use of self-help books and audiotapes as interventions for clinical problems. Aside from a lack of research support (Turkat, Feuerstein, & Ciminero, 1980), they can have negative consequences clinically. For example, June Chiodo and I reported on a case similar to that of Mr. P. (Turkat & Chiodo, 1980), who used self-help assertive books on his own initiative to improve his social skills. The result was that he came across in an awkward and aggressive manner which exacerbated his previously existing problems.

"busy work schedule"), had never kissed a girl, and reported difficulty in interacting with women suggest a variety of things that might elicit negative reactions from others. Further, the fact that Mr. P. interpreted his avoidance of dating as due to the possibility of "the girl's family breaking up because of me" is clearly grandiose (e.g., "I'm so important I can break up her family") and/or persecutory (e.g., "Her family will be against me") and certainly inappropriate since he doesn't even know the girl or her family well.

In short, understanding why Mr. P. wanted to learn assertiveness skills would most likely aid the clinician in detecting his paranoid behavior and lead to a more useful formulation of the problems that would dictate a treatment plan other than assertiveness training.

Presenting Complaints

In addition to Mr. P.'s report that others pick on him and his self-prescribed need for assertiveness training, he presented the following complaints: (1) avoidance of women, (2) social isolation, (3) fear of being murdered or harmed, (4) penile pain following sexual attraction, and (5) depressive feelings. In my experience, none of these complaints is atypical for a PP case except perhaps for penile pain.

Avoidance of Women. It is quite uncommon for a 26-year-old male in our society to be a virgin, and even more strange if he has never kissed a girl. It is not uncommon for some to be awkward in opposite sex encounters. Nevertheless, both of these complaints occur commonly in men in the mid-twenties who are PP cases.

Why should Mr. P. be so uncomfortable around women? Whether or not Mr. P. is a PP case, two hypotheses are tenable: (1) he has an anxiety problem and/or (2) he has a skills deficit. From our experience with PP cases it would seem likely that Mr. P. has both problems. Speculation on how these problems may have developed will be discussed below.

If Mr. P is a PP and if we assume the evaluative-uniqueness theory to be correct, then we would expect Mr. P. to view himself as special and to be hypersensitive to evaluation. Given these traits, sexual intercourse should be a frightening situation since the openness, closeness, and demands to perform are intensely scrutinized. These requirements for sexual intercourse are precisely what the PP fears. Accordingly, interactions with women (which hold the prospect for intercourse) are anxiety-generating and elicit awkward, uncomfortable behavior.

A good example of the PP's evaluative-uniqueness view toward a relationship with a woman is Mr. P.'s idea that if he went out with a girl this would lead to the breaking up of her family. If this is assumed to be true, then Mr. P. has no choice but to: (1) be anxious around a woman (since he "knows" he will cause her psychological harm if he gets involved) and (2) not to get involved (since the girl's family will break up and Mr. P. will be blamed). Mr. P. "knows" what will happen; therefore he should avoid women.

It is important to recognize that if we were to grant Mr. P. his assumptions (i.e., "I will break up her family") then we would come to the same conclusions (i.e., "I must avoid women") as he. Unfortunately, these assumptions are often incorrect and thus generate untenable inferences. A related example is the male PP's belief that he may be homosexual, a phenomenon that Freud believed produces paranoia. Interestingly, many male PPs report a fear of being homosexual; I believe that this is a consequence of and not a precursor to PP. Keep in mind that *PP cases make logical inferences based on faulty assumptions* in addition to *making faulty inferences based on minimal information.* If a male PP is anxious around women and avoids them, he must make some inference about why he does so. Mr. P.'s "I will break up her family" seems to work for him. However, would not "Maybe I avoid women because I'm really a homosexual" work as well? The fact that the male PP does not feel sexual attraction to males (many PPs will not think of this datum) does not seem to affect the homosexuality inference. An additional point of interest is that the 26-year-old male who avoids women is often accused by others of being homosexual.

Social Isolation. I have yet to see a PP case which did not involve social isolation as a problem. As in other cases, Mr. P. has numerous rationalizations as to why he is not to blame for this (e.g., "too busy at work"). Social isolation not only prevents Mr. P. from obtaining the rewards inherent in good social relationships, it restricts his ability to learn how to obtain such rewards. Further, social isolation affords the PP too much time to be ruminating (Cameron, 1963) which leads to thoughts which can seem quite far from reality.

To illustrate the kind of thinking a PP engages in while socially isolated, actual excerpts from a diary/journal that Mr. P. kept are presented below.

> I am afraid to show my feelings with girls, afraid that they will reject me. I guess I feel that if they reject me I will be in danger in some way. It bothers me when girls make implicit demands. I shouldn't make implicit demands. It's not fair. I shouldn't expect implicit demands to be met. I don't

have much desire to please! Why should I expect others to. By the same token I shouldn't criticize others for not meeting my implied demands. I feel very lonely and I don't know how to get involved with people. I am afraid of rejection from the people I want acceptance from. I feel as though I have nothing to give. I feel dry and empty, unwanted, useless, a useless dreamer. I want experience but I am afraid to initiate it. Afraid something bad or just not good will result and I'll get blamed. So I don't try. Most of the time I hide from my feelings, especially my anger. I never just do what I want to do. I rarely know what I want to do. I don't seem to think of anything to do or say. I am hurting inside and I just want to escape the pain. Work is like a drug. I am not sure I know why I hurt or what hurts. Sometimes I think about suicide, although I don't think I'd go for that. I am really very angry, but I don't know why. I like to hurt people by ignoring them. It helps me to relieve my anger. When I get around others I get depressed because I turn my anger inward. I feel worthless! I hate myself! I've wasted so many years to be perfect now that I have to throw it all away and start all over again. I feel cheated. I don't even know where to begin. I am afraid of failure, set-backs and more disappointment. I am very disappointed! Why are you disappointed! Why are you disappointed!—I mean in the area of friends and sex. I've never been any good at these. I am always driving to get ahead. But I won't do any good. It won't make me any friends. I may survive, but I'll be alone. I am afraid, I am afraid of bad experiences. I am angry at myself at being afraid, chicken, as if I could help my fear.

Failure to love. Fear of other people's failure to love. Fear of tragedy, of being a participant in it. Of not being able to stop it, of not being omnipotent and yet so many people come to church due to tragedy and I don't condemn them. I am afraid that someone like my parents will blame me for tragedies that I can't help! That is very unfair. I am afraid I will be criticized for not having dated much; there is something wrong with my heart, I am selfish. I am too busy to get involved with a girl. I am afraid I will be criticized for being Catholic.

I have fears about being accepted. Remember the overly critical environment I come from which makes me perfectionistic. I am always needing people to tell me I am okay. I concentrate sexually on too many girls at once. I act hard and tough when I am gentle and sensitive. Satan is slowly trying to kill me by getting me to commit suicide. The spirit spoke through me tonight but I don't know what it is about. I'll stay by Jesus—I am not going to let Satan convince me to commit suicide. Suicide is ultimate complete isolation compared to lonelinesss in present life. Helping someone who is overly dependent can increase their self-hatred and make them hate you. Watch out for the other guy's self-image. Don't hurt the other person's self-concept and you'll be okay. Even when you correct someone, watch their self concept. People don't understand me, fear me, are out to get me. If someone doesn't deal openly with me it means they assume my behavior to be pathological—beyond my control. When they do confront me, I should acknowledge the fact that they consider my behavior to be seriously pathological to deal with me overtly then I should proceed to present my side. If my behavior is not pathological I am within my rights to resent their overkill tactics and to complain to the proper authorities. Especially if I have not given them probable causes for their suspicion. Why do I sometimes feel inadequate? It's because I have learned to think that I need to take advantage of every opportunity available. People are not open with me because I am not open with them. I am not mature. Phony high standards are a way to dodge criticism. I won't call that girl because I am afraid she will reject me, punish me, and I'll get mad and hold a grudge. I am afraid I may not fit within her social crowd. Her friends may not like me. Maybe her phone is tapped and they can use that against me? Do I really want to break up her family? If I don't meet their standards, they might reject me. Besides, they may take advantage of me like my mother has exploited me all her life. God how I despise her. I have to be prepared. I have to be prepared. I have to be prepared: relaxed, groomed, financially comfortable, transportation, place to go, program for the evening. I know I have to give up my mysterious identity and become regular; but you are not normal. You are extraordinary. I don't want to get involved because I will get criticized and won't have any power. I am afraid other people will criticize me and use personal information against me. I avoid sex to get back at my mother because i hate her for taking away my books about sex. I won't be a suitable marriage partner. I am afraid I will be criticized if some woman is attracted to me and we have sex.

Fear of Being Murdered or Harmed. In the case description, Mr. P. reported a fear of being murdered or harmed which did not have a specific focus (e.g., Mr. Smith wants to kill me). Rather, he seemed to report various situations which might bring him harm (e.g., attacked by a dog) or death (e.g., murdered in a bar). Occasionally he inferred that Satan might be trying to kill him. Three important issues are raised by this complaint: (1) why Mr. P. feels he may be harmed or murdered, (2) why he speculates that Satan may be the cause, and (3) why he revealed these thoughts in an interview.

We already know that Mr. P. feels picked on by numerous people, co-workers, churchgoers, even strangers. If so many people are "against" Mr. P., he must be very cautious and hyperalert for signs of others' hostility. Therefore, since he expects others to attack him (whether by picking on him or otherwise), it is not too hard to imagine conditions which increase the seriousness of the attacks Mr. P. might expect.

Let us assume that the actions others can take to "be against" Mr. P. lie on a continuum. At one pole is a slight criticism. At the other pole is a group out to torture and murder Mr. P. As Cameron has pointed out, we all make inferences based on limited information and our affect strongly influences our inferences. Thus, on a good day when the secretary at work smiles, we think everything is fine; but on a bad day, we may think a pink slip (i.e., notice that we are going to be fired) is coming. In terms of Mr. P.'s inferences, we would expect the same: on a good (i.e., nonstressful) day he comes home from work, sees a notice that a package is waiting for him at the post office, and is eager to find out what it is; on a bad day, he might worry that there is a bomb in the package and will dread going to the post office.

Why would Mr. P. feel at times that Satan is trying to kill him? Clearly, we would expect such an inference only on a very stressful day. Further, such an inference may serve to make sense out of a range of seemingly persecutory events. For example, assume that Mr. P. has the following "data-base" for the day:

- The waitress at lunch was rude to him.
- The boss told him to improve on his work.
- The car broke down on the way home from work.
- On the way home from the gas station, a man with whom he had once had a fight "followed" his car for three blocks.
- The evening paper was not in the driveway (which was very unusual)
- The phone rang as he entered his house but had ceased ringing by the time he reached it.

Given these experiences, Mr. P. might conclude that many persons are acting against him and that some harm is likely to befall him. As he ruminates about this, he attempts to distract himself by reading the church bulletin, which reminds him of the devil. When he imagines that Satan is after him, what appear to be discrete persecutory events (e.g., boss, car, telephone) now make sense.[5] If the above illustration were to lead to a well-systemized, full-blown delusion, then we would be dealing with a paranoid disorder and no longer just a paranoid personality.

As for the third question, how likely is it that a PP case would reveal such unusual thoughts in the initial interview? In my experience it is most unlikely. However, the clinician can engage in an interview strategy which seems to increase the probability of a PP's revealing unusual thoughts. I call this strategy *stepwise questioning*, and it has two primary components: (1) making it seem safe to admit unusual thoughts and (2) progressively increasing the threat of a question. Here, the interviewer tries to establish that the patient feels set apart from others ("Do you ever feel misunderstood?" "Do you ever feel kind of different from others?" "Do you ever feel as if others were judging you?" "Do you ever feel that others seem especially interested in you?"), then assesses persecutory feelings ("Does anyone seem to give you a hard

---

[5] See Cameron's (1963) description of the pseudocommunity and his hypotheses about the functions it serves.

time?" "Do you ever feel like people are giving you a hard time in general?" "On purpose?" "Do you ever get the feeling that the cards just seem stacked against you?" "Do you ever feel at times that people really seem against you?") and then grandiose feelings ("Do you ever feel special compared to others?" "Do you ever feel that you are unique?" "How are you unique?" "Do you ever feel that you have certain talents or skills that others do not have?" "Do you ever feel that you have certain powers that others do not?" "Do you ever feel people are jealous of you?"). Critical to this line of questioning is that the therapist appear supportive and understanding and control the interchange in a matter-of-fact manner. Gentle requests for elaboration on replies, use of "why" questions and therapist disclosures (e.g., "when my boss gives me a hard time, sometimes I think that he's jealous. Do you ever feel this way?") seem helpful. Further discussion of stepwise questioning can be found in Turkat and Maisto (1985).

Penile Pain. Mr. P. reported that he would experience pain in his penis hours after feeling sexually attracted to a woman. On the face of it, this complaint seems psychogenic in nature but to err on the side of caution Mr. P. should be encouraged to have this problem checked medically. Nevertheless, one could speculate that this complaint might be attributable to Mr. P.'s basic psychological problems. For example, he is quite capable of creating interesting explanations for avoiding women (e.g., "I might break up her family") and this might be another (e.g., "Since I get pain in my penis from sexual attraction I had better avoid women"). This complaint could have other "useful" properties as well (e.g., "The therapist can't ask me to be involved with women if I get pain in my penis from it"). Further, the facts that Mr. P. reports a several-hour interval between sexual attraction and penile pain, that he is frightened of women, and that he interprets things in a self-referential and defensive manner suggest that penile pain may be a consequence of how Mr. P. spends this several-hour interval.

Depressive Feelings. In view of the myriad problems that Mr. P. presents, it is not surprising that he experiences depressive episodes as well. In my experience, depression appears to be a natural conse-quence of behaving in a PP mode and appears to clear once the major target problems have been alleviated. Of course, anyone who experi-ences suicidal thoughts during these episodes and reports such ideas as that Satan may be trying to kill him should be viewed seriously. As noted earlier, Mr. P.'s views on Satan may be hypothesized to be a pseudocommunity-type of inference to explain his isolation and his perceptions of varied sources of persecution. Since these persecutory experiences are viewed as consequences of his anxiety and social skill problems, amelioration of these latter difficulties should lead to a diminution of depression.

Physical Appearance

Mr. P.'s physical presentation at the initial interview was described as neat and conservative. Noteworthy is the fact that Mr. P. wore thick-lensed eyeglasses and that he was a bit chubby. In itself this information provides little for useful clinical inference formation. However, in my experience many male PP cases have physical appearance attributes which repel others (e.g., unstylish, ill-fitting clothes; unkempt hair). In the matter of helping Mr. P. get the better of his social isolation, treatment might include helping him lose weight, switch to stylish glasses or contact lenses, dress less conservatively, and so on.

Interview Behavior

Aside from Mr. P.'s concern about videotaping (which we discussed earlier), he was described as: (1) concerned about pleasing the therapist, (2) speaking in detail about things unrelated to the question, (3) spending considerable time thinking before giving answers, and (4) being highly motivated for treatment.

Since Mr. P. is hypersensitive to threat (a defining characteristic of PP), it makes sense that he would try to prevent the therapist from being a threat (e.g., being cold, asking pointed humiliating questions) by attempting to please him. Although PP cases are often viewed as hostile, I have found that most can be quite nonhostile in the therapy room.

Mr. P.'s speaking in detail about topics unrelated to the questions asked suggests a number of things. One must keep in mind that the nature of the question is vital. For example, if the interviewer is asking a question to which Mr. P. feels a truthful answer might prove very embarrassing, he might deliberately talk about other things with the hope that the clinician will move on to a less threatening question. On the other hand, Mr. P. has a unique way of thinking about things which might lead him to misinterpret the nature of a question. Yet again, Mr. P. may be a poor judge of when and how much he should drift off topic in conservations (an important social skill). Thus, when asked why he has no friends, Mr. P. might start off by stating that he is too busy at work and then expand on all of what being busy at work entails. Finally, most PP cases are perfectionists and thus when discussing a topic may speak at great length in much detail to avoid making an "error" and thereby prevent being misunderstood (a common complaint in PP cases).

The fact that Mr. P. spent considerable time thinking before replying suggests that he was being cautious in his answers, a common characteristic of PP. Perfectionists in general often have a similar style during interviews, paranoid or not (cf. Turkat & Meyer, 1982).

Finally, it should come as no surprise that Mr. P. seemed highly motivated for treatment, given his reason for seeing a therapist (i.e., assertiveness training) in the first place.

History

Earlier in this chapter, the evaluative uniqueness theory of PP development was presented. The brief historical information about Mr. P. which appears in the case description seems somewhat in line with this etiological theory.

Mr. P.'s father was described as paranoid, his mother was over-possessive and both as being hyperconcerned about social evaluation. Further, the family was viewed by the parents as special in that secret family information (e.g., Dad had pimples on his buttocks) had to remain in the family at all costs. Thus, Mr. P. had a good model for paranoid behavior (Dad) and a relevant early training ground (the overcritical environment, guarded family secrets, overconcern with social evaluation, avoidance of social interaction).

Missing from the case history (perhaps because there was none) is specification of a particular attribute of Mr. P. that earned him a unique status in his, his parents', and others' eyes. However, there are various bits of information which seem to fit. For example, he was the youngest of four children all of whom were described as intelligent but never having lived up to their potential (indicating high expectations). Mr. P. also seemed to despise his mother for treating him like a baby, resented the intense parental criticism which made him feel unintelligent and unworthy, and also reported fear of becoming an adult. These data suggest that Mr. P. was viewed by himself and his parents as being a baby—special as compared with his older siblings. Mr. P. seemed to think that he could never perform well as an adult and thus feared becoming one.

As a child, Mr. P. reported experiencing what seemed to be PP traits. For example, he felt that others were especially interested in him and were watching him; he was a loner; he was fearful of making mistakes and being blamed for things; he felt his teachers were against him. Although not explicitly stated in the case description, it seems likely that Mr. P. was socially isolated in high school and had much time alone to ruminate about his predicament as well as miss out on learning good social skills. Thus, by age 26 Mr. P. had no friends, was a virgin, had never kissed a girl, felt that others were against him and had brief periods in which he engaged in intense persecutory and grandiose thoughts.

Testing Clinical Hypotheses about Mr. P.

Based on the case description and the clinical speculation in the preceding pages, several hypotheses can be advanced concerning the formulation of the case of Mr. P.:

1. The core of Mr. P.'s problems is a hypersensitivity to others' evaluations which exacerbates and is perpetuated by Mr. P.'s social skill problems.
2. This central problem contributes to his social isolation, which in turn promotes his paranoid ideation.
3. These problems lead him to experience depressive episodes which in turn increase the intensity, frequency, duration, and pathological quality of his paranoid thoughts.

The main target for treatment, therefore, would be to reduce Mr. P.'s hypersensitivity to criticism and to reduce those social behaviors he performs which elicit criticism from others.

One way to test the major hypothesis would be to expose Mr. P. to criticisms, neutral events which could be inferred by him (but not by others) to be criticisms, and clearly neutral events and to evaluate his autonomic and subjective arousal, as was done in a similar case (cf. Turkat, Maisto, Burish, & Rock, in press). Another method is to compare Mr. P. to norms on a relevant standardized test, such as the FNE (Watson & Friend, 1969). To test his hypersensitivity and social skills problems simultaneously, Mr. P. could be videotaped and monitored physiologically (using a telemetric device) while interacting with confederates (male and female). In this experiment, several predictions could be made; a few are listed below:

1. Mr. P. should show more arousal to women than to men.
2. Mr. P. should show more arousal when evaluation (be it positive or negative) is introduced explicitly, especially by a woman.
3. Mr. P. should show selective attention of evaluative cues (particularly implicit ones) when asked to recall events in the interactions.

4. Mr. P. should show a good deal of self-referential thinking in terms of processing the confederates' cues (i.e., misinterpreting innocuous behavior by the confederates to have special meaning).
5. Mr. P. should act in an awkward, unskilled manner as judged by objective raters.

Treatment of Mr. P.

The major approach to the treatment of Mr. P. stems directly from the formulation and would focus on reducing Mr. P.'s hypersensitivity to criticism and changing his social behavior. More specific points are addressed below.

Anxiety Management. Here, a hierarchy would be created consisting of imaginary, analogue, and in *vivo* criticisms. Mr. P. would be taught methods by which to compete with the anxiety (e.g., relaxation training) and practice bidirectional control (cf. Turkat & Kuczmierczyk, 1980).

Social Skills Training. This would involve instructions, modeling, role playing, and videotaped feedback to ameliorate Mr. P.'s attentional, information-processing, response emission, and response-to-feedback deficits and excesses. In addition, efforts would be made to increase his physical attractiveness. Of particular importance is for him to learn how to act like others and to stop viewing himself as unique and special and acting in ways which indicate that he thinks so. Since Mr. P. is so sensitive to criticism, social skills training would have to follow anxiety management, since social skills training involves a good deal of criticism.

Therapeutic Relationship. In carrying out the treatment plan, it would be critical for the therapist to relate to Mr. P. in line with the formulation. Thus, at first the clinician would be totally accepting of Mr. P. and gradually would become more critical as Mr. P. progresses.

SUMMARY

The purpose of this chapter has been to review what is known about paranoid personality disorder and to illustrate how such a case is formulated clinically. As we have seen, considerable theory has been advanced for paranoid pathology, and three theories (Cameron, Millon, Turkat) for the PP exist. Hardly any research on PP can be identified, in part, perhaps, because of problems in diagnostic practice and because

PP individuals seem unlikely to volunteer participation in research. A case of PP was discussed in light of the evaluative–uniqueness theory and my clinical experience with PP cases. It appears that PP is a fascinating disorder which remains an enigma in terms of scientific criteria.

REFERENCES

Abelson, R. (1981). Going after PARRY. Behavioral and Brain Sciences, 4, 534–535.

Adams, H. E. (1981). Abnormal psychology. Dubuque, Iowa: William C. Brown.

Adams, H. R., & Calhoun, K. S. (1974). Innovations in the treatment of abnormal behavior. In K. S. Calhoun, H. E. Adams, & K. M. Mitchell (Eds.), Innovative treatment methods in psychopathology (pp. 1–15). New York: Wiley.

Agassi, J. (1981). Simulation? Behavioral and Brain Sciences, 4, 535–536.

American Psychiatric Association (1980). Diagnostic and statistical manual of mental disorders (3rd ed.). Washington, DC: Author.

Cameron, N. (1963). Personality development and psychopathology: A dynamic approach. Boston: Houghton-Mifflin.

Cameron, N. (1974). Paranoid conditions and paranoia. In S. Arieti & E. Brody (Eds.). American handbook of psychiatry (vol. 3, pp. 676–693). New York: Basic Books.

Carey, M., Flasher, L. V., Maisto, S. A., & Turkat, I. D. (1984). The a priori approach to psychological assessment. Professional Psychology, 15, 515–527.

Cerney, J. (1965). Chinese psychiatry. International Journal of Psychiatry, 1, 229–239.

Chalus, G. A. (1977). An evaluation of the validity of the Freudian theory of paranoia. Journal of Homosexuality, 3, 171–187.

Colby, K. M. (1975). Artifical paranoia: A computer simulation of paranoid processes. New York: Pergamon Press.

Colby, K. M. (1976). Clinical implications of a simulation model of paranoid processes. Archives of General Psychiatry, 33, 854–857.

Colby, K. M. (1977). Appraisal of four psychological theories of paranoid phenomena. Journal of Abnormal Psychology, 86, 54–59.

Colby, K. M. (1981). Modeling a paranoid mind. Behavioral and Brain Sciences, 4, 515–560.

Colby, K. M. (1983). Limits on the scope of PARRY as a model for paranoia. Behavioral and Brain Sciences, 6, 341–342.

Colby, K. M., Fraught, W. S., & Parkinson, R. C. (1979). Cognitive therapy of paranoid conditions: Heuristic suggestions based on a computer simulation model. Cognitive Therapy & Research, 3, 55–60.

Colby, K. M., Hilf, F. D., Weber, S., & Kramer H. (1972). Turing-like indistinguishability tests for the validation of a computer simulation of paranoid processes. Artificial Intelligence, 3, 199–221.

Derogatis, L. D. (1975). SCL-90. Copyright: Author.

Gunderson, K. (1981). Paranoia concerning program-resistant aspects of the mind—And let's drop rocks on Turing's toes again. Behavioral and Brain Sciences, 4, 537–539.

Kass, F., Spitzer, R. L., & Williams, J. B. W. (1983). An empirical study of the issue of sex bias in the diagnostic criteria of DSM-III Axis II personality disorders. American Psychologist, 38, 799–801.

Izard, C. E., & Masterson, F. A. (1981). Colby's paranoia model: An old theory in a new frame? *Behavioral and Brain Sciences, 4*, 539–540.

Kendler, K. S. (1982). Demography of paranoid psychosis (delusional disorder). *Archives of General Psychiatry, 39*, 890–902.

Kendler, K. S., & Tsuang, M. T. (1981). Nosology of paranoid schizophrenia and other paranoid psychoses. *Schizophrenia Bulletin, 7*, 594–611.

Lazare, A., Klernan, G. L., Armor, D. J. (1970). Oral, obsessive, and hysterical personality patterns. *Journal of Psychiatric Research, 7*, 275–290.

Lemert, E. M. (1962). Paranoia and the dynamics of exclusion. *Sociometry, 25*, 2–25.

Lindsay, R. (1981). How smart must you be to be crazy? *Behavioral and Brain Sciences, 4*, 541–542.

Lorr, M., Klett, J. C., & McNair, D. M. (1963). *Syndromes of psychosis.* New York: Pergamon Press.

Magaro, P. A. (1980). *Cognition in schizophrenia and paranoia: The integration of cognitive processes.* Hillsdale, NJ: Lawrence Erlbaum.

Magaro, P. A. (1981). The paranoid and the schizophrenic: The case for distinct cognitive style. *Schizophrenia Bulletin, 7*, 632–660.

Magaro, P. A., & Shulman, H. G. (1981). Colby's model for paranoia: It's made well but what is it? *Behavioral and Brain Sciences, 4*, 542–543.

Maher, B. A. (1981). Testing the components of a computer model. *Behavioral and Brain Sciences, 4*, 543.

Maher, B., & Ross, J. S. (1984). Delusions. In H. E. Adams & P. B. Sutker (Eds.), *Comprehensive handbook of psychopathology* (pp. 383–409). New York: Plenum Press.

Manschreck, T. C. (1979). The assessment of paranoid features. *Comprehensive Psychiatry, 20*, 370–377.

Manschreck, T. C. (1983). Modeling a paranoid mind: A narrow interpretation of the results. *Behavioral and Brain Sciences, 6*, 340–341.

Meissner, W. W. (1981). The schizophrenic and the paranoid process. *Schizophrenia Bulletin, 7*, 611–631.

Millon, T. (1969). *Modern psychopathology.* Philadelphia: W. B. Saunders.

Millon, T. (1981). *Disorders of personality DSM-III: Axis II.* New York: Wiley.

Millon, T. (1983). The DSM-III: An insider's perspective. *American Psychologist, 38*, 804–814.

Millon, T., & Millon, R. (1974). *Abnormal behavior and personality.* Philadelphia: W. B. Saunders.

Munro, A. (1982). Paranoia revisited. *British Journal of Psychiatry, 141*, 344–349.

Pfeiffer, V. W. M. (1962). Mental disturbance among the Sudanese. *Psychiatrica et Neurologia, 143*, 315–333.

Pfeiffer, V. W. M. (1963). Comparative psychiatric studies of different population groups in West Java. *Transcultural Psychiatric Research Review, 15*, 32–36.

Reid, W. H., & Riedler, J. F. (1981). Psychiatry and computers: An uneasy synthesis. *Behavioral and Brain Sciences, 4*, 547.

Shapiro, M. B. (1957). Experimental method in the psychological description of the individual psychiatric patient. *International Journal of Social Psychiatry, 111*, 89–102.

Shapiro, M. B. (1970). Intensive assessment of the single case: An inductive-deductive approach. In P. Mittler (Ed.), *Psychological assessment of mental and physical handicaps.* London: Methuen.

Shapiro, M. B. (1975). The requirements and implications of a systematic science of psychopathology. *Bulletin of the British Psychological Society, 28*, 149–155.

Shapiro, M. B. (1979). Assessment interviewing in clinical psychology. *British Journal of Social and Clinical Psychology, 18,* 211–218.

Silverberg, R. (1972). *If I forget thee O Jerusalem.* New York: Pyramid Communications.

Swanson, D. W. (1981). Is PARRY paranoid? *Behavioral and Brain Sciences, 4,* 548–549.

Swanson, D. W., Bonhert, P. J., & Smith, J. A. (1970). *The paranoid.* Boston: Little, Brown.

Torrey, E. F. (1981). The epidemiology of paranoid schizophrenia. *Schizophrenia Bulletin, 7,* 588–593.

Turkat, I. D., & Alpher, V. S. (1983). An investigation of personality disorder description. *American Psychologist, 38,* 857–858.

Turkat, I. E., & Chiodo, J. F. (1979). Detrimental effects of self-help intervention. *Clinical Behavior Therapy Review, 1,* 31.

Turkat, I. D., & Kuczmierczyk, A. R. (1980). Clinical considerations in anxiety management. *Scandinavian Journal of Behavior Therapy, 9,* 141–145.

Turkat, I. E., & Levin, R. A. (1984). Formulation of personality disorders. In H. E. Adams & P. B. Sutker (Eds.), *Comprehensive handbook of psychopathology* (pp. 495–522). New York: Plenum Press.

Turkat, I. D., & Maisto, S. A. (1985). Application of the experimental method to the formulation and modification of personality disorders. In D. H. Barlow (Ed.), *Clinical Handbook of psychological disorders* (pp. 503–507). New York: Guilford Press.

Turkat, I. E., & Meyer, V. (1982). The behavior-analytic approach. In P. L. Wachtel (Ed.), *Resistance: Psychodynamic and behavioral approaches* (pp. 157–184). New York: Plenum Press.

Turkat, I. D., Feuerstein, M., & Ciminero, A. R. (1980). Audiotape intervention: An empirical review. *Behavioral Engineering, 6,* 49–55.

Turkat, I. D., Maisto, S. A., Burish, T. G., & Rock, D. K. (in press). Evaluating case formulations of psychopathology. In H. Lettner & B. Range (Eds.), *Handbook of behavioral psychotherapy.* Sao Paulo, Brazil: Editoria Pedagogica e Universitaria.

Ullman, L., & Krasner, L. (1975). *A psychological approach to abnormal behavior* (2nd ed.). Englewood Cliffs, NJ: Prentice-Hall.

Watson, D., & Friend, R. (1969). Measurement of social evaluation anxiety. *Journal of Counseling and Clinical Psychology, 43,* 384–395.

6

HISTRIONIC PERSONALITY

The Case of Ms. H.

Ms. H. was a 32-year-old white, single woman who resided alone. She had never been married and had no children. She had recently broken up with her boyfriend. She was employed as a caseworker in a social agency.

The Referral

A co-worker had suggested that Ms. H. contact the psychologist. Both her physician and her mother had encouraged her in the past to see a psychologist. When asked what prompted her contact now, she replied, "I just felt bad and decided to call." While still on the telephone, Ms. H. made a dramatic, but veiled, suicide threat. She was equally dramatic in denying intent to harm herself when questioned about her comment. She denied current medications or previous contact with a mental health professional.

Physical Appearance

Ms. H. was a woman of average height and build. She had dark brown hair, hazel eyes, and a smooth complexion. She was very attractive. She dressed fashionably but made slight overuse of makeup and jewelry.

Presenting Complaints

Ms. H. complained of depression and gastrointestinal distress. She said these symptoms had been present for two months but that she had had similar episodes in the past.

Her depression involved "bad moods" accompanied by crying episodes, mild insomnia, boredom, low frustration tolerance, irritability, decreased activity, decreased interest, and occasional suicidal ideation. She denied attempts but acknowledged several threats in the past. She suggested inactivity and negative interactions with her mother as antecedents to her bad moods.

Her gastrointestinal complaints included stomach pain and diarrhea. She had seen a physician about this distress, and he had suggested that the symptoms were secondary to tension. She denied awareness of any antecedents.

Ms. H. also complained that her mother interfered in her business. Although her mother was often very helpful in times of distress and illness, Ms. H. reported frequent arguments between them. She believed her mother's moods to be capricious.

She described her job as unsatisfactory and boring. She was almost contemptuous of the clients seen by her agency. She had poor interactions with most of her co-workers in that the women were jealous of her and the men were not her social equals.

She had lost contact with her friends from the past. Their lives had changed significantly (i.e., marriage, children), so Ms. H. felt different from most of them. She had difficulty sustaining friendships. She spoke with pride about her ability to make anyone she was interested in notice and like her. Things always seemed to begin well enough. At first people were a lot of fun and appeared to want to be very helpful. Sooner or later, though, the other people seemed to have less time for her and to become boring. It appeared to her that the longer you knew someone the less considerate they became. Her relationships with men were characterized as initially intense and exciting. The relationships tended to be short-lived and usually ended as a result of her lack of interest or the man's involvement with another woman.

Parents

Ms. H.'s parents were divorced when she was an infant. She knew little if anything about her father. Despite having a part-time job to support herself and her daughter, Ms. H.'s mother always had plenty of time to give her attention and guidance. Ms. H. was the center of her mother's life. The mother was described as a very responsible parent, if emotional and opinionated.

Interview Behavior

The patient was doubtful about the usefulness of seeing a psychologist, but she said she was willing to let him prove himself. At the start of the interview, her expression was a constant smile, but her affect became more appropriate as the interview continued. Her mannerisms were occasionally seductive. She was generally cooperative. Her responses tended to be dramatic, with emphasis on the shortcomings of others. She was quick to excuse her own past behavior by referring to illness on her part or insensitivity on the part of others. She professed confusion about why people treated her the way they did and why she did not seem to be able to stay healthy and happy. At several points in the interview, Ms. H. offered simplistic explanations for all her problems and demanded to know if the interviewer agreed.

6

Histrionic Personality
A Behavioral Formulation

PHILLIP J. BRANTLEY and ELEANOR B. CALLON

INTRODUCTION

Histrionic personality disorders have been described as among the most interesting, yet least understood, of the personality disorders (Halleck, 1967). Individuals with personality disorders employ maladaptive strategies in their social behavior (Adams, 1981; Lion, 1978; Millon, 1981; Turner & Hersen, 1981). Those with histrionic disorders are difficult to treat, both medically and psychologically, mainly because these very strategies interfere with successful intervention (Halleck, 1967; Moskovitz, 1976; Peele & Rubin, 1974; Schmidt & Messner, 1977). The current diagnostic criteria (American Psychiatric Association, 1980) allude to the problems encountered by these individuals in their daily lives and to the challenges to be met by those who would intervene. Use of this diagnosis requires that the patient suffer significant impairment in social and/or occupational functioning or significant subjective distress. Current and long-standing behaviors are characterized by at least three of the following: self-dramatization; incessant drawing of attention to self; craving for activity and excitement; overreaction to

PHILLIP J. BRANTLEY • Departments of Psychology and Family Medicine, Louisiana State University, Baton Rouge, Louisiana, 70803. ELEANOR B. CALLON • Department of Psychology, Louisiana State University, Baton Rouge, Louisiana, 70803.

minor events; irrational, angry outbursts or tantrums. Interpersonal relationships (including those with persons offering professional help) are disturbed by at least two of the following: seen by others as shallow and lacking in genuineness; egocentric, self-indulgent, and inconsiderate; vain and demanding; dependent, helpless, constantly seeking reassurance; prone to manipulative suicidal threats, gestures, or attempts.

Histrionic personality disorders are said to be common (American Psychiatric Association, 1980). This diagnostic category was hidden under other labels until 1968 (Peele & Rubin, 1974) and the publication of the second edition of the *Diagnostic and Statistical Manual of Mental Disorders* (DSM-II) (American Psychiatric Association, 1968), making accurate data before that year impossible. Data on the exact incidence still are not available (Adams, 1981).

A survey of the history behind current conceptions of histrionic personality disorders follows the histories of classification in both medicine and psychiatry. It began with an attempt to understand medical presentations that have since been called hysterical. There followed a period during which these phenomena were associated with certain personality patterns that eventually came to be designated histrionic. The current understanding is that histrionic patterns are not necessarily associated with hysterical phenomena.

Examination of the etymologies of the two adjectives, *histrionic* and *hysterical*, both clarifies the current conceptualization and suggests the long and confusing history behind it. *Histrionic* is derived from the Latin *histrio (-onis)* referring to a stage player. The Latin word is derived from the Etruscan *hister*, meaning a buffoon. On the other hand, *hysterical* is etymologically linked to the Greek *hysterikos*, meaning suffering in the uterus. Use of the adjective *histrionic* emphasizes the self-dramatization and the lack of genuineness characteristic of individuals with such a disorder. Whitehorn (cited in Forrest, 1967) commented that all human beings play roles, but the person with a histrionic personality does so in such an unconvincing way that the role playing itself is the center of attention. *Hysterical* refers to the earliest assumptions regarding the etiology and gender linkages of a variety of disorders which were originally combined under the rubric *hysteria*.

The first references to hysterical personality (character) appeared in psychoanalytic literature (Marmor, 1953; Reich, 1950; Wittels, 1930). These authors were discussing the personality structure underlying conversion reactions. It was generally assumed that (1) all hysterics had similar personality structures and that (2) individuals exhibiting these personality characteristics either had had conversion symptoms in the past or would develop them at some time in the future.

Chodoff and Lyons (1958) were among the first to test these assumptions. A major problem was that no clear definition of hysterical personality had been offered. They abstracted a definition from the available literature. Then, they examined 17 patients whom they agreed had hysteria. Only three met the criteria included in their definition. Thus, the validity of the first assumption appeared questionable. Other studies also failed to support the assumption. Stephens and Kamp (1962) evaluated 100 patients with hysteria and found only 9 whom they considered to have hysterical personalities. Merskey and Trimble (1979) examined 89 patients with conversion symptoms. Only 17 were judged to exhibit hysterical personalities.

Direct testing of the second assumption is more difficult. One can determine whether or not individuals with hysterical personalities currently exhibit conversion symptoms or have done so in the past. It is more difficult to determine if they are going to do so in the future unless they are followed throughout their lives. Even then, someone committed to the assumption might argue that they probably would have, had they not died prematurely. Pollak (1981) reviewed the available evidence, however, and concluded that the assumption was not supported. Luisada, Peele, and Pittard (1974), for example, studied 27 patients diagnosed as having hysterical personalities; none of them exhibited conversion symptoms.

Chodoff and Lyons preferred Whitehorn's (cited in Forrest, 1967) term histrionic personality to the commonly used hysterical personality, mainly because of the association of the latter term with hysterical conversion reactions and because the former term more accurately described the behavior patterns exhibited by patients who fit their definition. The compilers of DSM-III (APA, 1980) concluded that hysterical "has many irrelevant historical connotations and suggests a relationship to conversion symptoms" (p. 379). They chose histrionic personality disorder as the preferred label.

The focus of this chapter is on the assessment process we employ, using histrionic personality disorder as our example. We will introduce our approach to assessment and case formulation by discussing the assumptions we make. We will provide a description of the systematic progression we try to use in all our assessments. That is, we will describe our data collection process. Our interview process will be described in detail—identification and referral information, problem identification and definition, and developmental analysis. We will discuss the circumstances in which we gather data from other sources and describe alternative sources. Then, we will describe how we put all of that data together to provide a case formulation for the individual patient. Ms. H.

will be presented as an illustrative case. We will discuss our approaches to treatment briefly, because our assignment is to discuss assessment and formulation. We will end with a brief summary of the whole process.

We try to adhere to an empirical approach in our work. Therefore, we will draw from the available literature to support our presentation. DSM-III has attempted to provide clear criteria for histrionic personality disorder. The publication of that work is quite recent—1980. Publications prior to that date may or may not be describing disorders that meet the current definition. Specific inclusion and exclusion criteria have been especially problematic for histrionic personality disorders. Zisook, DeVaul, and Gammon (1979), for example, argued that this is "one of the least sharply defined, yet most commonly used diagnostic entities" (p. 113). Zisook and DeVaul (1978) compared the diagnostic criteria suggested by three different sources available at the time they were preparing their report (APA, 1968; Chodoff & Lyons, 1958; Lazare, Klerman, & Armor, 1970). There was no overlap between DSM-III and the other two sources in terms used to describe the characteristics of the disorder. Chodoff and Lyons listed seven terms; Lazare, Klerman, & Armor, six. They agreed on three. In doing our literature review, we found a lot of confusion about terms, as we indicated in our brief discussion of the history of this disorder. The references cited in the remaining sections of the chapter are limited to histrionic personality disorder and features of that disorder. We do not use the term interchangeably with hysteria, hysterical conversion reaction, or Briquette's syndrome.

ASSESSMENT AND CASE FORMULATION

Our assessment and case formulation is directed toward designing treatment for an individual patient. We reject a homogeneous disorder model for histrionic personality disorders (or for any other disorder). We assume that treatment will differ from patient to patient. Therefore, we rely on idiographic, rather than nomothetic, assessment procedures. Our assignment is data-based, but the data gathered is selected and/or designed to answer specific questions about a particular individual. Normative data may be used for general description, but they cannot tell us what specific interventions are needed for a given patient. We do not find global psychological assessment of strengths and weaknesses very helpful in designing treatment programs. Behavior is our unit of study. That behavior may be motoric, biological, affective, or cognitive-perceptual.

The center of our assessment process is the interview. Our interviews are both more detailed and broader than those of many other clinicians. They are directive and specific. They are organized to allow the patient to demonstrate his or her psychopathology, to test hypotheses about the conditions under which that psychopathology surfaces and subsides, and to formulate a testable hypothesis about the etiology and/or maintainance of that pathology. The interview and other assessment procedures are systematic. We will describe them in detail and show how they lead directly to case formulation and treatment planning.

Identification and Referral Information

We begin the assessment process by gathering information about identifying characteristics and the reason for the patient's pursuit of psychological care. Basic demographic variables such as the patient's age, sex, marital status, place of residence, employment status, and current medications are obtained to provide a background or framework for conceptualizing subsequent data concerning the patient. This information may be obtained in the initial contact with the patient, provided by the referral source, or collected from available patient records. Although simple demographic facts rarely aid in making fine discriminations in patient diagnosis or case formulation, they do provide a starting point for assessment by steering the clinician away from areas of low probability. For example, psychotic disorders are of low probability among middle-aged individuals with stable employment and marriages unless there is evidence for a psychosis associated with an organic brain syndrome.

Although it is by no means a diagnostic determinant, patient gender has been shown to be a variable that influences the diagnosis of histrionic personality disorder. It is generally agreed that the disorder is far more common among women than among men. Reliable statistical data on differential incidence between males and females are not available. Slavney and McHugh (1974) reported a ratio of seven females to one male in their study of 32 patients diagnosed histrionic. Some reports have estimated that 92 percent of patients with this diagnosis are women (Winokur & Crowe, 1975). Luisada et al. (1974) reported a very rough estimate of one male histrionic personality disorder in 1,000 diagnoses, but they gave no comparative data on females.

The acceptance of histrionic personality disorder as largely a female phenomenon has raised concern that the diagnosis has been overused, particularly with seductive females (e.g., Lion, 1978). There is at least one report that inexperienced psychiatric residents tend to use this label for young, attractive, sexually provocative females regardless of the presence or absence of other histrionic symptoms (Lazare, Klerman, & Armor, 1966).

Evidence also exists for sex bias in the differential diagnosis between histrionic and antisocial personality disorders (Brantley & Sutker, 1984). Warner (1978) presented a hypothetical clinical profile to 175 mental health professionals. The profile included references to minor suicide attempts, failure to enjoy sexual relations, failure to sustain close relationships, and failure to feel affection for others. It described a person with an immature, narcissistic, and self-centered disposition who lacked remorse for an illegal act and presented in an excitable, self-dramatizing, and flirtatious manner. The sexual designation of the profile was randomly distributed with a male represented in 86 instances and a female in 87. The number of male and female professionals equalled the sex distribution of the profiles, but half of the male diagnosticians saw a male profile and half saw a female profile. The same was true of the female professionals. The diagnosticians were asked to choose from among eight diagnostic categories, including antisocial personality disorder and histrionic personality disorder. Both male and female professionals assigned the diagnosis histrionic personality disorder more frequently than any of the others. However, when the profile was presented as that of a female patient, it was judged as representative of a histrionic personality disorder 64 times and of an antisocial disorder 19 times. Apparently, diagnosticians are not averse to using the histronic diagnosis for males, but if the patient is a female the diagnosis is chosen more frequently than is the antisocial category.

Along with gathering basic demographic data, the clinician should determine, early in the assessment process, the circumstances leading to the patient's seeking psychological services. The primary symptoms or concerns, what factors prompted the patient to seek treatment, and who referred the patient are of particular concern. Such information frequently provides one of the first substantive clues concerning patient diagnosis and case formulation. As in the case of demographic data, referral information is certainly not sufficient for making major assessment decisions. Rather, this information can serve as a broad discriminator which allows the clinician to separate symptom groups or diagnoses which are highly probable from those of low probability. Knowledge regarding referral circumstances of various psychological disorders is necessary in making this distinction. For example, individuals with histrionic personality disorders appear in treatment for particular problems with a high frequency. Slavney and McHugh (1974) studied 32 patients whose diagnoses included histrionic personality disorder. Half of them were hospitalized following a suicide attempt.

Almost 80 percent presented with depression on admission. Kass, Silvers, and Abroms (1972) reported their work with five histrionic patients. Four were admitted following suicide attempts, and the fifth was admitted because of anxiety with a panic attack. Blinder (1966) reported an international study of 21 patients diagnosed histrionic personality disorder. In addition to suicide attempts and reactive depressions, this group included patients who sought psychiatric help for "nervousness" and chronic unexplained somatic complaints. The disorder has also been found at relatively high frequency among substance abusers (Slavney & McHugh, 1974) and among individuals with somatoform disorders (Millon, 1981). Hendler (1981) found histrionic personality disorder frequently enough to include a chapter on this disorder in his book on patients with exaggerated pain.

Another important consideration related to referral circumstances is whether patients are seeking help on their own accord or are being pressured or strongly encouraged to participate in treatment by others. Specifically, the question is whether patients perceive themselves as having a problem or appear for treatment only because a significant other such as a spouse, physician, employer, or legal authority insists that they need it. This issue should be clarified by the clinician because it can have a profound influence on patients' motivation to cooperate with assessment and treatment. Such information can also be of direct benefit to diagnosis and case formulation. For instance, given the well-established finding that individuals with personality disorders possess deficits in interpersonal performance and problem solving (Adams, 1981; Turner & Hersen, 1981), it is not surprising to find that many are seeking treatment for problems with significant others in their lives.

Finally, patients will often present with problems of a long-standing nature for which they have only recently considered seeking treatment. In these instances, the clinician should make a strong effort to determine what circumstances or factors prompted the patient to seek treatment at this time. Problems of a long-standing nature, such as the case with personality disorders, are typically very resistant to change. By determining the circumstances that were potent enough to motivate the patient to seek treatment, the clinician increases the probability of finding effective contingencies for behavior change and planning effective treatment.

Problem Identification and Definition

We consider construction of a complete list of patient problems one of the most crucial aspects of the assessment process. Before any attempt can be made to formulate a patient's case or to explain a presenting complaint, the clinician must be aware of the entire spectrum of patient problems. Failure to isolate a complete picture of patient complaints can result in misdiagnosis of the patient and an incomplete and inaccurate case formulation. Omissions in the patient problem lists are by far the most frequent errors we have observed in psychology graduate students during the initial stages of their training in patient assessment. Many behavior therapists who assess only the few complaints they will treat make this same error.

The patient's behavior during the interview is an important source of information about problems. The interview provides a situation during which the clinician can observe the patient's presentation to other people, responses to stressful interactions, and responses to various means of behavioral control. Peele and Rubin (1974) observed that the female patient with a histrionic disorder displays many characteristics typical of that disorder during the first interview: drama, exaggeration, effervescence, confusion between fact and wish. Halleck (1967) observed the patient's repeated attempts to control the interview, attention-seeking behavior, dishonesty in communication, self-portrayal as helplessly dependent, and reluctance to assume responsibility. Any of these behaviors during the interview are likely to be typical of many of the patient's other interactions and warrant further investigation by the clinician.

The clinical interview remains the most frequently used means of isolating patient symptoms or problems. Construction of a complete problem list requires that the interviewer ask the right questions. There is clearly a good deal of truth in the expression, "The best clinicians ask the fewest questions." The statement comes from the notion that a well-trained clinician is likely to ask highly relevant and useful questions, thus completing the assessment process in a short time and with little wasted effort. An interviewer's ability to ask relevant questions is highly contingent on knowledge of psychopathology and clinical diagnosis. Such knowledge enables the clinician to address significant aspects of patient problems and ensures that all pertinent areas of potential concern are addressed.

It is in the generation of a patient problem list that the DSM-III (APA, 1980) system is particularly useful. Although determining a patient diagnosis is not extremely important in case formulation or treatment planning, diagnostic descriptions are useful in that they help to insure that the interviewer asks the appropriate questions. Using the DSM-III diagnostic system as a guide, the clinician can be alerted to a variety of diagnostic possibilities depending on the initial complaints of the patient. Once the interviewer determines which diagnoses are highly probable, a systematic line of questioning can ensue. The clinician attempts to address the relevant diagnostic criteria of the highly probable diagnoses. By determining the presence or absence of the various diagnostic characteristics, the clinician is able to rule out possibilities gradually and to narrow the focus of questions to fewer and fewer diagnostic categories and criteria. Thus, rather than asking an extremely wide range of questions or trying to exhaust a list of all possible patient problems, the clinician uses a deduction, or elimination, process to direct questioning toward characteristics of fewer and fewer diagnostic categories. Once the possibilities have narrowed to one or a few categories, the clinician's knowledge of diagnostic criteria and psychopathology associated with particular disorders helps insure that all relevant problems and associated characteristics of a diagnostic category will be addressed. This is not to say that DSM-III is a perfect system or that diagnostic categories are independent of each other. Rather, we are recommending the use of this sytem as a rough guide to direct the early stages of the assessment process.

The assessment of histrionic personality disorder lends itself well to the system discussed above. For example, as we mentioned earlier, patients with histrionic personality disorder are often seen by mental health professionals in connection with suicide attempts and complaints of depression. Given these patient problems, the clinician must initially entertain a wide variety of possible diagnoses (organic affective syndrome, psychosis, major depression, bipolar disorder, dysthymic disorder, cyclothymic disorder, adjustment disorder, personality disorder, etc.). This list of diagnostic possibilities is typically reduced drastically with a few pieces of basic information (e.g., no apparent organic or psychotic signs, depression short-lived and not of a severe nature, depression accompanied by interpersonal problems). By entertaining characteristics of more severe disorders such as organic, affective, and psychotic first, the clinician can logically progress to less severe disturbances which are highly correlated with histrionic personality disorders.

Certain Axis I diagnoses have a high association with personality disorders; thus, when these are present, it behooves the clinician to entertain the possibility of an Axis II diagnosis that is of longer standing than the Axis I diagnosis. Millon (1981) discussed a number of diagnoses that frequently coexist with histrionic personality disorder. They are (1) anxiety disorders, (2) phobic disorders, (3) obsessive compulsive disorders, (4) somatoform disorders, (5) dissociative disorders, and (6) affective disorders. At this level, the clinician is still attempting to discard diagnostic categories by exploring general issues such as the presence of anxiety symptoms or physical complaints. As the assessment process continues, it will become less easy to eliminate diagnostic possibilities totally.

In addition to their high correlation with certain Axis I disorders, histrionic features often appear in mixed personality disorders with features of other disorders such as narcissistic, antisocial, and borderline (Millon, 1981). Therefore, one must assess for characteristics of several disorders. When this point is reached, it becomes important to make full assessment for all symptoms associated with the remaining diagnostic possibilities. Now, rather than eliminating entire sets of questions, the interviewer is asking all questions relevant to the remaining diagnostic possibilities. Thorough assessment for all relevant criteria of the remaining diagnostic categories insures that an exhaustive and complete problem list will, in fact, be obtained.

Along with identifying patient problems, the clinician must define or describe these problems adequately. To define patient complaints, the clinician must be able to describe the problem in a concise and accurate manner. Rather than using broad descriptors such as, "The patient is depressed," or suggesting vague personal characteristics such as impulsivity, more concise and specific problems should be noted. For instance, in the early stages of assessment the clinician might note several examples of a patient's decision-making style which suggest that the patient frequently makes abrupt decisions based upon little data without considering several obvious alternative courses of action. By listing the problem as stated above, rather than by a general descriptor such as "impulsive," the clinician is providing a clearer description of the patient's behavior, thus allowing for a more detailed formulation that will provide obvious and clearcut targets for treatment. Problem lists containing unspecific or highly general problems frequently lead to vague case conceptualizations which do not suggest a specific plan for treatment. Using the above example concerning impulsivity, it might be logical to attribute much of the variance in a problem list to a patient's so-called trait of impulsivity. However, there is no clear-cut treatment of choice for impulsivity. When the problem is expressed in more specific terms, however, clear-cut targets emerge (e.g., failure to generate an adequate list of alternative possible solutions to problems) which suggest a specific skills deficit amenable to problem-solving treatment protocols.

Another aspect of descriptive specificity is to list all problems separately. During the stage of generating the problem list, it may be seriously misleading to assume that any given problem is simply a symptom of a more general problem. For example, delayed sleep onset is frequently associated with depression. Yet, there is a wide variety of reasons for this difficulty (drugs, daytime inactivity and sleeping, etc.). By assuming that sleep difficulties are connected with a patient's report of depressed mood and are thus merely part of a syndrome of depression, the clinician may fail to assess the sleep problem adequately. In short, the clinician should not attempt to formulate patient problems too early, making assumptions based on limited data and speculation. Many problems on the list are likely to be related to a much smaller number of problems. Each must be described in detail before one can make conclusions about the existence of syndromes.

Ten classes of behavior characteristic of a histrionic personality disorder are listed in the DSM-III criteria. Adjectives, rather than behavioral descriptions, are used. If the purpose of the assessment is simply to make a diagnosis, then adjectives might suffice. If assessment is to lead to treatment, and if the clinician expects to be able to demonstrate treatment effects, then adjectives are insufficient. Specific behaviors characteristic of the individual must replace the adjectives. Illustrative samples of behaviors suggesting each of the adjectives listed in the criteria appear in Table 1. The examples, not intended to be an exhaustive list, are drawn from our own clinical work and descriptions we found in the literature (Halleck, 1967; Millon, 1981; Peele & Rubin, 1974; Schmidt & Messner, 1977; Spitzer, Skodol, Gibbon, & Williams, 1981).

Problem definition also requires that the parameters of patient problems be determined. Typical parameters include (1) when did the problem start, (2) what has been the course of the disorder, and (3) what are its possible antecedents and consequences. Again, the emphasis should be on specificity. Vague descriptions of problem parameters such as "I am always anxious" and "I never have any fun" should be avoided. They provide little information. Rather, attempts should be made to pinpoint the occurrence or exacerbation of problems and to quantify their perceived severity. The interviewer should attempt to isolate specific information about when a particular problem started. We gather the immediate history of the current episode of the problems during the problem identification phase of assessment. However, exhaustive histories should be confined to the developmental analysis phase. The reasons for that statement will become apparent in the discussion that follows.

Developmental Analysis

We are using the term *developmental analysis*, rather than *developmental history*, to emphasize how the data gathered during this phase of assessment are to be used. These data will form the basis for analyzing the complex interplay between the patient's behaviors and the major

Table 1. Sample behaviors Representative of DSM-III Diagnostic Criteria for Histrionic Personality Disorder

Criteria	Sample behaviors
Self-dramatization	Indiscriminate use of superlatives Overuse of *always* and *never* Exaggerated laughter Tears come easily Gestures beyond what is necessary to make point Exaggerated gestures Embellishes ordinary descriptions
Drawing attention to self	Turns most topics to discussion of self Dresses to call attention to self Dress is strikingly inappropriate for the occasion Makes inappropriate comments in serious discussions Calls attention to self during meetings by . . . (e.g., rustling papers, giggling or laughing at serious times, arriving late) Uses medical problems to gain attention and strive for attention from physicians
Craving activity and/ or excitement	Content of talk provides exciting stories of past misdeed of others, sexual material, etc. Continues to party after bar is closed and others want to go home Drug use or experimentation Dating or partying at higher frequency than the norm for age group Exposes self to danger unnecessarily Gets agitated when required to perform boring tasks for prolonged periods
Overreaction to minor events	Snaps at employees when delayed or when wishes are not possible Cries at minor disappointments Pouts when others prefer to do something different from patient's desire
Irrational angry outbursts or tantrums	Screams at spouse when unable to reach him or her at time expected Destroys own property when angry Screams at spouse or child when he has hurt himself Storms out of the house when disappointed or contradicted
Perceived as shallow and lacking genuineness	Uses charm rather than substance to negotiate with others Generous with praise Overtly seductive Others sense they are being conned, misled Enters relationships and activities enthusiastically and with promise but does not follow through when durability is required
Egocentric, self-indulgent, inconsiderate of others	Borrows from friends without returning items Breaks dates on whim or if something better comes along Ascribes personally directed malicious intent to child's normal misbehavior

Table 1. (continued)

Criteria	Sample behaviors
Vain and demanding	Frequent attempts to reschedule appointments and accuses professional of not caring about patients when this is not indulged
	Insists on being seen immediately, assuring professional, "You have never seen a case like mine"
	Expects others to rearrange their plans to help patient with minor inconveniences that he or she describes as a crisis
Dependent, helpless, constantly seeking reassurance	Disavows control over temper
	Disavows responsibility for behavior on the grounds, "How could I have done otherwise?"
	Blames others (e.g., parents, spouse) for own psychological problems
	Calls on others to handle situations that could easily be taken care of
	Does not stay alone overnight
	Has lived alone for only very short periods of time
	Frequently elicits approval from others
Manipulative suicidal threats, gestures, or attempts	Takes overdose of pills and immediately calls lover who has threatened to break off relationship
	Cuts wrists superficially when faced with minor disappointment
	Insists, "I can't live without you"
	Insists, "I'd kill myself if . . ."

variables that may influence them. The clinician is not simply gathering a standard set of facts, hoping that some pieces of information will emerge to "explain" the current behavior. Neither is the clinician attempting to write an exhaustive biography of the patient, a mistake commonly made by neophyte therapists. Instead, the purpose is to identify the variables associated with the patient's effective and problematic behaviors.

Some variables are potentially relevant to the developmental analysis for any patient. Informaiton about family background (age of parents at patient's birth, number of siblings, their age and sex, socioeconomic variables during early years, stability of residence, etc.) guides the clinician's search for the types of events and relationships one might reasonably expect to appear later in the patient's history. For example, the patient whose family moved frequently from community to community is not likely to have had the same friends throughout childhood and adolescence. If, however, the patient lived in the same area the whole time but had different friends over the years, the clinician will become curious about why. Did other people consider the patient's behavior so peculiar that they dropped the relationship? That might be the case with a young schizophrenic. Did other people tire of the patient's demandingness and abuse of the relationship? People with personality disorders are likely to have a history of that kind of disruption in their relationships. Educational and occupational variables serve as indicators of the patient's usual functioning and suggest points of change, whether in the direction of improvement or deterioration. The clinician becomes interested in what else was going on at the time when a patient who did well in school up through junior high barely passed high school or quit in the 10th grade. The situation in which a history of mediocre functioning dramatically improved would be of equal interest. What else was happening when this "late bloomer" flourished? The patient's medical history, including any known drugs, can suggest associated limitations or alterations in functioning. The clinician is interested in how the patient and his or her family dealt with medical crises or chronic illnesses. What was happening in terms of other normally occurring developmental events at the time? If there were any unusual stressors in the patient's life, it is important to know about them and to know what was happening with other normally expected events at the time.

Throughout all of the developmental analysis, the examiner is interested in the status of the behaviors contained in the problem list. For example, if mood disturbances are among the current problems, the clinician is curious about what the patient's mold was at various points along the way, especially at times when other variables were going exceptionally well or badly.

Family Background. There is no "typical" developmental profile for individuals with histrionic personality disorders. Descriptions in the literature are inconsistent, further supporting our thesis that the disorder is not a homogeneous one.

Peele and Rubin (1974) describe the typical patient with a histrionic personality disorder as the only or youngest child. The patient is often married to a much older individual, and the marriage is stormy and short-lived unless the spouse is very indulgent. Though earlier years are not recalled by the patient as unusual, the patient may have seemed more dramatic than other children. Unless in a field where modishness or dramatics paid off, the patient is likely to have performed below potential. Overuse of medications or alcohol is highly likely.

Zetzel (1968) suggests different histories for each of the several types of histrionic personality disorders she has seen in her practice. Many of one group were the eldest child, often the most gifted and the father's favorite. They often experienced loss or extended separation from at least one parent around age 4 or 5. Many have made notable achievements in areas other than their heterosexual relationships. The female is often a virgin or has been disappointed in her sexual experiences. On the other hand, the typical patient from another group is the youngest or the only child. She tends to be passive and inconsistent in academic and occupational performance. Friendships are unstable and openly ambivalent. She concludes that the patient from the third group probably experienced separation from at least one parent during the first four years of life. At least one parent had serious pathology, often associated with an unhappy or broken marriage. The patient may have suffered serious and/or prolonged physical illness in childhood. Sustained relations with either sex is absent.

Schmidt and Messner (1977) describe the patient as having been special to someone as a child—often "daddy's little girl" or "grandmother's little princess." The patient frequently describes a parent or some other close relative as having been volatile. Lazare (1971) says that the better functioning woman with a histrionic personality disorder is likely to have had a mother who was consistent, responsible, and engrossed in family life. The patient, however, may describe her as uninteresting, sexually frigid, and ridiculous in her pretense toward desirability. The family is likely to regard the patient as juvenile, inefficient, cute, dependent, and lovable. Halleck (1967) says the patient despairs of finding closeness with her mother during childhood and turns to the father.

Slavney and McHugh (1974) compared 32 patients with primary or secondary discharge diagnoses of hysterical personality (DSM-II nomenclature and criteria) with 32 controls, who were the next admission, matched for sex and age. They examined 50 variables covering reason for admission, family history, and personal history. Only four comparisons yielded statistically significant differences between the groups. Those diagnosed hysterical personality were more frequently admitted because of a suicide attempt and more frequently had a record of previous attempts. They were more likely to report a poor home atmosphere when young, describing their parents as separated, divorced, or having open extramarital affairs or fights. Those who were married at the time of admission more frequently described their marriages as unhappy. They found no differences between their groups with respect to birth order, sexual inhibition and behavior, family or personal substance abuse, frequent or unexplained vague illnesses requiring hospitalization or prolonged treatment, gynecological or other abdominal surgery, or marital status or history.

Apparently, there are few, if any, particular life circumstances that one can predict will be found in the developmental history of a patient with a histrionic personality disorder. It may be that what is missing in the history is more outstanding than what is present. For example, social adjustment during adolescence is usually impaired in the histories of patients with personality disorders. The histrionic may have been very popular, making "friends" easily. Closer examination of the relationships will, however, show that the ability to sustain intimate relationships with others may be absent.

Etiological Hypotheses. Theories about how an individual acquires the disorder or becomes vulnerable to it suggest other questions that might be examined during the developmental analysis. If we are to build a model that describes how a given patient developed the problems currently being exhibited, it is advantageous to know what possibilities have been suggested. Knowledge of psychopathology and etiological hypotheses prepares the clinician to be alert to the evidence presented by the patient under examination.

Biological Hypotheses. Histrionic personality disorders are said to be more common among family members than in the general population (APA, 1980). There is no evidence to support a hypothesis of direct genetic transmission of any of the personality disorders. The possibility of genetic influences does not require direct transmission of a specific disorder. Slater (reported in Shields & Gottesman, 1971), whose sample included monozygotic and dizygotic twins who had living same-sex co-twins, found insufficient evidence for direct transmission of histrionic personality disorders. Yet, almost 50% of the probands in his study had a co-twin who exhibited some psychopathology. Slavney and McHugh (1974) found no statistically significant differences between their two groups in parental drug abuse, alcoholism, or mental illness. They made no comparisons between either of these patient groups and members of the general population, so we do not have evidence for or against high concordance of mental disorders among family members.

The large discrepancy between males and females in the incidence of histrionic personality disorders led earlier workers to look for biological variables in the etiology of the disorder. Chodoff (1982) considered the data on brain and hormonal differences between the two sexes and concluded that there is insufficient evidence to support a biological basis for much of the behavior of women who are diagnosed histrionic. He agreed with Maccoby and Jacklin's (1974) argument that children learn to adapt to social stereotypes that have a basis in biological reality.

Millon (1981) speculates about possible biogenic factors on the basis of types of behavioral responses observed in histrionics. He says such behavior is suggestive of both high levels of energy and activation and of low thresholds for autonomic reactivity. The histrionic's propensity for expressing both positive and negative feelings easily and intensely suggests high degrees of sensory irritability, excessive sympathetic activity, or lack of cortical inhibition. He suggests that a neurally dense or abundantly branched limbic system could result in intensely and easily expressed emotions. Low thresholds for reticular activation may be the substrate for excitability and diffuse reactivity. Other possibilities include ease of sympathetic arousal, adrenal hyperreactivity, and neurochemical imbalances. Millon is careful to point out that none of these hypotheses has been tested. Jordan and Kempler (1970) examined one physiological response system in female undergraduates diagnosed either hysterical personality or not. They found no differences between the two groups in galvanic skin response (GSR) during no threat, academic threat, and sex-role threat conditions; both types of threat produced heightened GSR in all subjects.

Psychoanalytic Hypotheses. Two major psychoanalytic hypotheses have been offered. The first emphasizes unresolved oedipal conflicts, which become prominent during the phallic stage around ages three to five or six. The second emphasizes a fundamental lack of trust developing from the experience of severe maternal deprivation during the oral stage (in the first two years of life) and resulting in repeated unsuccessful attempts to establish intimacy throughout life (Halleck, 1967). Little evidence, other than clinical observation, is offered to support these hypotheses. Lazare et al. (1966, 1970) attempted to differentiate among oral, obsessive, and hysterical personality patterns. They concluded that they had done so, but methodological flaws leave both the internal and external validity of their studies in question. We found no studies that would differentiate among normals, histrionics, and other disorders on the basis of these traits. Neither did we find any studies differentiating various groups of histrionics suggested in the psychoanalytic literature.

Sociological Hypotheses. Several writers offer a sociological explanation for the marked imbalance between the sexes in the incidence of histrionic personality disorders. They propose a variety of cultural factors increasing the probability of histrionic behaviors in women.

Chodoff and Lyons (1958) speculate that histrionic behavior is a caricature of femininity. Chodoff (1982), using historical data, concludes that women are predisposed to histrionic behavior by the roles and expectations placed on them within cultures that regarded them as inferior and subservient.

Halleck (1967) argues that social position requires females to be indirectly aggressive. Therefore, when they are adapting to actual or perceived deprivation of love, they are more likely than males to adopt the highly dependent roles characteristic of histrionic personalities. Men who adopt the same kinds of roles are ridiculed for effeminacy. Consequently, he concludes, social expectations increase the probability that women with this background will become histrionic and that men will become antisocial.

Compton (1974) examined each of seven character traits said to be characteristic of histrionic personalities. She concluded that there is little distinction between histrionic and feminine traits. In each case, she argued for the adaptiveness of the trait in a male-dominated society that considers women inferior.

Indirect evidence, at best, is all that can be gathered to test sociological hypotheses. It is true that not all women in any society have ever been described as histrionic, even though reports such as those of Chodoff and of Compton imply that most, if not all, women have histrionic features. The evidence on sex bias (Warner, 1978) in the differential diagnosis between antisocial and histrionic personality disorders more nearly approaches hard evidence for sociological explanations than anything else reported.

Behavioral Hypotheses. Both the psychodynamic and the sociological hypotheses ascribe a major portion of the variance in behavior to learning. Reich (1950) listed the "character of the persons who exert the main educational influence" (p. 189) as one of two most important conditions for character differentiation. Zetzel (1968) pointed to the significance of the child's effort to gain approval and to avoid disapproval from each parent in developing particular strategies for working out relationships within the family and with others. Halleck (1967) says that the histrionic "learns to approach her father (and later other men) with a fearful and angry demandingness which coexists with her search for love and affection." He adds, "As the hysteric learns to exaggerate her image of irresponsibility, she increases the likelihood that others will take care of her" (p. 753). The authors cited in this paragraph describe histrionic personality disorders as representing maladaptive patterns of behavior to solve problems of living or to cope with interpersonal situations.

From a behavioral point of view, the unit of study in any form of psychopathology is behavior, including cognitive-perceptual activity, emotional responses, overt behavioral responses, and nervous system activity. Behaviorists prefer to look directly for principles of learning involved in the acquisition, maintenance, generalization, and extinction of behaviors unless genetic or constitutional factors can be shown to account for the major portion of the variance in these behaviors (Skinner, 1953). We may use learning theory terminology to reinterpret Halleck's comment, for example. Having others take care of her is a reinforcer for the child being described. Exaggeration of her image of irresponsibility has, in the past, been paired with presentation of this reinforcer and can be viewed as an operant (a means of operating on the environment to elicit reinforcement). As additional pairings between this operant and reinforcer occur, the probability that this class of behavior (exaggeration of her image of irresponsibility) will be emitted to elicit reinforcement (being taken care of) is strengthened. This sequence increases the probability that the operant will be used again.

A learning theory model attempts to explain how behaviors that are emitted by the organism come to serve as operants. If new skills are to be added to the individual's repertoire, they must be shaped by discriminant reinforcement of successive approximations of the desired quality or quantity of behavior; however, each behavior involved has been emitted previously. Discriminant reinforcement increases the probability that the behavior will be emitted again. Noncontingent (nondiscriminant) reinforcement increases the probability of random emission of desired and undesired behavior. The social learning model (Bandura & Walters, 1963) attempts to account for the addition of new behaviors (never before emitted) to the individual's repertoire through vicarious learning from models, literature, television, movies, and so forth.

All except the last of the classes of behavior suggested by the diagnostic criteria for histrionic personality disorder can easily be seen as within an individual's repertoire from a very early age. It is extremely probable that these behaviors are followed by positive consequences from time to time. Even the last, suicidal threats and gestures, is within the realm of possibility when you consider that for most people illnesses and injuries are usually followed by several of what Skinner refers to as generalized reinforcers—attention, affection, submissiveness of others, and sometimes tokens such as gifts. Models for all of the behaviors are certainly available in anyone's environment. Why, then, does everyone not become histrionic? How do these behaviors become characteristic of only a few people rather than everyone? It has been suggested that what appears to be a problem of excesses in behavior, as in histrionic personality disorder, may indeed be a problem of deficits. That is, an inflexible pattern of behavior results from failure to expand one's repertoire of responses. That would represent a skills deficit. Another possibility is that the histrionic behaviors attract other people's attention quickly and dramatically and lead more immediately to whatever the individual is trying to gain from the environment. Nonhistrionic behaviors may be ignored or infrequently responded to in the individual's environment. In this kind of situation, there could be a motivational deficit for using nonhistrionic operants.

Millon (1981) uses learning principles to describe several possible lines of development the end result of which could be a histrionic personality disorder. He offers three features characteristic of the learning history of the future histrionic: (1) minimal criticism or punishment, (2) positive reinforcement contingent upon performance of parentally approved behaviors, (3) irregularity in positive reinforcement. He says these experiences "appear to create behaviors that are designed primarily to evoke rewards, create a feeling of competence and acceptance *only* if others acknowledge and commend one's performance, and build a habit of seeking approval for its own sake" (p. 152). Daily exposure to interactions with a histrionic parent provides modeling for exhibitionistic and dramatic behavior. Sibling rivalries in which cuteness, charm, attractiveness, and seduction are the most effective strategies for securing parental attention increase the probability that such strategies will be used in general. He also points out that aesthetically pleasing girls and likable or athletic boys often learn to rely on these talents for gaining special recognition. The development of other talents is neglected, so that later in life, childish exhibitionism and adolescent and flirtatious styles of relating become predominant. Finally, he suggests that the parents who adopt a laissez-faire policy (because of vacillation in themselves or preoccupation with other matters) do not teach their children stable sets of values. They are likely to produce children who "size up each situation as they face it and . . . guide themselves in accord with the particulars of the situation, and no other" (p. 154). Histrionic patterns of behavior are maintained because the individual's preoccupation with the external world prevents the development of skills for integrating experience and the development of memory traces for evaluating experience.

We employ a biological-behavioral conceptualization. We are acutely aware that in the case of histrionic personality disorder specific empirical support for this hypothesis is little better than for any other. The current evidence is indirect. Turner and Hersen (1980) reviewed studies demonstrating that operant techniques (e.g., contingency management and social skills training) have been employed to modify behavioral deficits and excesses identified as specific to individuals with personality disorders. Bandura and Walters (1963) demonstrated experimentally the acquisition of a number of responses in presumably normal individuals through observational learning. Using a given procedure to modify a behavior does not mean it was acquired that way in the first place. Demonstrating acquisition in a particular manner does not mean that this would account for its generalization or for its becoming a major strategy in one's behavioral repertoire. On the other hand, it appears quite likely that models, extraneous reinforcement, and inconsistent reinforcement have played major roles in developing the behavioral excesses and deficits we find. Our approaches to formulation and treatment are built around hypothesis testing. If our formulation is incorrect, our error is soon uncovered by failure to obtain the expected results.

Interviewing Techniques. So far, we have been describing the content that might be expected to appear in the analysis of the histrionic's history. We now turn to the techniques used in gathering this information. The problem is to gather relevant data, first, to support the diagnosis of histrionic personality disorder and, second, to suggest appropriate treatment. This analysis, important in any case, is crucial for the diagnosis of a personality disorder. The examiner must, by definition, find that the patient's presenting problems are current replications of long-standing behavior patterns and not simply unusual responses to some recent stressor (APA, 1980).

The clinician must take special care in gathering data for the developmental analysis. It is based on retrospective data and subject to all the problems associated with that kind of information. The patient will be guilty of selective memory. How the patient describes past events is highly dependent on how the clinician asks the questions. Questions must be asked in a manner such that the clinician, rather than the patient, makes the inferences about the past. "Tell me about your social life in high school" invites the patient to make several inferences. "Whom did you date?" "What did you do on dates?" "How frequently did you date?" leave the clinician free to draw conclusions about the patient's social functioning and success in maintaining relationships with members of the opposite sex.

The wording of questions must be designed to elicit the kinds of information needed to make the developmental analysis rather than to allow the patient to ramble on with many irrelevant details, however interesting they may be. People with histrionic personality disorders are particularly prone to providing health care professionals with dramatic and exciting stories about whatever the patient thinks the examiner finds interesting (Peele & Rubin, 1974). That, after all, is part of the pathology. It is necessary to allow patients to demonstrate their pathology during the assessment interview. However, once it has been established that dramatic embellishment with little respect for factual information is a problem for this patient, the task of the interview changes. It then becomes essential to control those behavioral excesses and deficits in order to complete the task at hand.

Many clinicians examine each area of functioning separately. That is, they inquire about developmental milestones, medical history, family relationships, educational functioning, and occupational functioning, each as a separate category, and gather all the information they want with respect to one before moving on to the next. We prefer a chronological history to a categorical one. A major goal of the developmental analysis is to establish a time line for the items on the problem list. We are looking for the beginnings, exacerbations, and abatements of these problems over time. We are trying to determine not only the antecedents and consequences of a particular behavior within one category of functioning, but the similarities in antecedents and consequences across problems and years. When we get to the formulation stage, we want to be able to establish whether the behavioral excesses and deficits we have identified represent lack of skill or alterations in motivation. A time line approach gives us a clearer picture of fluctuations than a categorical approach would.

The problem list tells us what areas must be covered in our chronological examination. The histrionic's irrational, angry outbursts are likely to alternate with periods of charm and seemingly genuine concern. Syndenham (cited in Veith, 1977) described this behavioral pattern in 1848: "All is caprice; they love without measure those whom they will soon hate without reason" (p. 26). The goal of a developmental analysis is not simply to document that such swings occurred in the patient's past. Instead, the goal is to be able to make reasonable hypotheses about the circumstances in which the patient exhibits each of these behaviors. We find that a chronological approach offers us a higher probability of discovering the sequences of events that are associated with the fluctuations in these behaviors.

Data from Other Sources

Along with interview data, valuable and often necessary information may be obtained from other sources. Frequent sources of additional assessment data include the following: interviews with persons familiar with the patient, results of psychological tests, direct observation of the patient's behavior, patient recording or monitoring of ongoing events, patient responses to questionnaires and checklists, audio-video recordings of patient behaviors in analogue assessment situations, and psychophysiological procedures. Such procedures often provide corroborative evidence for the data obtained from patient interviews and may provide information that is difficult or impossible to obtain from interview assessment (e.g., the specific antecedents of mood changes).

Our selections among alternative sources for assessment rest heavily on the perceived completeness and accuracy of the data obtained in the clinical interview. In some instances, we may determine that a case formulation can be made based on interview data alone. It is unusual, however, when treatment planning and therapy can be conducted without using some alternative data sources.

Selection involves a variety of issues. The amount of resources such as therapist time and availability of equipment and materials is certainly a major factor. The issue or question that the clinician wishes to assess is equally important. Since assessment methods vary in their ability to address certain questions, the clinician must be aware of which procedure or instrument is best for particular decisions. Frequently, clinicians use particular procedures because of their own familiarity with them. Others use a variety of procedures consistently to provide a large amount of data. The use of multiple assessment methods is viewed as useful and advantageous by many clinicians who advocate a need to obtain redundant validity across sources. Problems arise, however, when methods fail to agree on key issues. Our use of alternative procedures is dictated far less by our fondness for particular methods or a desire to collect vast stores of data. We suggest the use of particular procedures when they are appropriate for answering the questions we could not answer adequately in the patient interview.

There are no procedures which we routinely use with individuals whom we suspect of having a histrionic personality disorder. This is because there are no widely accepted measures of this disorder for either clinical or research use (Pollak, 1981). In fact, most research using standardized psychological tests has not involved the entity of histrionic personality disorder as spelled out in DSM-III. For instance, this diagnostic category was not one of the original criterion groups used in the development of the MMPI. Behaviors that are among the diagnostic criteria for histrionic personality disorders are included in the descriptions for several MMPI profiles, but in no case are enough listed to meet the full DSM-III criteria. Although clinical lore sometimes associates the disorder with a 4–3 MMPI profile, strong experimental support is absent for this claim.

Despite the fact that no test measures the entity as defined, a wide variety of self-report instruments are used to measure the behavior of individuals so labeled. Traditional tests such as the MMPI often yield normative data for assessing the severity of depression, anxiety, or somatization in the histrionic patient. Shorter inventories, such as the Beck Depression Inventory (Beck, 1972), the State-Trait Anxiety Scales (Spielberger, Gorush, & Lushene, 1970), and a variety of marital satisfaction scales are also used to quantify target behaviors. Self-report instruments are also useful in assessing changes of behavior during subsequent treatment.

Behavioral assessment techniques are also frequently useful in assessing specific complaints of histrionic patients. For example, self-monitoring can often provide highly detailed information concerning ongoing behavior. The type of self-monitoring procedure will vary across patients, depending on the particular behaviors you wish to monitor. A sample form is provided in Figure 1.

This particular monitoring form is designed to aid in answering several questions. It can give the clinician an estimate of the patient's activity level, an idea of the types of activities in which the patient engages, a record of social contacts, and an indication of mood changes over time and across situations. This form can be easily modified to include other targets deemed useful for adequate assessment. Anxiety ratings or frequent cognitions can be added as additional categories for recording. The clinician could also elect to record medication intake

Date Time	Activity	With Whom	Mood

Mood rating guide:

        1   2   3   4   5   6   7

worst mood   best mood

Figure 1. Sample self-monitoring form.

or severity of specific physical complaints. The frequency of recording and numbers of categories should be determined largely by the ability level of the patient and by the limitations of the patient's daily routine. The actual selection of categories is, again, based on what targets the clinician determined during interview to be important in the assessment of the patient. The monitoring period should be long enough to allow adequate sampling of the range of target behaviors, and in most cases monitoring should continue until patterns or frequencies of target behaviors are perceived to stabilize. Given the format of the above figure, a monitoring period of one to two weeks would be indicated. Monitoring may be continued throughout assessment and treatment, although there are data suggesting that self-monitoring procedures are susceptible to fatigue effects over periods in excess of three months (Mooney, 1962; Sudman & Lannom, 1978; Sudman, Wilson, & Ferber, 1974).

Since individuals with histrionic personality disorders usually encounter problems in social functioning, procedures other than patient interviews are often necessary to isolate specific deficits and excesses in their interpersonal behavior. Interviews with significant others can often provide valuable data. Again, the need for specificity in questioning must be stressed. The interviewer must elicit detailed accounts of past interactions involving the patient and the significant other. Besides the global content of past interactions, the clinician should attempt to obtain specific descriptions of the patient's verbal and non-verbal communication style (e.g., tone of voice, gestures, eye contact, use of sarcasm). Needless to say, interviews with significant others also provide a sample of the social behavior of individuals with whom the patient interacts.

Analogue procedures involving videotaped role playing are often useful in assessing social functioning. Care must be taken, however, in the selection of scenes used with histrionic patients. Simply using standard scenes, such as meeting a stranger in a dentist's office, may not provide clues to the particular social skills deficits the patient has. For instance, many histrionics perform well in highly superficial social situations. Their inappropriate behavior is more likely to occur in more intimate interactions or in situations wherein they are being ignored or denied a request. Scenes must be selected which represent problem areas in social functioning identified from the interview. By targeting these areas for analogue assessment, the clinician helps insure that a detailed description of social deficits and excesses will be obtained. In some instances, analogue procedures may be enhanced by including significant others in the role play. For example, it might be very useful to observe the patient and spouse in a situation in which strong differences of opinion must be resolved. The optimal situation, of course, is direct observation. This option is rarely available, however.

Formulation

Case formulation is a hypothesis about the acquisition and maintenance of the behavioral excesses and deficits that are interfering with the patient's functioning. A complete formulation requires that all the information gathered during assessment be tied together to present a picture of how the behaviors that resulted in the patient's being in treatment began and are being maintained.

Several conceptualizations of probable causes have been suggested in the etiological hypotheses outlined in the previous section. Genetic formulations examine the involvement of gene-transmitted constitutional differences in predispositions to a category of traits (Kaplan, 1976; McGuffin & Reich, 1984). Biological formulations include genetics but are broader. They examine biological events which may or may not be genetically based. These biological events may include alterations in neurotransmitter functioning, hormonal changes, nervous sytem activity, sequelae of disease or injury, sex differences, endocrine changes, and so on (Ader, 1981; Fowles, 1980). Psychoanalytic conceptualizations focus on influences from the patient's early experiences in the family as the individual develops routine ways of coping with reality (Easser & Lesser, 1965; Reich, 1950). Behavioral hypotheses emphasize learned behavior through classical conditioning, operant conditioning, and social learning (Bandura & Walters, 1963; Skinner, 1953; Turner & Hersen, 1980). None of these hypotheses proposes that the factors being emphasized are the only influences on the behavior of the individual. Multiple causation of behavior is a commonly held assumption. We expect the formulation of any individual case to incorporate data from several domains—biological, behavioral, affective, cognitive, perceptual.

It is important to remember during the formulation phase that causal factors may or may not be equivalent to maintaining factors. One obvious example is that severe acute illness can interfere with a man's sexual functioning. Once the physical crisis has been resolved, the sexual dysfunction should disappear. However, some men, distressed about the loss of function, develop performance anxiety and begin to monitor their performance so closely that the monitoring maintains the dysfunction. One can conceive of a possible example involving behaviors characteristic in a histrionic personality disorder. A person may have acquired manipulation skills of flattery and superficial pampering because these behaviors originally served as operants to assuage a parent with a volatile and unpredictable temper. Negative reinforcement (avoiding or escaping attacks from this parent) maintained the behaviors. The behaviors may have generalized to other situations through intermittent positive reinforcement in that they are often seen initially as attractive by other people. If the person had multiple short-term relationships because of frequent changes of residence and/or serial parents, the opportunity or necessity for learning the skills for sustained relationships may not occur. In this scenario, the behaviors are already being maintained by factors other than the original cause.

Our formulations are an attempt to create a model of the patient's behaviors. We have no evidence that all individuals diagnosed histrionic personality disorder can be represented by any one model. Equally important, the object of the formulation is to dictate treatment, and that requires understanding of the details of the individual case. A global or general model will not suffice for us. We do not expect that the same treatment plan will be appropriate for all histrionics.

Our first step in building the model is to complete the time line that was begun as part of the developmental analysis and to account for all the items on the problem list. Biological factors that may increase the probability that these problem behaviors will be acquired and maintained are noted. Sources of modeling for these behaviors are incorporated into the time line. Types of reinforcement for these behaviors and schedules of reinforcement are included. Sources of limitations on the individual's behavioral repertoires are located on the time line. The fluctuations in behavioral excesses and deficits under particular types of stressors are recorded. The result of this step in model building is a rather complex, detailed picture of each problem, its initiation and the factors associated with its fluctuations. Patterns become apparent. The temporal associations among problems become clear. It is now possible to see which items on the problem list are associated with each other and what the nature of the associations are.

At this point, we can make hypotheses about whether a particular problem is part of a larger syndrome, the consequence of other behaviors, or the antecedent of other behaviors. For example, we said in our discussion of problem identification that it was too early in the assessment to draw conclusions about a problem such as delayed sleep onset. Those conclusions are now appropriate. It should now be clear whether this problem is one of several symptoms of an affective disorder or the result of excessive stimulation from overactivity or drugs, excessive rumination, or uncontrolled anxiety. If the delayed sleep onset is part of a depressive episode, it should also be clear whether the depression is a consequence of the breakup of yet another relationship entered into impulsively without examining the other person's history of disregarding the rights and feelings of others. Such a depression is not unusual among histrionics. If that is the case for a given patient, successful treatment of the personality disorder should eliminate the depression. We would not expect treatment of the depressive episode to eliminate the personality disorder or to prevent recurrence of the depression.

The model for each patient is represented schematically in a diagram. The diagram is a synthesis of the more detailed time line. It summarizes the patterns that recur in the time line. It is a hypothesis about the sequence of conditions and problems that resulted in the patient's being in treatment. A sample diagram will be presented in our discussion of an illustrative case.

The model, as we mentioned previously, will dictate treatment. The point of intervention, if the model is correct, is the earliest step in the model that can be changed. We cannot alter genetic makeup or change an adult's parents (reparenting is not one of our treatment modalities). If, however, we find that the individual's first choice of responses under interpersonal stress is tantrum behavior and that this leads to disrupted relationships which lead to depression which leads to acting out, then we want to increase the patient's repertoire of responses to interpersonal stress. If we find, instead, that the patient's unreasonable demands on relationships lead to interpersonal stress which leads to . . ., then our job is to alter the demands.

The model will not only identify the logical point of intervention, it will identify the independent and dependent variables necessary to test the hypothesis it represents. For example, if the point of intervention appears to be to alter the patient's unreasonable demands in relationships, our problem list, further assessment, and developmental analysis will have operationally defined unreasonable demands. Altering these behaviors will be the independent variable. The dependent variables will be the other complaints and problems. If our hypothesis is correct, these should change in the desired direction as the unreasonable demands are altered and replaced by realistic demands and expectations in relationships. To the extent that we have omitted or distorted relevant information in our observations, we run the risk of developing an inaccurate mode or intervening at the wrong point in the model. One of the maxims we live by is, "It is dangerous to start

treatment without a full assessment." The dangers are symptom transfer, no change or benefit, or exacerbation of the problems that already
exist. Full assessment is defined as a thorough and complete behavioral
analysis. Formulation is the act of interpreting the data from that analysis in terms that can be translated into specific treatment strategies.

ASSESSMENT AND FORMULATION IN THE CASE OF MS. H.

The case synopsis presented at the beginning of this chapter gives
a good overview of Ms. H.'s history and problems. Indeed, the material
provided in that summary is sufficient to make the diagnosis. Our
assignment was to describe our approach to assessment and formulation. Therefore, what follows is a detailed description of the process
we used in our work with this patient. Some redundancy is inevitable.
However, we are attempting to present the reader with as full an account
as possible of how we arrive at our treatment hypotheses.

Identification and Referral Information

Ms. H. was a 32-year-old white, single woman who resided alone
in a condominium which adjoined her mother's residence. She was
currently working as a caseworker in a social agency. The patient referred
herself by telephone contact, with complaints of depression and gastrointestinal distress. She displayed rather strong emotion when stating
her complaint of depression ("I'm not sure I can take it any longer") to
the extent that the psychologist inquired further concerning suicidal
ideation. The patient strongly denied that she actually wished to harm
herself and agreed that she would refrain from making any drastic life
changes or major decisions prior to our visit. Ms. H. said that she had
been given the name of the psychologist by an associate at work several
weeks prior to her contact and that she had never seen a mental health
professional despite past encouragement by her mother and her physician. When asked what prompted her contact at this time, she replied,
"I just felt bad and decided to call." She denied the use of any current
medications.

Comments: These data provide a few basic guides. The patient is
apparently educated, has no previous psychiatric contact, is holding a
job, and is purchasing a home. This suggests that she probably possesses
strengths in terms of adequate intelligence and adaptive functioning.
Such data point away from severe pathology of psychotic proportions.
Complaints of depressed mood and GI complaints are associated with

a wide variety of psychopathology (i.e., affective disorders, anxiety disorders, somatoform disorders, personality disorders, substance abuse, adjustment disorders, psychological factors affecting physical illness, factitious disorders). At this point in the assessment process, the clinician should entertain all these possibilities for the sake of thoroughness. The fact that significant others have encouraged treatment in the past suggests that the patient has experienced significant, possibly similar, psychological problems before. Demographic data raise a noticeable question about why a 32-year-old woman is unmarried and living in close proximity to her mother. These data are particularly suggestive of a long-standing personality disorder and/or difficult life circumstances which may have created adjustment problems. Some of the patient's interaction style with the psychologist also signals the need to entertain a potential personality disorder diagnosis. For example, the patient was emotional and dramatic in describing her complaints. She definitely got the clinician's attention with her implied threat of suicide. The patient's decision-making style in reference to her reason for contact with the psychologist shows a lack of well-thought-out action.

Patient Behavior in the Interview

The patient arrived promptly for the assessment interview. She appeared tense. She immediately volunteered that she had been having second thoughts about keeping her appointment. She added, however, that she had been told by a friend that the psychologist was very good and she had decided to test this claim. Ms. H., an attractive woman, was dressed fashionably but with slight overuse of makeup and jewelry. She wore sunglasses which she removed and held in her hands throughout most of the interview. She smiled almost constantly at the beginning, but her affect became more appropriate as the interview continued. Her behavior was rather seductive at several points in the interview (i.e., she made intense eye contact while smiling, then looking away). She was cooperative in answering questions. However, she often went into great detail, giving unsolicited but related information in responding to questions. The interviewer had to interrupt her responses on several occasions. She also made repeated attempts to explain or justify episodes of her behavior that were brought out during the interview. Most of her explanations for unpleasant experiences involved how other people had let her down or had otherwise behaved inappropriately. References to illness and physical distress were offered to excuse poor

.performance in certain situations; for example, "I can't function well prior to my period."

Problem Identification and Definition

The initial part of the interview was used to allow the patient to elaborate on her presenting complaints. Her depressive moods were described as having been short-lived but frequent during the past two months. Her "bad moods" typically lasted several hours, but they occasionally lasted as long as a couple of days. She was uncertain about antecedents (time of day, situations, monthly period) of her depressed mood although she agreed she generally felt better when she was active and felt worse when she was around her mother. When asked to identify any significant life event approximately two months ago, she volunteered that she had ceased dating a boyfriend of 6 months. She also admitted experiencing depressive episodes at other times in her life. She reported "crying episodes" during the past few weeks. Mild insomnia was mentioned as a chronic condition since childhood. She denied any change in its frequency or severity during the past few weeks. She reported no change in appetite or weight. Other complaints included boredom, a low tolerance of frustration, and frequent feelings of anger. Ms. H. acknowledged a decrease in daily activities and a reduced level of interest in hobbies and work. Social activities, in particular, were at low frequency and all of those involved her mother. She reported no dating in the past two months. Ms. H. expressed doubt and pessimism about her plans for the future. Although she endorsed suicidal ideation ("I felt like jumping off a bridge"), she reported the frequency as low. She reported no previous suicidal attempts, but she admitted having threatened suicide during past disputes with other people.

Ms. H. also presented with complaints of frequent gastrointestinal pain and diarrhea. While describing this chronic condition, she recounted that at least two physicians had diagnosed her problem as due to tension. Tranquilizers had been prescribed several years ago, and these helped the condition for a short while. The frequency and severity of her GI complaints were reported to have increased during the past four to six weeks. She agreed that she had been more tense and agitated in general during the past few weeks. The tension and agitation were described as restlessness, racing thoughts, quick to feel upset or frustrated. She vacillated between tears and anger. She had frequent thoughts of her own, and others', failures. Other somatic complaints included tightness in her chest and tachycardia. Again, she expressed uncertainty about antecedents to her increased tension. She did recount that her latest bout of extreme agitation and somatic distress followed an argument with her mother. She also suggested that her tension was associated with her "bad moods" and with her monthly period.

Given the apparent lack of social activity, attention was given to aspects of Ms. H.'s current social functioning. She admitted that she was having problems with her mother. She reported frequent arguments, followed by periods of mutual silence. She acknowledged that she sometimes slammed doors or threw things during these arguments. She stated that her mother was bothersome and complained that her parent often meddled in her affairs. Her mother, a divorced woman of 51, had been married only once, for 4 years, to the patient's father. She was currently involved with a married man she had been seeing for several years. She worked as a secretary for a governmental agency. Ms. H. described her mother as moody, selfish, and hostile. She did admit, however, that her mother was sometimes helpful and attentive during times when Ms. H. "felt bad." Ms. H. stated that her major reason for living in her current situation (i.e., in a condominium adjoining her mother's residence) was financial. She added emphatically, "If I were better off, I would move immediately." She demanded to know if the interviewer thought that her mother was her main problem and if moving would solve her problems.

Ms. H. reported few if any social contacts other than her mother and the people she interacted with at work. She stated that she rarely interacted socially with people from her office. She revealed a dislike for most of her fellow employees. She described several of the female employees as inferior to her in terms of their choice of dress, their family backgrounds, their choice of conversation topics, and so on. She stated that she did not get along well with most of the women at work. She attributed this to the women's jealousy of her, especially because of her ability to elicit attention from male supervisors. She also spoke poorly of her male supervisors and co-workers. She said that some of the men at work had made sexual advances toward her, but she insisted that she could never allow herself to become involved with "men of their type." She spoke in derogatory terms about the people her agency served (i.e., poor, black), constantly referring to their inferior breeding and life-style. Ms. H. described her job as unsatisfactory in general and suggested that this could be her major problem.

Ms. H. insisted that she had grown apart from the friends she once had. She said that her friends of the past had either moved away or had gotten married and experienced big life changes. She expressed feelings of being different from most people she encountered. She considered herself to be more honest and consistent in behavior than most other people. She admitted that she was possibly too outspoken to suit most people's taste. She described her relationships as disappointing, overall, and expressed confusion in trying to understand the behavior of other people. She insisted that she often went out of her way to please others, particularly men, but that people rarely returned her efforts. Ms. H. had much difficulty in describing what she expected from her social relationships, especially in regard to heterosexual relationships. Most of her descriptors involved such qualities as good humor, excitement, sensitivity to her needs, a desire to please her, good financial status, artistic interests.

Comment: This part of the interview reveals a number of current problems which are listed in Table 2.

Problems 1 through 11 would suggest that Ms. H. is experiencing mild to moderate levels of depression. It would appear that her depression was triggered by a breakup with her boyfriend and is possibly being maintained by her current life-style and circumstances, for example, decreased activity, no dating, problems with mother. Problem number 13 (GI complaints) seems to be related to periods of high arousal which in turn appear to be related, again, to the above-listed life circumstances. These periods of high arousal resemble episodes of anger

Table 2. Problem List for Ms. H.

1. Depressed mood	21. No friends
2. Crying episodes	22. Seductive
3. Delayed sleep onset	23. Manipulative suicide threats,
4. Lowered frustration tolerance	tantrums
5. Frequent angry feelings	24. Overly dramatic expressions of
6. Boredom	emotion
7. Reduced activity level	25. Outspoken, overly opinionated
8. Reduced social activities	26. Unrealistically high expectations in
9. Reduced interest in usual activities	relationships
10. Suicidal ideation	27. Difficulty in understanding or
11. Uncertainty about self and future	predicting others
12. Increased tension and/or agitation	28. Makes fast decisions based on
13. Increased GI problems	limited data
14. Tachycardia	29. Blames others or illness for
15. Tightness in chest	difficulties
16. Problems with mother	30. Often sees self as different,
17. Problems with men	sometimes better than others
18. Problems with social contacts	31. Dissatisfied with living arrangements
19. Problems with co-workers	32. Dissatisfied with job
20. No dating	33. Dissatisfied with social relationships

or frustration rather than intense anxiety. Ms. H. does not seem particularly distressed about her physical complaints (GI symptoms, tachycardia, tightness in chest) and does not appear to be so impaired by their presence that she is missing work or using illness as an excuse to avoid socializing.

One of the most striking aspects of the problem list is that the patient does not appear to be functioning well socially with anyone. This is, by far, the strongest evidence we have at this point for a potential diagnosis of a personality disorder. Coupled with this alienation is the fact that the patient views her interpersonal difficulties as the fault of others. She refused to entertain the notion that she may be behaving inappropriately. Instead, she would suggest that everybody else is to blame for her interpersonal difficulties. Indeed, virtually every problem listed which involves probable social skills deficits on the part of the patient was inferred by the interviewer. These inferences were based on the patient's descriptions of her social interactions and on her behavior during the interview. The patient's history of social behavior should be of prime importance during the developmental analysis. Specifically, the interview should address whether or not the patient's social problems are of long standing. If so, the interviewer must determine the factors which are relevant to their cause and maintenance.

Other key concerns in the developmental analysis should be the patient's history of depressive episodes and physical illness. In addition, since the problem list does contain symptoms which are associated with anxiety disorders (i.e., GI distress, agitation, tachycardia, tightness in the chest), the interviewer should entertain the possibility of long-standing problems with anxiety.

Developmental Analysis

Ms. H. was an only child whose parents divorced when she was less than a year old. She knew little if anything about her father. She was told, at age 10, by her mother that he traveled extensively as part of his job and that his involvement with another woman had prompted her parents' divorce. Ms. H. stated she was close to her mother. She was also close to her maternal grandparents, who lived nearby. They visited regularly and assisted Ms. H. and her mother financially.

Ms. H. described her mother as a highly emotional and opinionated individual. She stated that her mother had "spoiled" her and tried to give her everything she desired as a child. She stressed that her mother was a very responsible parent who put much effort into teaching Ms. H. how to "think and behave properly." She explained that her

mother "planned all her activites" during her childhood and early adolescence. Although her mother worked part-time as a secretary, she
consistently altered her work schedule to maximize her time with her
child. Throughout Ms. H.'s childhood and early adolescence, her mother
had only infrequent social contacts with female friends. She dated
rarely. Ms. H. recounted that her mother, in fact, often complained of
the shortcomings of men.

Ms. H. insisted that she had responsibilities early in life. She had
chores around the house and was encouraged to manage her own money.
She described herself as an obedient child who was rarely punished.
When punishment occurred, it consisted of loss of attention. She
responded with tantrums followed by pouting. Overall, she described
her early history as "happy, except during the occasions when my
mother was in one of her moods."

Ms. H. reported that she was very active socially in high school.
While making above-average grades, she participated in a variety of
extracurricular activities, e.g., was a member of social clubs and a cheer-
leader. She started dating at age 15 and dated a wide variety of boys
throughout high school, although she never dated any individual on a
steady basis during her teen years. She admitted that she experienced
problems with her female peers, insisting that they were jealous of her
popularity with teachers and male peers. She did insist that she had
one or two close female friends with whom she remained close until
her midtwenties. She described her friends as less attractive, less popular, than she was. She said she taught them things.

Following graduation from high school, Ms. H. entered an out-of-
state university. She said she was unable to complete her freshman
year because of illness, that is, repeated infections and GI distress. She
returned home and worked at a state agency job which was arranged
by her mother's boyfriend (a married state official). She was unable to
recount details of her first few months of college but admitted that she
was not pleased with her choice of universities. She particularly did
not like her fellow students. She returned to college the following year
at a university located close to her hometown. She described her subsequent college experience as positive overall. During her sophomore
year, she had her first steady boyfriend and her first sexual experiences,
which she described as initially satisfying. Her first steady boyfriend
was a university athlete whom she described as being from a good
family but lacking in "desirable social graces." They engaged in numerous joint activities during the first several months of their relationship.
As time went on, however, she perceived a decrease in his concern for
her and her desires. She responded with episodes of anger and by

frequently refusing to participate in things he wanted to do (parties, sex). Their relationship lasted approximately two years and ended because of his involvement with another woman. She denied significant depression after their breakup. Specific questions about her behavior at the time, however, suggested that she may, indeed, have been depressed. She endorsed having had decreased activities, social withdrawal, and increased GI problems. These symptoms apparently lasted at least six months subsequent to her breakup.

Following graduation from college, Ms. H. took her first job acquired by her own efforts. It was in a state agency. Her postgraduate work history has included jobs in three state agencies. Although she reported that most of her job changes had involved moves for more money and/ or higher rank, she admitted that her latest change had been prompted by problems resulting from her involvement with a male supervisor.

During the next several years, Ms. H. dated on a sporatic basis. She tended to alternate between periods of active dating and sexual activity and periods of relative social inactivity. Again, on the basis more of behavioral descriptions than her own admissions, it would appear that Ms. H. had experienced frequent episodes of depression which were consistently associated with decreased social activity. Her history of heterosexual involvement appeared particularly related to her depression behavior. Almost without fail, her most severe depressive episodes followed breakups in heterosexual relationships of moderate duration, that is, a few months. Ms. H. stated that she became very tense and irritable during these episodes. Her GI complaints increased, and she found it difficult to motivate herself to get out of bed each day. She reported almost constant crying episodes during periods when she was alone. It was during one of these more severe episodes about five years before that she had bought her condominium adjoining her mother's residence. She denied any connection between these events and protested that her purchase was strictly a financial move to gain tax benefits from owning her own home.

When asked to recount details of her past heterosexual relationships, Ms. H. spoke very negatively of the men with whom she had been involved. She consistently pointed to their inadequacies and failures as the reason why she was unable to continue her involvement. She implied that she had attempted to help each of them to better himself (offering suggestions for personal growth and exposure to cultural activities). None of them had appreciated her concern. There was considerable variability in the backgrounds and occupations of her men (a businessman, a student, a professor, a fellow caseworker). However, two of the four individuals with whom she reported having been the closest were married during the period of their involvement. Her most recent relationship was with a man who was legally separated. She met this man at a local crafts fair, and she initiated their first interaction. She described in detail her initial infatuation and the exciting first three weeks of their relationship. Again, however, she recounted that despite her constant efforts to please the man, he soon became selfish and unconcerned with her needs or desires. Ms. H. confessed that it was he who suggested that they should break up. She responded with a rather ambiguous suicidal threat which apparently delayed the split for a few weeks. Their relationship lasted approximately six months, after which he returned to his wife.

Comment: Ms. H. has a long-standing history of interpersonal difficulties. Both of her major complaints, depression and GI distress, appear to be related to periods of interpersonal unrest. Her developmental account does not tend to support a prolonged anxiety disorder. It would appear that Ms. H. has not experienced a wide variety of severe physical complaints throughout her life, ruling out a somatization disorder. Her social history suggests that she possesses many skills appropriate for superficial interactions but has difficulty in sustaining prolonged and intimate relationships, particularly with men. Ms. H. clearly meets the criteria for histrionic personality disorder and evidences features of narcissistic and (to a lesser degree) dependent personality disorders.

Further assessment should be done to obtain normative data on her level of depression and to provide a baseline. The mother's role in Ms. H.'s social development is evident. Direct information from the mother may prove valuable. The hypothesis that the patient's GI distress and depression are related to interpersonal distress and inactivity should be tested further by having the patient monitor these symptoms along with her daily activities and social interactions.

Further Assessment

The severity of Ms. H.'s depression was assessed further with the Beck Depression Inventory (BDI; Beck, 1961). Her responses suggested that she was experiencing mild to moderate levels of depression. Her responses were consistent with interview data regarding parameters of depression (sleep problems, crying episodes). She denied suicidal ideation at the time of completing the questionnaire. The BDI was chosen because it requires little time for administration and provides normative data on depressive symptoms. Furthermore, it is well suited for repeated administrations and allows for monitoring of depressive symptoms over time.

With permission from Ms. H., a brief interview as conducted with her mother. Her mother appeared well dressed, outgoing, and articulate. She talked constantly and was very opinionated concerning Ms. H. She stated her support of her daughter's pursuit of therapy and added that she had attempted several times in the past to persuade her to follow this course. She said that she had talked with Ms. H. almost daily since she moved into an adjoining condominium. She admitted, however, that recently she had become reluctant to call her daughter because of her frequent angry outbursts. She mentioned an incident a few days prior to the interview. Apparently, in the middle of a conservation, Ms. H. threw a flower pot across the room, in the general direction of her mother. When asked about the subject of their conservation, the mother reported that they were talking about the men Ms. H. had chosen to date in the past few years. In particular, they were discussing the shortcomings of her most recent boyfriend when Ms. H. allegedly told her mother to "shut up" and threw the flower pot. The mother's presentation of this and other scenarios was dramatic. She protested that her daughter's behavior was extremely inappropriate in light of the fact that what the mother was saying about these men was true.

Much of the developmental information given by Ms. H. was corroborated by her mother's report. The mother insisted that she had done her best to raise and care for Ms. H. She stated that she had attempted to be especially sympathetic to her daughter's problems during the past several months. In general, she, too, attributed the interpersonal difficulties encountered by Ms. H. to others.

Self-monitoring procedures involved the patient's hourly recording of her activities, social interactions, mood, and GI distress. Ms. H. complied with this procedure for only five days. On day six, she chose, instead, to write lengthy narratives about her daily experiences. These entries contained dramatic accounts of her negative interactions with her coworkers, mother, and a male telephone contact. When asked why she discontinued the monitoring procedure, she replied, "It was boring." Although only a few days of prescribed data recordings were obtained, the data suggested that her depressed mood and physical distress were negatively correlated with her general activity level and positive social interactions. They were positively correlated with unpleasant social contact.

Comment: A baseline level of mild depression was documented. Along with corroborating the patient's developmental account, the mother confirmed her influence on the development and maintenance of the patient's style of social interaction. Self-monitoring procedures added support to the hypothesis that both the patient's depressed mood and GI distress were associated with activity level and social reinforcement. Her noncompliance suggested that she was easily bored with routine activities.

Case Formulation

Ms. H.'s early history suggests that as an only child and grandchild she received a high level of reinforcement from her mother and grandparents. She was showered with attention and special favors from a mother who adjusted her work schedules and social life to remain in constant contact with her child. This high level of reinforcement provided by her mother proved extremely effective in motivating Ms. H. to adopt the beliefs and behaviors which her mother advocated and modeled. In fact, Ms. H.'s early behavior so closely resembled her mother's that the possibility of inherited characteristics cannot be excluded. Certainly, the absence of her father (who may have had a few characterological problems of his own) only added to the strength of her mother's influence. Her mother spent much time instructing Ms. H. in so-called proper social behavior. Many of these skills (proper dress, easy conversation, etc.) appear appropriate and were socially reinforced. However, there was a clear tendency toward excess in behaviors which would later be labeled as seductive. Along with these behaviors, the mother modeled and reinforced extreme demands for attention and compliance from others. When Ms. H. failed to receive a desired response from her mother or others during her childhood, she responded with manipulative displays of anger (tantrums). If this was not effective, she responded by withdrawing socially and remaining inactive for short periods of time (pouting). Since she did manage to get her way on an inconsistent basis with these tactics, the use of these behaviors was powerfully reinforced by an intermittent schedule of reinforcement.

Ms. H.'s mother both lacked close involvements with other adults and chose to remain very close to her daughter throughout the grade-school years. This close friendship with her mother appeared to be the primary source of social reinforcement for Ms. H. during this time. This state of affairs also served to maintain many of her earlier inappropriate social behaviors, for example, displays of anger and social withdrawal when denied attention or requests by others. Her superficial social skills were effective in gaining acceptance for her in extracurricular school organizations and activities. Her only substantial friendships, nonetheless, were with two girls who, possibly because of their lack of popularity and physical attractiveness, chose to tolerate the opinionated comments (and other excesses) of Ms. H.

Her early dating history shows a pattern of short-term dating without sustained or intimate involvement with any one individual. Again, this pattern demonstrates that her looks and superficial charms were effective, but her lack of skills, particularly her excessive demands for attention and social reinforcement, prevented intimate or sustained involvement. Certainly, her mother's constant complaints about men during Ms. H.'s childhood did not promote heterosocial attachment. Given her mother's strong support and her success in the above social situations, Ms. H. was able to maintain an acceptable level of reinforcement throughout high school.

Her personality disorder became a problem for her, however, when she moved out of state to attend college. Removed from the support of her mother, she was unable to obtain the high level of social reinforcement to which she was accustomed. Relying on previously reinforced patterns of behavior, she responded to others' lack of attention with anger and social withdrawal (pouting). This resulted in an extended period of heightened arousal, causing her first episode of GI distress. When repeated attempts failed to elicit high rates of attention and support from her peers, Ms. H. experienced her first significant depression and chose to withdraw permanently from this environment and return home. Once again in close proximity and frequent contact with her mother, Ms. H. managed to obtain adequate social reinforcement, and her symptoms of depression and somatic distress subsided. This consequence of her behavior, however, provided added reinforcement for her social skills deficits.

Ms. H. experienced her first sustained heterosexual involvement during her sophomore year in college. As with previous relationships, she initially used her superficial skills to obtain high levels of social reinforcement and attention from her boyfriend. At the same time, she significantly decreased her contact with her mother. With the passage of time, however, her boyfriend began to reinforce these superficial skills at lower rates. Ms. H. responded to this decrease in reinforcement by increasing her demands and acting out to gain attention. This behavior led, in turn, to increased tensions in the relationship and eventually to its termination, which was accompanied by GI symptoms and depression. Ms. H. increased her interactions with her mother and easily gained support and comfort through those contacts. This pattern of behavior toward men has been consistent, with minor variations, throughout all her heterosexual relationships. Each time the cycle occurs, it appears to end with increased somatic complaints and depression. Her current

GI distress and depression are no exception. The mother's role in supporting her daughter's maladaptive social behaviors is also obvious across the various relationships.

A summary of this pattern of behavior is diagrammed in Figure 2. Factors in the patient's early history which are hypothesized to have shaped an inappropriate style of social interaction are outlined. These factors are also seen as influencing her methods for solving problems. These patterns of thinking and behaving continue to be reinforced by the patient's mother. Her social skills deficits and problem-solving methods are causing interpersonal difficulties with everyone with whom she interacts. She responds to her interpersonal difficulties with autonomic arousal and withdrawal from others. Her high level of autonomic arousal and her lack of social contact, with a subsequent decrease in reinforcement, result in her present complaints of depression and somatic distress.

TREATMENT

There is no widely accepted treatment for histrionic personality disorder. The clinical literature contains a limited number of treatment accounts and no controlled outcome studies. Theoretical arguments have suggested preferences for either psychoanalysis or behavior therapy, but empirical support remains lacking.

Moskovitz (1976) sought the commonalities among several published reports claiming some degree of success in treating patients with histrionic personality disorders. The approaches included short-term insight-oriented (anxiety-producing) psychotherapy (Leibovich, 1974), behavior modification (Kass et al. 1972), and informational-educational treatment (Halleck, 1967; Peele & Rubin, 1974). He found that the authors (1) define the goals of therapy explicitly to the patient from the start, (2) focus on the here and now, (3) advocate relatively brief therapy, (4) specify a carefully designed structure controlled by an active therapist, (5) provide the patient with personal feedback, and (6) use the patient's relationships as the focal point of therapy. Unfortunately, data do not exist to allow for isolation of the most effective components or to specify particular changes produced in patients as a result of these general treatment strategies.

Our approach to treatment would suggest that there is no treatment of choice for patients with any particular diagnosis. Individual variations in symptoms within diagnostic groups, not to mention the variations in causal and maintaining factors, would dictate that treatment

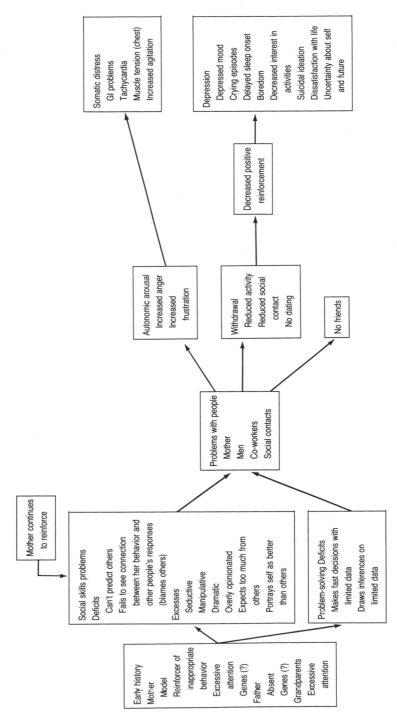

Figure 2. Diagram of the formulation for Ms. H.

programs must be tailored to fit a particular patient. This is not to say we believe in using psychoanalysis for some patients and behavior modification for others. We do not change our theoretical orientation according to patient types. Instead, we employ the same empirical approach in treatment that we use in assessment. Behavior (motoric, biological, affective, cognitive-perceptual) remains the unit of study and the target for change. Treatment planning involves construction of an individualized program which specifies which behaviors are targeted for change and describes the procedures best suited for producing the desired change.

Targets for treatment are dictated by a detailed and concise case formulation. The case formulation illustrated previously in Figure 2 shows a variety of potential targets for intervention. Using this case as an example, we could select several behaviors from numerous problem areas, increased anger, GI distress, reduced activites, the tendency to be overly opinionated. Indeed, a choice can be made to intervene directly with practically all the problems listed in the case formulation. Such an approach might be viewed as thorough but certainly time-consuming. A more efficient method would be to treat problems which the formulation identifies as most important or influential in relation to all other problems. Again, using the diagram of the sample case formulation, we see a progression of problem areas with arrows suggesting that problems further to the left side lead to problems toward the right. Such a chain of events suggests that greater impact will be realized if change is produced in areas designated as being earlier in the chain. Conversely, changes produced in targets on the far right should produce the least beneficial effects. In the case of Ms. H., our formulation suggests that only temporary or partial relief of the patient's presenting complaints would be obtained by intervening directly on these symptoms; i.e., somatic distress and depression. Moving a bit further toward the left of the diagram of problem areas, we see that intervention might be aimed at decreasing autonomic arousal and increasing activities and social reinforcement. This point of intervention also has its shortcomings as can be seen from the repeated attempts of the mother of Ms. H. to relieve her daughter's distress. The mother's ability to intervene successfully, which has diminished over repeated episodes, produces only a temporary effect and serves to reinforce other maladaptive behaviors which occur earlier in the formulation. The major point we are making is that initial targets for treatment should be those designated as early as possible in the chain of problems in the case formulation. This is the point at which the greatest impact can be made in the most efficient and effective manner. In the case of Ms. H., the formulation would dictate intervention directed at changing long-standing social interaction skills and problem-solving methods. It would also suggest that an outside factor, the behavior of the mother toward Ms. H., is also a major target for change.

Once the initial target areas for intervention have been chosen, the task becomes one of selecting the most appropriate therapy procedures. In selecting specific behavioral change techniques, therapists often make use of a wide variety of procedures described in clinical treatment literature. Many published protocols exist which are designated as treatment programs for specific disorders. Packaged training programs abound for problem areas such as social skills, assertion, self-management and self-control, and problem solving, to name a few. Although these prescribed programs may prove useful in providing ideas for treatment planning, we do not recommend their general use. Again, we stress that treatment procedures must be tailored to the specific needs of the patient. Borrowing basic paradigms and methods (e.g., counterconditioning, modeling) from published works is acceptable. When using these techniques, however, the therapist should use material (examples, subjects of conservation, stimuli for hierarchies) which are highly relevant to the patient being seen. In the case of Ms. H., a broad-based social skills program would not be our choice for intervention for her social skills deficits. We would certainly borrow a variety of general procedures (modeling, shaping, self-monitoring, videotaped role-playing), but the specific training materials and particular sample situations chosen for use in her therapy would be based on her past and, particularly, on her present life circumstances. We believe that the use of material highly relevant to the patient helps to insure that the patient will recognize the subtleties of the problem at hand and that this promotes generalization of therapeutic gains to the patient's daily functioning.

A final issue is patient motivation for treatment. It goes without saying that if a patient fails to comply with treatment demands treatment will be of little benefit. We do not assume that all of the responsibility for treatment compliance rests on either the patient or the therapist. We do believe that both must contribute substantial energy and expertise. For the therapist, the most crucial aspect of ensuring patient compliance in treatment is to make certain that an accurate assessment and case formulation is obtained. This is true for several reasons. First, the therapist's presentation of a detailed and convincing formulation helps assure the patient that the therapist is, in fact, competent to handle the problems involved. Second, a detailed formulation clearly spells out the targets for change and allows for a more obvious and precise therapy contract between patient and therapist. Finally, a detailed assessment and formulation informs the therapist of how others have successfully motivated the patient. This knowledge often proves essential in keeping the patient in treatment as well as increasing the probability of compliance with treatment.

REFERENCES

Adams, H. E. (1981). Abnormal psychology. Dubuque, IA: William C. Brown.

Ader, R. (Ed.). (1981). Psychoneuroimmunology. New York: Academic Press.

American Psychiatric Association. (1968). Diagnostic and statistical manual of mental disorders (2nd ed.). Washington, DC: Author.

American Psychiatric Association. (1980). Diagnostic and statistical manual of mental disorders (3rd ed.). Washington, DC: Author.

Bandura, A., & Walters, R. H. (1963). Social learning and personality development. New York: Holt, Rinehart, & Winston.

Beck, A. T. (1972). Depression: Causes and treatment. Philadelphia: University of Pennsylvania Press.

Beck, A. T., Ward, C. H., Mendelson, M., Mock, J., & Erbaugh, J. (1961). An inventory for measuring depression. Archives of General Psychiatry, 4, 561–571.

Blinder, M. (1966). The hysterical personality. Psychiatry, 29, 227–235.

Brantley, P. J., & Sutker, P. B. (1984). Antisocial behavior disorders. In H. E. Adams & P. B. Sutker (Eds.). Comprehensive Handbook of Psychopathology (pp. 439–478). New York: Plenum Press.

Chodoff, P. (1982). Hysteria and women. American Journal of Psychiatry, 139, 545–551.

Chodoff, P., & Lyons, H. (1958). Hysteria, the hysterical personality and "hysterical" conversion. American Journal of Psychiatry, 114, 734–740.

Compton, A. S. (1974). Who's hysterical? Journal of Sex and Marital Therapy, 1, 158–174.

Easser, B. D., & Lesser, S. R. (1965). Hysterical personality: A re-evaluation. Psychoanalytic Quarterly, 34, 390–405.

Forrest, A. D. (1967). The differentiation of hysterical personality from hysterical psychopathy. British Journal of Medical Psychology, 40, 65–78.

Fowles, D. C. (1980). The three arousal model: Implications of Gray's two-factor learning theory for heart rate, electrodermal activity, and psychopathy. Psychophysiology, 17, 87–104.

Halleck, S. L. (1967). Hysterical personality traits: Psychological, social, and iatrogenic determinants. Archives of General Psychiatry, 16, 750–757.

Hendler, N. (1981). Diagnosis and nonsurgical management of chronic pain. New York: Raven Press.

Jordan, B. T., & Kempler, B. (1970). Hysterical personality: An experimental investigation of sex-role conflict. Journal of Abnormal Psychology, 75, 172–176.

Kaplan, A. R. (1976). Basic human genetics. In A. R. Kaplan (Ed.), Human behavior genetics (pp. 5–32). Springfield, IL: Charles C. Thomas.

Kass, D. J., Silvers, F. M., & Abroms, G. M. (1972). Behavioral group treatment of hysteria. Archives of General Psychiatry, 26, 42–50.

Lazare, A. (1971). The hysterical character in psychoanalytic theory—Evolution and confusion. Archives of General Psychiatry, 25, 131–317.

Lazare, A., Klerman, G. L.., & Armor, D. J. (1966). Oral, obsesssive, and hysterical personality patterns. *Archives of General Psychiatry, 14,* 624–630.

Lazare, A., Klerman, G. L., & Armor, D. J. (1970). Oral, obsessive, and hysterical personality patterns: Replication of factor analysis in an independent sample. *Journal of Psychiatric Research, 7,* 275–290.

Leibovich, M. A. (1974). Short-term insight psychotherapy for hysterical personalities: Stages of the therapeutic process. *Psychother Psychosom, 24,* 67–78.

Lion, J. R. (1978). Personality disorders. In G. U. Balis (Ed.), *Clinical psychopathology* (pp. 333–357). Woburn, MD: Butterworth.

Luisada, P. V., Peele, R., & Pittard, E. A. (1974). The hysterical personality in men. *American Journal of Psychiatry, 131,* 518–521.

Maccoby, E. E., & Jacklin, C. N. (1974). *The psychology of sex differences.* Stanford, CA: Stanford University Press.

Marmor, J. (1953). Orality in the hysterical personality. *Journal of the American Psychoanalytic Association, 1,* 656–671.

McGuffin, P., & Reich, T. (1984). Psychopathology and genetics. In H. E. Adams & P. B. Sutker (Eds.), *Comprehensive handbook of psychopathology* (pp. 47–75). New York: Plenum Press.

Merskey, H., & Trimble, M. (1979). Personality, sexual adjustment, and brain lesions in patients with conversion symptoms. *American Journal of Psychiatry, 136,* 179–182.

Millon, T. (1981). *Disorders of personality.* New York: Wiley.

Mooney, H. W. (1962). *Methodology in two California health surveys.* (PHS Publication No. 942, Public Health Monograph No. 72). Washington, DC: U. S. Government Printing Office.

Moskovitz, R. A. (1976). Epithelializing an epithet: Therapies of the hysterical personality disorder. *Diseases of the Nervous System, 37,* 65–67.

Peele R., & Rubin, S. I. (1974). The hysterical personality: Identifying and managing one of the problem patients of medical practice. *Southern Medical Journal, 67,* 679–682.

Pollack, J. M. (1981). Hysterical personality: An appraisal in light of empirical research. *Genetic Psychology Monograph, 104,* 71–105.

Reich. W. (1950). *Character analysis.* London: Vision Press.

Schmidt, D. D., & Messner, E. (1977). The female hysterical personality disorder. *Journal of Family Practice, 3,* 573–577.

Shields, J., & Gottesman, I. I. (1971). *Man, mind, and heredity: Selected papers of Eliot Slater on psychiatry and genetics.* Baltimore: The Johns Hopkins Press.

Skinner, B. F. (1953). *Science and human behavior.* New York: The Free Press.

Slavney, P. R., & McHugh, P. R. (1974). The hysterical personality. *Archives of General Psychiatry, 30,* 325–539.

Spielberger, C. D., Gorush, R. L., & Lushene, R. E. (1970). *Manual for State–Trait Anxiety Inventory (Self-Evaluation Questionnaire).* Palo Alto, CA: Consulting Psychologists Press.

Spitzer, R. L., Skodol, A. E., Gibbon, M., & Williams, J. B. W. (1981). *DSM-III case book: A learning companion to the diagnostic and statistical manual of mental disorders.* Washington, DC: American Psychiatric Association.

Stephens, J. H., & Kamp, M. (1962). On some aspects of hysteria: A clinical study. *Journal of Nervous and Mental Disease, 134,* 305–315.

Sudman, S., & Lannom, L. A. (1978). *A comparison of alternate panel procedures for obtaining health data.* Urbana-Champaign, IL: University of Illinois Survey Research Laboratory.

Sudman, S., Wilson, W., & Ferber, R. (1974). *The cost-effectiveness of using the diary as an instrument for collecting health data in household surveys* (Report to the Bureau of Health Services Research and Evaluation). Urbana-Champaign, IL: University of Illinois Survey Research Laboratory.

Turner, S. M., & Hersen, M. (1981). Disorders of social behavior: A behavioral approach to personality disorders. In S. M. Turner, K. S. Calhoun, & H. E. Adams (Eds). *Handbook of clinical behavior therapy* (pp. 103–124). New York: Wiley.

Veith, I. (1977). Four thousand years of hysteria. In M. J. Horowitz (Ed.). *Hysterical personality*. New York: Jason Aronson.

Warner, R. (1978). The diagnosis of antisocial and hysterical personality disorders. *Journal of Nervous and Mental Disease, 166,* 839–845.

Winokur, G., & Crowe, R. R. (1975). Personality disorders. In A. M. Freedman, H. I. Kaplan, & B. J. Sadock (Eds.), *Comprehensive textbook of psychiatry* (Vol. 2). Baltimore: Williams & Wilkins.

Wittels, F. (1930). The hysterical character. *Medical Review of Reviews, 36,* 186–190.

Zetzel, E. R. (1968). The so-called good hysteric. *International Journal of Psychoanalysis, 49,* 256–260.

Zisook, S., & DeVaul, R. A. (1978). The hysterical personality: I. The healthy hysteric. *British Journal of Medical Psychology, 51,* 363 368.

Zisook, S., DeVaul, R. A., & Gammon, E. (1979). The hysterical facade. *American Journal of Psychoanalysis, 39,* 113–123.

7

GERIATRIC ORGANIC SYNDROMES

The Case of Mrs. R.

Mrs. R. was a right-handed, 78-year-old, white widow who lived alone in a small southeastern community. She had a high school education and had completed two years of college with a major in history. She had been widowed since 1965, after having been happily married to a prominent attorney and politician for 37 years. Her son died of cancer in 1968; her 45-year-old married daughter lived in another city, approximately 250 miles away.

The Referral

Mrs. R. had been admitted recently to a short-term psychiatric unit of a private general hospital for evaluation and possible placement in a long-term care facility (e.g., nursing home). Referral information cited episodes of possible delirium, primarily during evening hours while in the hospital (i.e., "sundowning"), as indicated by disorientation, memory disturbance, and "wandering the halls." Data sources also revealed increasing social isolation, possible delusional and/or hallucinatory phenomena, and mood disturbance. A recent CT scan, however, showed only mild cerebral atrophy. In light of these data, the patient was referred by her attending physician for neuropsychological and behavioral evaluations in order to clarify and validate functionally the provisional diagnosis of primary degenerative dementia, senile onset, and to offer placement recommendations.

Physical Appearance

Mrs. R. presented as a relatively well developed, healthy, elderly Caucasian woman of average height and weight who was in no apparent distress. Personal hygiene was adequate and she was dressed appropriately in a brown, flowered dress. The patient also wore subtle make-up, five gold and silver rings, and earrings which complemented her attire and her short, silver-gray hair. Mrs. R. walked with a cane and wore bifocal glasses with a hearing aid over the left ear. Medical records cited moderate hearing impairment and a 70% loss of vision in the right eye. Besides arthritis and mild hypertension, no other health problems were recorded.

Presenting Complaints

Mrs. R. reported initially, "I wound up in the psycho ward because my daughter thinks I'm not able to take care of myself. How would she know, I only see her once a year." Apparently, this first psychiatric hospitalization was prompted when the patient's maid contacted the daughter after she found Mrs. R. lying on the floor, disoriented, sobbing, and seemingly intoxicated.

Mrs. R. said that since her husband's death in 1965 she has lived alone in the family house. She reported feeling "unable" to part with the house and its "memories." Prior to her husband's death, Mrs. R. said, she was a "very active" woman, involved primarily in community activities (e.g., garden club), raising children, and entertaining her husband's professional and political acquaintances. After his death, however, "things really began to change. For one thing, I found out who my real friends really were." Specifically, she said, friends and acquaintances, particularly those who were still married, "seemed to begin avoiding me and seemed uncomfortable" even during casual, informal meetings (e.g., at church, at the market). "After the funeral, the only real friends I had left were a few widows like myself." She cited two widowed friends in particular who offered her much support and who were "good coffee mates" during subsequent years. Mrs. R. indicated, however, that in 1980 her best lady-friend passed away,and another widowed friend was forced to move to a distant city to live with her children.

Since that time, Mr. R. has had few regular social contacts, except for a maid who "visits" (i.e., cooks and cleans) twice a week for four hours each day. "I even stopped going to church, because I couldn't hear what they were saying and because I would get these funny feelings that people were saying bad things about me and my husband." She explained, "As the years go by, I trust fewer and fewer people. . . . I'm not even sure about my family anymore." Finally, she admitted, "The only place I feel safe is at home."

It was noted that Mrs. R. was not a member of a seniors group and had no close relatives in the immediate area. Leisure activities were also reported to be minimal. Mrs. R. found reading "too difficult" because of the vision problem. "Even listening to the radio is a chore— I can't hear what they are saying half the time and besides, what I do hear I don't like . . . it bothers me and it scares me." Although once an avid seamstress, she has had to discard this activity because of arthritis and poor vision. "I guess I spend most of my time just thinking."

Mrs. R. reported memory problems which "have really gotten worse" in the last two years: "I've gotten terrible with names. I forget addresses and phone numbers, and I even forget the names of my grandchildren!" The patient also reported "not being concerned enough" to remember days or weeks. It was interesting to note, moreover, that during informal memory testing on the Mental Status Examination, the patient remarked, "This isn't interesting enough to remember . . . tell me a good sexy story instead."

In regard to possible hallucinatory activity, Mrs. R. reported "hearing funny things all the time: I try to ignore them, but they're there a lot of the time." Specifically, she described hearing (1) voices talking to her, (2) music and "beating," and (3) "motors running."

Mrs. R. reported a long history of moderate alcohol consumption. "I began drinking with my husband and especially during our many parties." Prior to this hospitalization, the patient was consuming approximately two to three ounces of vodka per day—"It's the one thing I have to look forward to." She also reported the "occasional" use of several prescriptions for "nerves" and "trouble sleeping." "My doctor says to take one when I need it."

The patient also admitted to feeling depressed: "I think I've been depressed since my husband died. . . . I think I've learned to live with it, though."

Parents

She described her father as an "old southern gentleman and a fairly wealthy lawyer for those days." Mrs. R. indicated that she had been very close to her father, who was "always loving" and supportive and "always took care of his family." Her mother was described as a "socially conscious but very loving" woman who was "very committed to her family and her husband." Both parents were described as moderate users of alcohol. Although no family history of psychiatric illness was indicated, the patient cited "one uncle and one aunt" whom she considered alcoholics.

Interview Behavior

Mrs. R. was very cooperative and displayed a good sense of humor throughout the interview. Even at her advanced age, she exhibited a reasonable energy level and a certain zest. Because of her hearing impairment, however, questions had to be expressed loudly and in short, concise sentences to maximize comprehension. It was notable that she was easily distracted by extraneous stimuli, including a running fan (which she described as frightening), fluorescent lighting, and people conversing in the hallway. It was also necessary at times to refocus the patient's attention on the interview because she appeared preoccupied; on two occasions, refocusing was achieved only by calling her name loudly and by the use of touch.

7

Formulation of Geriatric Organic Syndromes

VICTOR J. MALATESTA

INTRODUCTION

Biobehavioral disorders associated with advanced age have received scant systematic attention in the behavior therapy literature. Although the feasibility of a behavioral approach to the unique problems of later life has been supported and demonstrated repeatedly (Barnes, Sack, & Shore, 1973; Cautela, 1966, 1969; Cohen, 1967; Hoyer, 1973; Hoyer, Mishara, & Riedel, 1975), these proposals have been embraced by only a handful of clinical scientists. Even today, O. R. Lindsley's important treatise, *Geriatric Behavioral Prosthetics*, published in 1964, remains generally unknown to the scientific community. Behaviorally oriented writers such as Cautela and Mansfield (1977) and Richards and Thorpe (1978) later attempted to organize efforts in the geriatric domain, but, as was the case with earlier endeavors, their impact on the field of behavior therapy was modest at best.

In response to society's growing awareness of the "Graying of America," however, psychology has begun to address its role in the field of aging, as indicated by the recent "Older Boulder" conference (Santos & VandenBos, 1982; see also Poon, 1980). Within the area of behavioral psychology, perhaps our most celebrated researcher and

VICTOR J. MALATESTA • The Institute of Pennsylvania Hospital, University of Pennsylvania School of Medicine, Philadelphia, Pennsylvania 19139 theorist has joined the ranks of senior citizens, and he too is now directing his expertise to the challenges faced by older adults (Skinner, 1983; Skinner & Vaughan, 1983). In conjunction with these developments, recent work by Hussian (1981), Lewinsohn (Lewinsohn & Teri, 1983; Lewinsohn, Teri, & Hautzinger, 1984), and others (e.g., Patterson & Jackson, 1981) is fostering a recognized and, finally, utilized behavioral psychology of aging. Even the 1984 edition of the *Annual Review of Behavior Therapy* makes mention for the first time of this growing interest in the field of aging (Wilson, Franks, Brownell, & Kendall, 1984).

Data available on behavioral geriatrics, however, tend to mimic mainstream behavior therapy with its often naive technological approach to intervention in which a targeted problem (e.g., anxiety) is simply matched with a specific behavioral technique—one typically employed with and developed upon younger adult populations (e.g., relaxation training). Behavioral efforts have also avoided systematic inquiry regarding the relationship between age-related cortical-sensory changes and environmental factors on information-processing skills and their potential psychopathological concomitants. The powerful behavioral tool of functional analysis, therefore, has not been applied to the organic brain syndromes of later life. Furthermore, a focus on formulation of complex geriatric disorders from a scientific behavioral perspective, one that is operationally sensitive to the interplay of organic, environmental, and person variables, has been conspicuously absent. Using the presented case as a vehicle, this chapter will attempt to illustrate the process and procedures of behavioral formulation as relevant to the conceptualization, clinical experimentation, and consequent treatment planning of particular cases involving organic brain syndrome. Before proceding with the case, however, early discussion will focus on the problem of geriatric avoidance in clinical psychology and on the prerequisites for accurate behavioral formulation of clinical geriatric cases. Pertinent issues of the aging process and response-system idiosyncrasies of older men and women will also require initial attention.

The Problem of Geriatric Avoidance

Scientific and clinical avoidance of geriatric problems is not unique to behavior therapy but is clearly a characteristic of clinical psychology in general. Related health fields, such as medicine and social work, although sharing a modicum of geriatric ambivalence, have demonstrated concerted development in the field of aging. Even experimental psychology, with its hybrid empirical perspective, has shown systematic interest and growth in the multidisciplinary field of gerontology (e.g., Birren & Schaie, 1977; Botwinick, 1978). With few exceptions, however (e.g., Gentry, 1977; Lewinsohn et al, 1984; Storandt, Siegler, & Elias, 1978), clinical psychology has been slow to have a notable impact upon the multiple biomedical and psychosocial needs of our older women and men, whose numbers are increasing rapidly. Even a cursory review of the major journals in clinical psychology indicates that not a single periodical is devoted exclusively to the problems of aging (APA has recently announced the publication of a new generalist journal, *Psychology and Aging*, which is forthcoming in 1985). Moreover, a major journal for behavioral outcome research, *Behavior Therapy*, issued by the Association for the Advancement of Behavior Therapy, published only three articles on aged patients between 1975 and 1980, "and in none of the studies were the unique issues of treating elderly patients discussed" (Steuer & Hammen, 1983, p. 286). As a consequence, the interested scientist-practitioner must necessarily venture outside the domain of clinical psychology and consult specialized sources in those fields cited above, that is, medicine (*Journal of the American Geriatric Society*; *Journal of Geriatric Psychiatry*), social work (*Journal of Gerontological Social Work*), experimental psychology (*Experimental Aging Research*), and gerontology (*Journal of Gerontology*, *The Gerontologist*). Finally, it should be noted that two new journals on aging have appeared, and although both are targeted for a wide practitioner audience of several mental health professions, each provides an important data source for the clinical geropsychologist (*Clinical Gerontologist*, *International Journal of Behavioral Geriatrics*).

Several explanations can be offered to account for clinical psychology's slow involvement in the field of aging. Most important, a very strong aura of therapeutic pessimism continues to dominate the thinking of researchers and clinicians alike in their attempts to understand and manage the unique problems of later life. A still stronger pessimism is associated with therapeutic efforts to help older men and women who are regarded as "brain-damaged," as the labels of senility, dementia, and organicicity obviously imply. In dealing with older patients, brain-impaired or not, it is tempting to conclude that treatment is nonfruitful (e.g., Wershow, 1977). Often this conclusion represents a lingering remnant of traditional psychoanalytic thinking, which posited that older patients were unsuitable candidates for psychologically based treatment, that is, unsuitable for psychoanalysis—the then dominant therapeutic model that still, today, requires mammoth investments of time and money, two commodities which older people possess in only limited quantities. In other cases, this conclusion is based upon the continued reliance on "custodialism" (Kahn, 1977), the predominant model of geriatric mental health care that reflects strong negative expectations and self-fulfilling prophecies about aging. Custodialism, as the term implies, is a highly fatalistic and regressive therapeutic approach to which the majority of our extended care facilities (e.g., nursing homes) continue to subscribe (see Kahn, 1977, for an interesting exposé).

A closely related reason for clinical psychology's geriatric pessimism concerns the fact that, until recently, most data on older adults were derived from institutionalized state hospital patients who typically displayed long histories of severe mental disorder with continued hospitalization (Barry, 1977). Because of the well-known iatrogenic effects of long-term institutionalization (Ullman & Krasner, 1975), a highly distorted and pessimistic picture emerged which then portrayed older people as helpless, dependent, and nonresponsive to therapeutic effort. It was not reasoned that relatively healthy, noninstitutionalized older adults, who, incidentally, represent the great majority of our elderly population, might present a different and more positive picture. The absence of age-appropriate assessment techniques and the dearth of relatively brief but effective treatment strategies, together with the absence of a true-life-span developmental psychology, make it not surprising that traditional clinical psychology has been slow to develop the specialty of clinical geropsychology, as intended by Gentry (1977) and others (e.g., Lawton & Gottesman, 1974).

A Reorientation

In order to confront the problem of geriatric avoidance and to develop a fruitful investigative plan, we must address two problems. First, it is necessary to overcome our therapeutic pessimism, which is deeply rooted in a Cartesian dualism and which prevents us from conceptualizing geriatric disorders, particularly the organic syndromes, from an active behavioral perspective. This mechanistic or dichotomous way of thinking, which has been questioned only recently by our medical colleagues (see Engel, 1977), isolates the biophysical from the psychological realm of experience and dictates that morphological changes in the brain due to aging exert a purely unidirectional and noninteractive effect on the behavioral, cognitive, and emotional aspects of daily functioning. Seemingly organic behavior, such as disorientation, memory dysfunction, and paranoid beliefs, are thus conceptualized as simple manifestations of cortical degeneration and neuronal cell loss which typically accompany aging (Brody & Vijayashankar,

1977). Appropriate treatment, when feasible, must therefore be directed at affecting brain integrity, directly (e.g., midbrain shunting to relieve hydrocephalus) or indirectly (e.g., choline acetyltransferase administration, hyperbaric oxygen therapy). However, since biomedical therapeutic technology in the area of brain degeneration remains in its infancy, available treatment usually involves palliative care, medication to control emotional behavior, and ultimately institutional placement.

Beginning with Rothchild's early work (1941), however, accumulating data have seriously challenged the validity of the dualistic notion and have demonstrated that a circular or interactive model may be most appropriate in understanding and managing the complex biobehavioral disorders associated with aging (Bakal, 1979; Ernst, Beran, Safford, & Kleinhauz, 1978, Hussian, 1981; Schwartz, 1982). In this model, a one-to-one relationship between organic deterioration and behavioral-cognitive change is not assumed and instead represents just one possibility. Investigative focus is directed alternatively at intervening variables which may interact with cortical status to produce onset and/or maintenance of characteristics common to organic brain syndrome. As will be discussed later, such variables may include sensory changes, attention deficit, environmental isolation, and iatrogenic drug effects. Using this interactive model, morphological change alone is not always sufficient to produce functional impairment unless mediated by environmental changes and/or cognitive and behavioral variables. These factors may ultimately compromise cortical integrity, thus "causing" functional deficits which would otherwise not be manifested given morphological change alone (see Ernst et al., 1978).

A second area of discussion emphasizes the required capabilities, coordinated efforts, and multidiscipline input necessary for effective evaluation and management of geriatric biobehavioral syndromes. For no other age group is the importance of a well-organized, interdisciplinary team approach more appropriate. Moreover, it does not suffice that each team member do his or her "own thing" in the geriatric arena; rather, each professional must be thoroughly familiar with the respective fields and be able to impart the mechanics and purposes unique to their expertise. Interdisciplinary communication and exchange are thus primary goals. Although the clinical psychologist is not typically designated the geriatric team leader by the health care system (this may be changing, at least in the area of chronic pain management; see Tollison, 1982), it is often the psychologist who is delegated to a position of decision making (i.e., formulation), particularly regarding thorny cases of differential diagnosis and treatment (e.g., dementia versus depression, organic versus functional psychosis). To fulfil this role successfully, he or she must understand, evaluate, and synthesize data from numerous sources. The clinical psychologist must also be cognizant of the various patterns of aging—not only chronological aging as reflected in biological maturation and degeneration, but also psychological and behavioral aging (e.g., response style, sensory thresholds, changes in coping resources), and social aging (e.g., retirement, widowhood; see Eisdorfer, 1969). Since these types of aging rarely coincide, the process of data integration and decision making becomes even more complicated.

Thus, to assess, formulate, and manage successfully the syndromes of later life requires a working knowledge in (a) the biomedical substrates of aging; (b) neuropathology and radiographic imaging techniques (e.g., computed tomography); (c) psychopharmacology, especially geriatric idiosyncrasies in drug absorption, elimination, potentiation, and so forth; (d) life-span developmental theory; (e) neuropsychology; (f) rehabilitation (e.g., physical therapy, cognitive retraining, self-care skills training); (g) the range of social services and habitational placement possibilities (e.g., home health care, congregate housing); and (h) sociocultural specificities (e.g., ethnic and religious concerns). Although this list of knowledge areas is staggering in many respects, two areas of clinical psychology, namely, behavioral medicine and neuropsychology, have already demonstrated that similar data integration, team utilization, and decision making are both possible and productive. Moreover, the emerging field of lifespan developmental psychology is gaining momentum and is thus offering an integrated framework and guiding perspective with which to conceptualize the tasks and challenges of later life (See Baltes & Schaie, 1973; Goulet & Baltes, 1970; Nesselroade & Reese, 1973).

Suitability of a Geriatric Behavioral Approach

Behavioral methods are not totally foreign to geriatric settings. Behavior modification programs, which relied upon token economies and other contingency management techniques, were initially designed to treat institutionalized mental patients. Since these patient-populations typically included a number of older individuals, "quite accidently, psychology acquired a history of successfully treating the aged along these lines [of behavior therapy]" (Gottesman, 1977, p. 5). As noted earlier, behavioral medicine and neuropsychology, the latter of which utilizes behavioral methodology and is beginning to court behavior therapy (e.g., Goldstein, 1979), have already gained a respectable place in the assessment and treatment of health-related disorders, many of which reflect the medical concerns of older adults (Blanchard, 1982; Lezak, 1983). Since older adults account for over 65 percent of health care expenditures in the United States (Pieper, 1977), and since the "most serious medical problems of today that plague the majority of Americans are ultimately behavioral" (Stachnik, 1980, p. 8), it is unavoidable that the older population will fall increasingly under the rubric of behavioral health technologies.

The behavioral approach is ideally suited to a systematic investigation of the organic brain syndromes associated with advanced aging. A primary emphasis on psychiatric diagnosis and inference is avoided, and instead, initial clinical activity is directed at (1) an exhaustive identification and listing of specific problem areas, each of which can be operationalized, and (2) an examination of functional relationships among organic, environmental, and organismic (cognitive, motoric, and autonomic) variables. Subsequently, this information, which is typically obtained from the interview and from other data sources (e.g., medical records, family members, observation), is organized and categorized. Hypotheses are stated, and a tentative formulation is developed which attempts to integrate the data within a unified but testable construct. With the goal of identifying and then validating a behavioral mechanism of the disorder when appropriate (Turkat & Meyer, 1982), the formulation is then tested in the more formal assessment situation, but not necessarily under the guise of a standardized psychometric battery of tests. Rather, tests are selected and mini-experiments are designed to determine the validity of the formulation. When the tentative formulation is not empirically supported, new hypotheses are developed and another formulation is derived and tested. Ultimately, the validated formulation will serve as a guide in developing in individualized treatment plan and in monitoring therapeutic progress and outcome. In contrast to both the psychoanalytic and the organic approach, the behavioral method is action-oriented, specific, optimistic, and inclusive. A strict reliance upon organic mediators as the only possible formulation is avoided, as is a focus on intrapsychic conflict and untestable constructs. Similarly, the approach is more consistent with the immediate needs and distinctive qualities of older adults, the majority of whom prefer a practical and commonsense solution to their problems. Finally, since the behavioral formulation undergoes empirical validation, the information derived can be utilized in understanding similar cases and in designing a systematic research program to investigate particular parameters of the organic brain syndrome.

BACKGROUND I: PRINCIPLES AND ISSUES OF THE AGING PROCESS

The presented case description of Mrs. R. highlights many of the unique challenges which confront today's older women and men. Multiple problem areas, each cutting across organic, psychological, and social boundaries, interact to produce functional impairment of a significant degree to attract the attention of concerned others and to warrant at least temporary placement within a protective environment. In order to appreciate the complex interplay of these factors, it is necessary to embark on a brief discussion of important principles and issues related to the aging process. Subsequently, attention will focus on an overview of geriatric response-system idiosyncracies by employing Adams's (1981) behavioral classification system as a framework.

Demographics

It is widely known that average life expectancy has increased substantially during the twentieth century and that as a consequence older Americans aged 65+ are becoming a more dominant and visible population group in the United States. In 1900, for instance, 4% of the population was over 65 years of age. Today, there are 23.5 million older men and women who now comprise 11% of the population total. Moreover, if present trends continue, the older segment of our society is expected to increase 35%, representing 32 million by the year 2000 (U.S. Department of Health and Human Services, 1980). Unfortunately, although advances in biomedical technology have permitted many people to reach older ages, society has been much slower to come to grips with their psychological, economic, and social idiosyncrasies. Relevant to the presented case, the need situation is undoubtedly more acute for the older woman, for whom widowhood is an epidemiological certainty (Malatesta, 1980 a,b). That is, because of gender differences in life expectancy and because older men show higher rates of marriage and remarriage, older widowed women outnumber widowed men 5 to 1 (DHHS, 1980). As a consequence, there are approximately 7.2 million widows above the age of 65 and fewer than 1.3 million widowers. Widowhood for females is also lengthened by developmental changes in life expectancy which accompany advanced age. That is, although the average age at which widowhood occurs is 56 (Lopata, 1971), fewer than 5% of women ever remarry (Cleveland & Gianturco, 1976), even though at age 65 they can be expected to live at least 17 more years (DHHS, 1980). As a consequence, older women represent a high-risk group for development of biobehavioral dysfunctions since their chances for health problems and stressful life complications (e.g., death of spouse, living in isolation, decreased income, relocation, disability), as well as the duration of such, are so much greater than for men. Not surprisingly, depression has its highest incidence in women 45 years and older (Hendricks & Hendricks, 1977); suicide becomes an increasingly utilized alternative (the elderly represent 31% of recorded suicides in the United States; see Vital Statistics of the U.S., 1974), and organic deterioration becomes a more likely consequence of this advanced age. Still, only 5% of people above the age of 65 are institutionalized (Federal Council on Aging, 1981); the great majority, regardless of their particular liabilities, are community-dwelling, functional adults.

Misconceptions about Aging

There is a pervasive tendency in our society, as reflected in the therapeutic pessimism discussed earlier, to attribute negative characteristics to older people. Similar to prejudice toward other types of minority groups, older adults are chronic victims of stigmatization, or "ageism," which affects virtually every aspect of their lives (Butler and Lewis, 1974). Ageism is displayed in a variety of myths about older individuals and their behavior, ranging from issues about sexual expression (e.g., Malatesta, Chambless, & Pollack, 1983; Pease, 1974; White, 1982) to misbeliefs about activity, health, and learning ability (see Palmore, 1977). Many of these widespread misconceptions have borrowed from traditional media portrayals of the stereotyped elderly person who is seen as feeble-minded, egocentric, and senile. Others are related to (1) our perceptions about the aging process, as derived from our parents' developmental crises, and (2) ambivalent attitudes regarding our own aging which may be less than optimistic. Although geriatric specialists have devoted investigative attention to the problem of ageism (cf. Benedict & Ganikos, 1981), the professional community is unenlightened regarding this attitudinal barrier and thus has been slow to recognize and correct its negative beliefs about older adults.

Individual Differences

One component of the ageism issue is reflected in the widely held belief that older people represent a relatively homogeneous class when compared to younger age groups. In actuality, however, nothing could be further from the truth. When normal individual variability as displayed in early life becomes augmented by the inherent differences in individual aging patterns, the result can be stated as a truism: *Variability increases with age.* Thus, patterns of behavioral, emotional, and physiological function become more diverse and more difficult to predict solely on the basis of chronological age (Barry, 1977). The age variable becomes a decreasingly useful predictive index, and as a consequence, to generalize about older adults represents a risky, error-laden endeavor. Not surprisingly, the clinical implications of this functional variability with age are immense. Assessment devices which utilize normative standards for accurate interpretation become of questionable utility. A technological approach to treatment intervention, already viewed as tenuous with younger age samples, becomes highly inappropriate and counterproductive with older adults. Moreover, group clinical data tend to be cohort-specific, providing at best only a rough and unstable guide for one's attempts to apply specific findings to the individual geriatric patient. As such, the suitability of a behavioral approach to geriatric assessment becomes even more apparent, and the challenge of accurate case formulation becomes more acute.

Research Methodology in Aging

Research in the field of aging can be characterized, on the one hand, by oversimplification and overgeneralization of findings, but, on the other hand, by methodological complexity and profound experimental variability. Regarding the former, the majority of experimental data on aging patterns and behaviors has been derived from cross-sectional studies. In this well-known design, two or more different age groups are compared at one point in time across a specified dependent variable, which might be reaction time, recognition memory, or level of depression. The results of such studies, though often cited as evidence of aging decline and deterioration, actually provide information only relevant to *age differences* on the particular variable. Too often, researchers have viewed such findings as indicative of *age changes.* For example, if memory for a word list decreases systematically across age samples, then this must mean that memory decreases with age. However, this is an unjustified inferential leap since such data tell us only that memory for this word list is different across age groups and is probably more a function of age-group differences in education, response style, and so forth. Furthermore, the results of cross-sectional studies leave unclear whether the obtained effect is a function of (a) the *age variable*—factors related to the aging process and maturation; (b) the *cohort variable* which includes cultural and educational history and essentially covaries with age and time of birth; or (c) the *time of measurement or period variable*, which addresses a potential confusion of age and environmental influences (e.g., measuring widowhood sexuality during a time of sexual permissiveness). Although these effects are concurrent, they do not necessarily represent similar sources of variance.

In order to begin a proper differentiation of these effects and to measure age changes, some researchers have relied upon the longitudinal design which assesses the same subject group over a number of time periods while thus controlling for the effect of cohort. However, the period effect in this design remains confounded with the age variable, and only a time-lag comparison which measures different cohorts at various times can rectify this problem. In an attempt to differentiate more efficiently, Schaie (1965) proposed three different design models, each composed of a varying combination of the cross-sectional, longitudinal, and time-lag designs. A full discussion is beyond the scope of this chapter, but the reader is encouraged to consult Schaie (1965, 1967) as well as other sources regarding experimental design models appropriate for aging research (Baltes, 1968; Baltes & Goulet, 1971; Botwinick, 1978; Wohlwill, 1970).

The important point, however, is that longitudinal studies and other research involving complex design strategies are costly and require tremendous logistical support over several years' duration. Because of such constraints, geriatric longitudinal data are sparse, and the preponderance of cross-sectional studies has been frequently overinterpretated and overgeneralized, thus contributing to the already distorted and incomplete picture of aging behavior. With this in mind, the following section offers an overview of geriatric response-systems which will provide a foundation for analysis and formulation of the presented case.

BACKGROUND II: GERIATRIC RESPONSE SYSTEMS

Biological Response System

Chronological aging is associated with variable but progressive deterioration in all major biological subsystems (e.g., renal, cardiac, pulmonary, hepatic) and in all vital functions (e.g., basal metabolic rate, neural conduction velocity, cardiac output). The various systems age at different rates and are influenced by individual disease processes which are only correlated with chronological age (thus confusing discrimination between normal and pathological aging; see Estes, 1977).

The net result, however, is impaired coordination of physiological and behavioral functions with a progressive decrease in the older person's capacity to (1) adapt and readjust to both internal and external changes that accompany daily activity and ordinary life stresses and (2) mobilize physiological and psychological resources necessary for smooth execution of complex behavioral sequences which require coordinated and sustained input (e.g., physical exertion, problem solving; see Shock, 1962).

Central to age-related changes in the biological response system are cellular death and tissue loss which ultimately may be most deleterious to the central nervous system (Hayflick, 1975). At a biochemical level, neuronal cell loss is exacerbated by decreases in cerebral blood flow and arterial oxygen saturation that are not due to age per se but to arteriosclerotic effects on cerebral circulation and metabolic rate (Strub & Black, 1981). The autonomic nervous system, which also shows age-related alterations, modulates with CNS changes to induce additional disruption and further jeopardize biological, behavioral, and cognitive self-regulation (Frolkis, 1977).

Pharmacological Influences. Within the biological response system, the older individual's potential for disregulation is exemplified by geriatric idiosyncrasies in pharmacological response (Lehmann, 1972). Age-related changes in physiological functions (e.g., reduced renal blood flow, urinary retention, decreased muscle mass) produce idiopathic drug responses, which include alterations in (1) drug absorption rate, (2) drug distribution throughout the body, and (3) detoxification and drug elimination rate. These changes increase the likelihood of drug toxicity and thus may cause or exacerbate (existing) behavioral and cognitive impairments (Hollister, 1977). The presence of physical disease, which may itself produce system disregulation and require corrective medication, can exert an additional effect on drug activity. Moreover, being subject to multiple system pathologies, the older adult is very likely to have many drugs prescribed, thus compounding the difficulties. For instance, one study found that hospitalized medicare patients were receiving an average of ten prescription medications (Fann, 1973). Nonprescription agents such as laxatives, antacids, and aspirin, were not even included in this analysis.

As a consequence, polypharmacy is a constant problem in the elderly which may result in (1) undesirable side effects, some of which may be irreversible; (2) quasi-organic phenomena which further cloud the assessment picture; and (3) misattribution of drug side effects (e.g., hallucinations can be a side effect of benzodiazepine administration in the aged). Paradoxical drug effects are also more common among older adults, and their medication habits reflect a variety of potential problems: omission errors (forgetting to take medication), self-medication ("My doctor says to take one when I need it"), and poor awareness of drug–food and drug–drug interactions which can undermine and/or cancel principle drug action (see Goethe & Penberthy, 1980, and Salzman, Hoffman, & Schoonover, 1983, for thorough reviews on aging and psychopharmacology).

Mention should also be made of alcohol, which is the "foremost substance of abuse" by the elderly and which has just recently attracted investigative attention (Mishara & Kastenbaum, 1980; National Institute on Alcohol Abuse and Alcoholism, 1982; Schuckit, 1977). Not only do older adults display a more variable pattern of alcohol metabolism, but they also reach higher peak blood–alcohol levels as compared to younger people who have consumed similar amounts of alcohol (Vestal, McGuire, Tobin, Andres, Norris, & Mezey, 1977). First, idiosyncratic response to alcohol may interfere with the older person's ability to self-monitor alcohol ingestion in relation to perceived effects, thus increasing the likelihood of overintoxication. Second, prescription medications can be expected to interact adversely with alcohol to produce drug potentiation, toxicity, and a wide range of behavioral effects, which, again, may present as a quasi-organic state. Finally, cortical changes which accompany aging may further potentiate the effects of alcohol and result in confusion and disorientation. Indeed, alcohol-induced organic syndromes have been reported (Butters & Cermak, 1980; Mishara & Kastenbaum, 1980), and studies show that preexisting organic dysfunctions can be exacerbated by any number of chemical substances (Hollister, 1977).

The susceptibility of the biological response system to pharmacological adversities is thus maximized in later life. In essence, the drug variable can operate as a mechanism in cases that present with organic symptomatology. Close examination of pharmacological influences thus represents an important component in accurate behavioral assessment of geriatric brain syndromes (drug assessment guidelines are provided by Hussian, 1981; and Salzman et al., 1983).

The Central Nervous System. Although all somatic cells have a finite life span, it is only the neuron that is incapable of being replaced through cell division (i.e. proliferation). Since the individual neuron is thus subject to the accumulation of intraneuronal metabolic errors which occur naturally over time, "neuronal depopulation," as described by Vogel (1977), appears to be a fact of life. One result is that at age 30 one can anticipate an estimated 0.8 percent annual decrement in total neurons. Forty years later, microscopic analysis of the aging brain may reveal evidence of senile plaques and granulovascular change in the hippocampus and frontal cortex, neurofibrillary tangles, diffuse lipofuscin pigment degeneration, and neuroaxonal dystrophy of the nucleus gracilis (Berry, 1975; Sinex, 1975). Whether or not these changes result inevitably in senile dementia remains an open question which is tempered by Terry and Wisniewski's (1975) conclusion that the difference in the brains of normal and demented elderly is in degree only. Other data, however, raise questions about this conclusion (Ernst *et al.*, 1978; Schneck, Reisberg, & Ferris, 1982; Tomlinson, Blessed, & Roth, 1970). Finally, Botwinick (1981) indicates that, at this time, the favored position is that "the degenerative organic brain state is not part of normal aging and is thus pathological or abnormal" (p. 139).

From a clinical perspective, however, microscopic and histological analysis of brain tissue is usually not feasible. The clinical alternative is to evaluate the degree of cerebral atrophy resulting from neuronal loss and from degeneration of other brain tissue. Although electroencephalography (EEG) continues to be employed as a measure of cortical activity (VanderArk & Kempe, 1973; Wilson, Musella, & Short, 1977), the advent of neuroradiographic imaging techniques, most notable the CT scan (computerized transverse axial scanning) and most recently the PET scanner (positron emission tomography), has revolutionalized the biomedical assessment of geriatric organic conditions (Bondareff, Baldy, & Levy, 1981; Jacoby & Levy, 1980; Jaffee, 1982).

Briefly, the CT scan involves examination of the cranium in successive layers and angles by a narrow beam of x-rays which results in approximately 30,000 readings (taken by each CT detector) which are then computer-processed. Images of the different densities of internal brain structures are provided, thereby permitting visualization of intracranial anatomy. The procedure is safe and noninvasive and provides a reasonably clear measure of cerebral atrophy and other brain changes through images of the ventricles, the bony structures, the brain tissues, the subarachnoid spaces, and of any collections of blood or tumor mass in most cases.

There are organic conditions, however, in which the CT scan as well as other biomedical procedures are not effective in assessment (See Wells & Duncan, 1977). Moreover, measures of cerebral atrophy bear a variable and inconsistent relationship to the degree of behavioral and cognitive dysfunction observed (Marquez, 1983). Neuropsychological assessment, therefore, represents a viable adjunct which has gained prominence in recent years (Albert, 1981; Filskov & Boll, 1981; Golden, 1981; Lezak, 1983; Parsons & Hart, 1984). The techniques of neuropsychological assessment will be discussed later, and the reader interested in neuroradiology is referred to Gonsalez, Grossman, and Palacios

(1979), Hanaway, Scott, and Strother (1979), and Traveras and Wood (1976).

Organic Brain Syndromes and Organic Mental Disorders. In light of demographic changes in life expectancy discussed earlier, the diagnosis of an organic disorder is an increasingly common clinical problem in geriatric settings (Mortimer & Schumann, 1981). Although the DSM-II (American Psychiatric Association, 1968) definition of organic brain syndrome was overly restrictive (Fauman, 1977), DSM-III (APA, 1980) has broadened the general category of organic disorders by making a distinction between organic brain syndromes and organic mental disorders. This diagnostic distinction, however, is based entirely upon etiology. That is, *organic brain syndrome*, of which there are ten different kinds, refers to a constellation of behavioral and cognitive symptoms *without reference to etiology*. In contrast, the term *organic mental disorder* is used to designate specific organic brain syndromes in which the etiology is known or presumed (See Parsons & Hart, 1984; Steel & Feldman, 1979 for detailed explanations). Included under this category are primary degenerative dementia (Alzheimer's disease), multi-infarct dementia, and the substance-induced withdrawal/intoxication states.

In actual clinical practice, the differentiation between and among organic brain syndromes and organic mental disorders is often confused, even though a few research studies have reported that accurate classification is possible (e.g., Seltzer & Sherwin, 1978). As a consequence, use of a nonspecific diagnosis such as organic brain syndrome or dementia often remains the rule rather than the exception. Moreover, diagnosis of an organic mental disorder, such as primary degenerative dementia of the Alzheimer's type (which is the most common of the dementias), can only be confirmed in autopsy when pathognomonic changes in brain tissues are demonstrated. Thus, in clinical practice, this becomes a presumed diagnosis or diagnosis by exclusion, that is, when all other possibilities in diagnosis have been in some way eliminated. The diagnostic picture becomes even more complex and imprecise when we note that in the later stages of disease process most degenerative conditions cannot be functionally distinguished (See Lezak, 1983). Still, research and discussion in this area abound (Coyle, Price, & DeLong, 1983; Glenner, 1982; Miller & Cohen, 1981; Schneck et al., 1982; Storandt, 1983; Wells, 1979), and increasing attention has focused on the syndrome of pseudodementia and its differentiation from other organic conditions (Caine, 1981; Malatesta, 1985; McAllister, 1983).

Most important, however, clinical diagnosis of geriatric organic disorders should not be regarded as the end point in the assessment process, as it is often assumed to be. Rather, in light of the diagnostic difficulties and uncertainties which beset this area, behavioral analysis and specific problem listing offer a less pessimistic approach which is more sensitive to accurate case formulation and active treatment planning. In this manner, our clinical attention is focused on concrete problem areas and related intervening variables which can be operationalized and manipulated, thereby generating a testable formulation from which to design a practical intervention strategy. In contrast, to focus on an ambiguous organic diagnosis only blinds us to treatment possibilities while "absolving the caretaker from the responsibility of actually providing therapeutic treatment for the elderly patient" (Ernst et al., 1978, p. 469).

Perceptual and Motor Response Systems

In his behavioral classification scheme, Adams (1981) defines the perceptual and motor response systems as activities involving detection, recognition, and discrimination of environmental stimuli, as well as the motor behaviors necessary to act upon and modify stimulus input. Although variability remains the norm, the aging process tends to exert a uniformly progressive effect upon all sensory subsystems (e.g., vision, audition, pain), such that acuity becomes dull, thresholds rise, and discrimination becomes increasingly more difficult. Aging research in perceptual-motor behaviors, however, has concentrated primarily on age differences and not on age and maturational changes. Similarly, relevant data are often confounded since a variety of other factors tend to modulate with and intensify pure age effects (e.g., age-related hearing impairment and degree of lifetime noise exposure).

From the perspective of sensory reception, the older adult, in effect, is gradually cut off from the world and yet is expected to maintain function despite an increasingly deprived and distorted stimulus environment. Within the visual mode, for instance, near-distance sight becomes progressively impaired (presbyopia), and the lens of the eye gradually yellows and clouds, thus causing complicated problems with lighting (e.g., glare, dark adaptation) and color discrimination (e.g., colors at the dark end of the spectrum, blue, green, and so on are filtered out). Hearing loss is initially more pronounced with high-frequency sounds (presbycusis) but gradually includes frequencies within the range of speech (Bergman, 1971). The perception and comprehension of speech becomes even more compromised with the presence of background noise or other distractions to which older persons are more susceptible (Elliott, 1982). Moreover, hearing impairment has been shown to generate paranoia in the experimental situation, and this finding has special relevance to older adults (Zimbardo, Andersen, & Kabat, 1981). Although governed by many factors (e.g., medication, cigarette smoking), the other senses show similar age decrements, and as a consequence foods lose their flavor, erogenous tissues exhibit decreased sensitivity, odors may be less reliably identified (e.g., the smell of something burning in one's home), and a decreased sense of balance and proprioception becomes a growing problem. Gross and fine motor movements as well as complex psychomotor behaviors (e.g., operating an automobile) reflect similar age-related deterioration which is compounded indirectly by common disease processes associated with aging (e.g., arthritis). Indeed, motor disturbances tend to produce restrictions in ambulation—thus further curtailing the potential stimulus environment of the older adult (See Birren & Schaie, 1977; Botwinick, 1977, for comprehensive reviews of aging and perceptual-motor changes).

Age-related changes within the perceptual-motor response systems may have far reaching implications for the development of psychopathology in the elderly. Ernst and his colleagues (1978, 1979), for instance, have paralleled the progressive sensory-motor restrictions and perceptual isolation of the aged to the well-known effects of sensory deprivation demonstrated in the experimental situation (Hebb, 1955; Heron, 1957; Zubek, 1969; Zuckerman, 1979). Citing a variety of animal and human data, they argue that stimulus isolation can result in morphological brain changes which then may result in additional alterations in behavior.

Since external stimuli become less readily available and/or distorted, and because one's active attempts to seek and attend to such stimuli are repeatedly punished, it is reasonable to argue that attending behaviors may be gradually extinguished over time. As a consequence, it is possible that internal sources of stimulation, which remain more readily available (thoughts, images, somatic responses), gain greater relative salience, thus affecting in a negative manner the process of information selection (see next section). However, with restricted external feedback by which to validate and correct the meaning of internally produced stimuli, the likelihood of cognitive and somatic distortion is considerably enhanced.

It is not surprising, therefore, that for the sensory-impaired elder a deprived stimulus environment can function as a breeding ground for depressive symptomatology, paranoid reactions, confusion and disorientation, and other maladaptive behaviors. Indeed, the "sundowning" effect, which is characterized by night-time confusion and agitation, is due in part to the decreased availability of familiar stimulus input associated with the evening hours. Under normal daytime conditions, environmental input serves an orienting function for the individual, and cases of sundowning have been remediated by simple provision of a night-light. Finally, it is not surprising that the sundowning effect tends to be more common, as well as more pronounced, in unfamiliar environments (e.g., hospitals, nursing homes).

Age-related alterations in this area also have a variety of practical implications for therapeutic design of "prosthetic" environments, the goal of which is to maximize sensory opportunities, minimize sensory-motor liabilities, and thereby facilitate functional adaptations to these progressive disabilities. For example, in light of the changes in color perception noted earlier, which pill and tablet colors facilitate more rapid discrimination, thus minimizing one type of medication error? In the hospital environment, which color contrasts for floor and wall coverings minimize visual confusion and aid best in ambulation? The possibilities are endless, and the interested reader should consult Skinner and Vaughan (1983) for a compendium of practical ideas and suggestions.

Cognitive Response System

Divided into four major components, the cognitive response system involves behaviors which indicate the processing of information (Adams, 1981): *Information selection* is closely related to perceptual activities and involves attending, orienting, focusing, and scanning of both internal and external stimuli. *Information storage and retrieval* are synonomous with learning and memory, and *conceptualization* and *reasoning* include the sorting and classification of information and the derivation of hypotheses from selected data respectively. These last two components deal explicitly with what we call intelligence. It should be noted that the cognitive response system is concerned with the *processes* of cognition. It thus has minimal relationship to cognitive-behavioral approaches which deal only with the *content* of such processes (i.e., thoughts, attitudes).

Selective literature reviews in the field of gerontology indicate that aging is characterized by a progressive decrement in the ability to suppress irrelevant stimuli (Layton, 1975). Referring to a general perceptual deficit, this hypothesis does not require existence of a neuronal mechanism but is based upon observed manipulation of environmental stimuli. For instance, older adults display greater decrements in speech perception under conditions of extraneous noise when compared to their younger counterparts (Elliott, 1982). Simple sensory deficits do not explain this increased susceptibility. Moreover, research in other areas supports a similar idea, namely, that older adults are less well able to filter out, inhibit, and ignore irrelevant information in their cognitive responses (see Botwinick, 1978). As such, the process of information selection is directly affected, and it is reasonable to assume that environmental variables (e.g., social isolation) will heighten this susceptibility. Pronounced changes in sensory function, discussed earlier, should exacerbate the problem, thus leaving the person at risk for development of a specific disorder in information selection.

It is hypothesized, therefore, that a form of attention deficit disorder may represent the end result of this interplay of variables, particularly if remaining skills in accurate stimulus selection are not afforded adequate maintenance. Whether referring to an attentional response atrophy or response inversion (i.e., greater focus on internally produced stimuli), this form of attention deficit is viewed as a primary mechanism in particular cases of geriatric brain syndrome. Elaboration of this behavioral formulation will constitute the basis of the case to be presented.

Although experimental research on attentional processes has been slow in finding its way into the clinical situation (e.g., Neill, 1977), a few researchers have suggested that attention deficit disorder need not be restricted to the childhood years (e.g., Horowitz, 1981; Wender, Reimherr, & Wood, 1981). However, it is only recently that the role of attention deficit in adult psychopathology has been recognized. Adams, Malatesta, Brantley, and Turkat (1981), for instance, successfully treated a case of adult schizophrenia based upon a behavioral formulation of attention deficit. Treatment was aimed directly at this hypothesized mechanism, and problem remediation was maintained at six-month follow-up.

Although several kinds of attention deficit may be identified (e.g., impaired selective attention, perseveration or mental inertia, impaired vigilance, and hemi-inattention or unilateral neglect), the present hypothesis is most concerned with selective attention, and not with the other types which are more commonly associated with significant brain impairment (See Howard, 1983; Lezak, 1983). Attention deficit in the present context is also differentiated from those phenomena observed in cases of acute delirium.

The processes of information storage and retrieval have received attention in the aging literature. Although controversy and uncertainty remain, learning studies, for example, have shown that classical conditioning is generally slower with older adults and that the processes of habituation and extinction occur more rapidly (implications abound for use of conditioning therapies with the elderly). Data also indicate that operant conditioning is less effective unless stimulus information is presented at a slower rate and unless response latency variables are eliminated (i.e., self-paced). Memory studies reveal that storage mechanisms remain relatively intact but that retrieval processes show age-related decrements. Sensory memory is impaired, whereas primary memory (short-term recall) remains relatively intact (as long as amount of material to be learned does not exceed primary memory capacity of 5–7 items). However, secondary or new long-term memory, which requires some organization of information, reveals variable decrements which are to least partially related to the inadequate use of mediational techniques (Hulicka & Grossman, 1967). Measures of secondary memory are also influenced by the *meaningfulness* or relevancy of the information to be learned and recalled. In other words, older adults tend to be more selective in what they are willing or motivated to learn.

Older individuals also tend to *fatigue* faster and are more cautious in the testing situation, preferring to make errors of omission (e.g., "I don't know that answer") rather than of commission. Clearly, these extra-test factors have very important implications for accurate interpretation of assessment data derived from psychometric instruments (see Albert, 1981). The potential for inaccurate and distorted test data is maximized when employing pencil and paper measures and when using test stimuli which are irrelevant to the older adult (e.g., recall Mrs. R.'s comment, "this isn't interesting enough to remember . . . tell me a good sexy story instead"). For a thorough discussion of these response variables in relation to learning and memory in the nonimpaired older adult, the reader is encouraged to consult Botwinick (1978, 1981; Botwinick & Storandt, 1974), Craik (1977), and Hussian (1981). See also Weingartner *et al.* (1981) on the subject of senile dementia and memory dysfunction.

A final note concerns the intellectual changes associated with normal aging. In general, intellectual functions which are not heavily dependent upon rapid perceptual-motor responding or abstract reasoning abilities (especially involving mental flexibility) tend to show minimal age-related deterioration. Included here are verbal skills, expressive and receptive language functions, concrete reasoning, and fund of knowledge. While measures of problem-solving ability seem to show age-related alterations, test performance is at least partially dependent upon (a) the meaningfulness and relevancy of the task (e.g., see Arenberg, 1968), (b) stimulus–response characteristics of the task (e.g., rate of stimulus presentation, response latency), and (c) the degree of interference imposed by irrelevant or competing information. Overall, intellectual functioning in the later years has been heavily researched (Botwinick, 1977; Craik & Trehub, 1982; Lezak, 1983).

Emotional and Social Response Systems

There is general consensus that social activity and social-familial support variables exert an important moderator effect on mood state and overall well-being of individuals across the life span. The social response system has been implicated similarly in several behavioral formulations of affective disorder, primarily depression (see Carson & Carson, 1984). Since the older adult is increasingly dependent upon environmental factors for optimal psychological functioning, the relationship between social and emotional variables is intensified in later life. Therefore, aging is associated with an increased interdependence between the social and emotional response systems. Given the omnipresent nature of this relationship as presented in both the gerontological and behavioral literature, current discussion will focus only on selected areas of investigative inquiry. The concept of personality in relation to aging will not be addressed, nor the variety of theories and models that have attempted to account for psychological adjustment patterns of older adults to the multiple life stresses of advanced age. For informational purposes, however, Hamlin's (1967) utility theory, Atchley's (1977) continuity theory, and Hussian's compensatory model (1981) are perhaps most consistent with a behavioral approach, despite the fact that minimal research has been generated by these attempts. In contrast, a long battle between activity theory (Havighurst, Neugarten, & Tobin, 1968) and disengagement theory (Cumming & Henry, 1961) has created very active research pursuits, even though both formulations have been critized repeatedly as being inadequate. Finally, although various stage theories have enjoyed widespread acceptance in the gerontological literature (e.g., Erikson, 1963; Erikson & Erikson, 1978), their relevance to the behavioral approach has not been realized.

Adaptation to the multiple losses associated with aging has been viewed as one of the major psychological tasks faced by older adults (Pfeiffer, 1977). Inadequate or unsuccessful coping with these stresses has long been implicated as a primary cause of psychopathology in the later years. Although appealing from an anecdotal perspective, research on coping and life stress has not necessarily confirmed the importance of this relationship to the mental health problems of the elderly. This is an intriguing clinical area that has been said to reflect a "primitive" research methodology, the problems of which have been comprehensively addressed by Lazarus and DeLongis (1983). Not only is the majority of relevant data of a cross-sectional nature, but also the few longitudinal studies available suggest that "variability, rather than clear central tendencies, is the rule in both the sources of stress and the types of coping engaged in among the elderly" (Lazarus & DeLongis, 1983, p. 245). Relevant theory and research, however, has not accounted for this variability of response. Moreover, the emphasis on life events as an adequate description of stress is naive and does not include the "minor annoyances" (Skinner & Vaughan, 1983) or the "daily hassles" (Lazarus & DeLongis, 1983) that may represent a more irritating and personally significant source of stress. In this regard, many of us are unaware of the daily hassle involving the "fear of victimization" which plagues the nearly 75 percent of elderly individuals who live in urban areas (Hendricks & Hendricks, 1977). One unfortunate consequence produced by this fear is additional restrictions in activity level (e.g., avoiding use of public transportation).

In comparison to issues facing stress research on the elderly, the definition and measurement of coping reflects even greater ambiguity. Nevertheless, coping is viewed as a key concept in various theories addressing successful life adjustments of older adults (e.g., Havighurst, 1968b; Pfeiffer, 1977; Solomon, Faletti, & Yunik, 1982). Some clarity has been provided, however, by Lazarus and DeLongis's (1983) distinction between two basic functions of coping: problem-solving and regulation of emotion. Finally, other writers have emphasized coping history and the cumulative effects of repeated stressors in understanding the older adult's ability to handle current life demands (Hendricks & Hendricks, 1977)

Comment

The preceding overview and introduction to the aging process has been necessarily cursory and incomplete. Many important areas have been either omitted or only touched upon. Its purpose, however, has been twofold: first, one hopes, to stimulate the reader's interest in this frontier area of clinical possibilities and potentials; and second, to provide some appreciation for the muliplicity of variables and their profound interactions that comprise an accurate understanding of the older adult. In light of the interdisciplinary nature of the field and since variability among aged individuals is paramount, it is easy to see why generalizations derived from research and clinical data are often inaccurate, premature, and possibly counterproductive to management of the individual geriatric patient. As a consequence, the geriatric clinician is provided with only the roughest of guidelines with which to conduct his or her clinical work. The input of organic and sensory variables adds to this complexity, as does the interactive role of cognitive and environmental factors. Existing methods in gerontology, however, have only begun to integrate this multiplicity of variables into a testable framework useful for clinical decision making. The field of clinical geropsychology remains in its infancy and the role of behavioral treatment and formulation remains unexplored. This is unfortunate, for behavioral methods could yield broad benefits to clinical geropsychology by fostering an empirical understanding of selected clinical cases. The data base derived from such case work could eventually lead to a systematic research program designed to answer basic questions about the various geriatric organic syndromes. With these goals in mind, the remainder of this chapter is devoted to the case of Mrs. R.

CASE ANALYSIS

Preliminary Comment

It may be wise for the reader to review the case description of Mrs. R. at this point and to formulate his or her own ideas and hypotheses regarding relevant clinical issues. Since a variety of questions remain unanswered by the data provided in the description, it will be necessary to make certain assumptions as we proceed with the case analysis.

Biomedical Assessment

Ethically, a geriatric biobehavioral disorder remains outside the domain of the mental health professional until various organic factors have been reliably assessed and identified by medical personnel. Although neuropsychological assessment may represent one exception to this rule, it can also be argued that organic factors, in principle, can never be fully ruled out. Nevertheless, reflecting our need for good working relationships with geriatric-trained physicians (i.e., internist, neurologist, psychiatrist), the medical work-up constitutes an essential prerequisite for the behavioral assessment and formulation of most geriatric cases. Unfortunately, this is an assessment area of which most phychologists profess ignorance. This lack of familiarity, however, tends to promote clinical avoidance of such cases and often undermines and/ or impedes our understanding of clinical phenomena displayed by older adults. Although it may be argued that the medical evaluation is more important in cases of suspected organic involvement, it is important to emphasize again the essential role of health variables and other organismic factors that impact upon most geriatric cases. For instance, I have had geriatric cases referred to me for anxiety management that ultimately revealed the primary influence of neurological and metabolic factors. Adherence to the requirement for biomedical assessment, therefore, insures that diagnostic errors regarding organic influences are kept to a minimum.

The medical data base should be derived from three essential subareas of assessment: (a) a thorough medical and health history, (b) physical examination, and (c) laboratory evaluation which includes neuroradiological procedures. This assessment phase has been outlined and described by Brocklehurst (1978) and Reichel (1978). The laboratory work-up should include the usual aids such as blood count, blood chemistry, and urinalysis, as well as tests devoted to assessment of the vascular system to check for cerebrovascular insufficiency related to the heart or major vessels, hypertension and hypotension, cardiac arrhythmias, and congestive failure. Special assessment procedures should also be included to evaluate individual disease processes when applicable (e.g., diabetes; see Table 1).

Since the case referral for Mrs. R. was provided by a physician working within an in-patient psychiatric setting, it is assumed that necessary biomedical assessments have been conducted. Thus, medical conditions related to vitamin deficiency, drug or alcohol toxicity, and so forth have been ruled out as primary mechanisms of the presenting problems. The only positive finding, therefore, is the CT scan, which revealed mild cerebral atrophy. Given the patient's age, however, and in the absence of other CT findings (e.g., ventricular enlargement), the diagnostic picture thus far is not strongly suggestive of an organic mental disorder such as primary degenerative dementia. Neuropsychological assessment would probably clarify support for or against this conclusion. In the absence of other evidence, however, and unless subsequent analysis reveals conflicting data, it is hypothesized that the presenting clinical phenomena represent some form of an organic brain syndrome and not an organic mental disorder as suggested by the referring physician. This represents an *a priori* hypothesis and does not imply that a contrary hypothesis (one in favor of OMD) would preclude behavioral analysis. Finally, despite the patient's history of alcohol consumption, we have no evidence of alcohol-related liver impairment; however, subtle but significant neuropsychological deficits related to sustained alcohol use may be operative even though undetectable by CT scan (see Goldstein & Shelly, 1982; Leber & Parsons, 1982).

Table 1. Biomedical Assessment: Laboratory Evaluation

Procedure	Designed to reveal
A. Urine studies	
1. specific gravity	renal dysfunction
2. glucose	diabetes
3. ketones	diabetes, malnutrition
4. casts	renal disease
5. albumin	renal damage
6. differential	infection
7. sodium	hyperactivity of adrenal cortex
	pituitary malfunction
	Addison's disease
8. WBC	infection
9. heavy metals	toxicity
10. protein electrophoresis	renal damage
B. Blood studies	
1. hemoglobin, RBC, HCT	anemias
2. WBC	infection
3. sedimentation rate	inflammatory process
4. creatinine	renal dysfunction
5. total bilirubin	liver disease
6. SGOT	liver damage
7. calcium	renal, thyroid dysfunction
8. glucose	diabetes, pancreatic dysfunction
9. BUN	malnutrition
10. drug screen	drug toxicity
11. folate level	anemia due to alcoholism
12. VDRL, RPR	syphilis
13. T_3, T_4	thyroid disease
14. B_{12} level	vitamin deficiency
C. X-rays	
1. chest	chronic lung disease
	infectious processes
2. skull	lesions, abcesses, tumors
	fluid changes
3. CT scan	intracranial masses
	focal or diffuse cerebral atrophy
	cerebral infarction
	hydrocephalus

The Clinical Interview

The critical first step in conducting a geriatric assessment is the initial clinical interview (more than one if necessary, of course). It is this first formal contact with the patient which will determine to a great extent whether or not reliable and sufficient data are available to proceed with an objective assessment and, just as important, whether or not the patient becomes "invested" in the assessment process. Clinical interviewing for geriatric biobehavioral disorders is a highly complex procedure which can be deceptively clear-cut but which clearly demands considerable judgment, flexibility, and keen observation. The interviewing of older patients, however, represents another area wherein clinicians not trained in geriatrics often feel quite incompetent and thereby providing another reason for clinical avoidance of such cases. Quite frequently, interview techniques normally utilized with younger patients are inappropriate and counterproductive when used with older adults. There is also greater need for use of ancillary interview procedures when working with the elderly. Unfortunately, the majority of clinical training programs continue to provide only limited direct experience with older patients, and clinical supervisors who have expertise in gerontology are few in number (see Cohen & Cooley, 1983; Lewinsohn et al., 1984; Smyer & Gatz, 1979). Conducted in a professional manner, however, the clinical interview will represent the cornerstone of the geriatric assessment and will provide the materials necessary for conducting a functional analysis of the presenting problems.

In addition to the goals of problem specification and functional analysis, the aim of interviewing for geriatric organic syndromes is (a) to establish communication between patient and therapist and to determine the extent to which adjunctive interview procedures will be employed (e.g., nursing staff, significant others); (b) to generate a detailed list of problems; (c) to conduct a brief neuropsychological screening examination; (d) to generate and test hypotheses about the development and maintenance of the presenting problems; (e) to arrive at a tentative formulation about the case; and (f) to develop an experimental plan for the formalized, objective assessment which follows (or to request or conduct a complete neuropsychological assessment).

Preparing for the Clinical Interview. Most clinicians are unaccustomed to preparing for an interview since our experience with younger patients dictates that most relevant information can be obtained without difficulty during the interview process. Moreover, the experienced clinician can usually exercise sufficient flexibility and judgment to handle successfully a diverse assortment of patient types. In working with older adults, however, the typical interview format is appropriate in only a small portion of cases. These cases usually include those "young-old" individuals (i.e., age 55–75) who are reasonably healthy, well-functioning community dwellers, who are encountered in an out-patient setting. Even then, modifications in the interview procedure are often required in order to maximize validity and reliability of obtained data.

In attempting to assess cases suspected of organic brain syndrome, the clinician is more often faced with an "old-old" adult (i.e., age 75 + ; see Neugarten, 1975) who has significant health problems and sensory loss and who may appear disoriented, confused, and restless. Memory problems and focusing difficulties may further complicate the situation. Such individuals are usually in-patients who have recently encountered a crisis of one form or another. Consequently, they may also present in a state reflecting distrust, opposition, or bewilderment. It should be obvious, therefore, that the clinician, unprepared for such an encounter, is also more likely to appear confused and bewildered, as well as uncertain about the control, content, and direction of the interview.

In light of such very real possibilities, the clinician should attempt to learn as much as possible about the patient prior to the actual clinical interview. Bearing in mind the multiplicity of variables that interact with and influence the older person's behavior, the following information sources are useful, if not essential, for interview preparation: (1) a complete review of medical records, including current data (e.g., lab findings), health history, sensory problems, pharmacology, diet and nutrition (contact with the patient's primary care physician may supplement these data); (2) a complete review of developmental social data, including family history, education, occupational history, ethnic background, negoiation of life-span milestones (e.g., marriage, retirement); (3) analysis of environmental and ecological variables, including living situation, financial status, activity level, and social supports; and (4) contact with nursing personnel and significant others, sometimes including neighbors, clergy, and former work colleagues.

In this manner, the clinician is ready to organize as well as modify the interview format according to the unique needs and liabilities of the individual patient. Also, the clinician has already developed a broad information base from which to begin generating a list of problems, developing hypotheses, and ruling out areas of unnecessary inquiry. Moreover, the clinician will be more likely to convey confidence, authority, and understanding in this first contact with the patient. Communication and trust will be facilitated, and the patient will be more likely to cooperate fully with the assessment process.

Conducting the Interview. A number of important issues deserve discussion regarding the execution of the geriatric clinical interview. First, in attempting to help compensate for sensory deficits so commonly seen in older adults, I routinely use a blackboard throughout the actual interview (Meyer & Turkat, 1979). As clinicians, we often assume that our patients accurately understand, encode, and organize relevant information that is exchanged during the interview. We also tend to assume that this processing of information occurs in a manner similar to that of the therapist, and that mutually congruent conclusions are drawn from the same data presented. Confidence in this assumption, although marginal at best with younger adults, is seriously compromised in clinical work with the elderly. This is especially the case when one is dealing with an older person who displays OBS symptoms. To overcome such difficulties in information processing, the blackboard provides a visual aid which insures that important data are processed in multiple channels. Relevant problem areas and developmental data, for instance, can be listed and displayed for mutual discussion and clarification. Use of the blackboard also tends to elicit greater and more appropriate verbal behavior from the patient, thus providing more useful feedback for the clinician regarding hypothesized target areas and tentative formulation. Indirectly, the blackboard also provides a second focal point for the patient—a discriminative stimulus which facilitates attention and concentration.

Similarly, I often provide the patient (and/or spouse, nursing staff), at the close of the session, with a typed or audiotaped summary of the highlights of the interview. This summary is usually quite brief, consisting of a problem list, a graphic diagram, or a few "buzz" words related to content of the interview. In other cases, a brief audio cassette tape seems more effective (in one instance, a mildly demented, retired musician received prepared audiotapes consisting of important assessment data set to music). These aids, despite their simplicity, tend to help compensate for memory difficulties while offering the patient a continuing focus for future assessment sessions. Use of other devices is limited only by the clinician's flexibility and creativity.

A second area concerns duration of the clinical interview. Typically, I prefer to conduct brief sessions of 15–30 minutes duration, sometimes several during a single day. Scheduling occurs during the patient's "best" time—that is, the time of the day when he or she tends to be more lucid, clearly oriented, and refreshed. Logistically, such provisions are more readily incorporated when working with an in-patient setting. However, the telephone can be a valuable adjunct in working with elderly out-patients. Brief sessions can be conducted over the telephone in order to complement face-to-face interactions and to provide contiguity (interestingly, confused patients often respond quite well to the telephone, perhaps finding it easier to focus on one stimulus source).

Multiple interview sessions scheduled over short time durations allow the clinician to (a) conduct continuous assessments over time, (b) test for reliability and consistency of obtained data, whether pertaining to actual test findings (e.g., memory) or self-report information, and (c) compensate for problems of patient fatigue associated with advanced age and disability.

Variations in the setting of the interview may be extremely important in working successfully with the older adult patient. Data obtained from the preinterview work-up should permit the clinician to decide, for instance, where best to conduct the interview (e.g., office, hospital room, patient's home). Similarly, preinterview information will determine whether or not the presence of a third party during the actual interview (e.g., spouse, nurse, daughter) might increase cooperation while minimizing fear and distrust. In other cases, the clinician may decide to rely primarily upon significant others rather than on the patient for provision of assessment data. This alternative may be more apropriate when the patient's symptoms of disorientation and confusion are too severe and unyielding to allow interviewing to be conducted effectively.

Finally, the clinician may decide on the basis of preinterview data to employ other aids to interaction (i.e., increase focusing while decreasing distractibility). Since marked age differences between older patient and younger clinician are so common, the judicious use of therapeutic "hooks" can sometimes help to establish a connection between parties, particularly if other efforts have failed. I have used such aids as: (a) the gender variable (as is true of many people, certain patients, especially if confused, "work" better with either a male or female therapist; (b) the ethnic factor (my Italian heritage has been a deciding variable in selected cases); (c) the display of cohort-relevant or person-specific stimulus objects, such as selected antiques, photos, crewel work (another geriatric patient who had performed as a musician during his younger days was inadvertently engaged when he noticed my interest in music from a displayed wall-sticker which said, "Support your Local Musician"); and (d) brief self-disclosures regarding my older relatives who encountered problems similar to those of the patient.

The above list serves to point out the need for extreme flexibility on the part of the interviewer. The geriatric clinician must be ready to modify, improvise, self-disclose, and circumvent in any manner a multitude of potential barriers. In essence, the interview is adjusted to fit the patient uniquely, not vice versa. The interviewer is thus continually varying his or her style to meet the demands of the particular situation. The case description of Mrs. R., for instance, exemplifies the judicious use of physical touch in maintaining a focus upon the assessment. Similarly, the interviewer's use of a loud voice and short, concise sentences to aid comprehension are notable examples. The patient's periodic distractibility and response to extraneous stimuli during the interview (e.g., describing a running fan as frightening) would be important foci for assessment. As such, the following questions would need to be answered through selective hypothesis testing: How does the distractibility response vary? For instance, an operant component (i.e., secondary gain) is often suggested if the patient "tunes out" during discussion of personally relevant topics (e.g., Mrs. R.'s alcohol consumption, relationship to daughter). On the other hand, a strong stimulus-deprivation or stimulus-distortion component is suggested if distractibility varies as a function of setting (e.g., interviews at patient's home or at the hospital), time (e.g., night-time disorientation), and overall quality and content of the stimulus environment (e.g., describing a running fan as frightening is not an uncommon response and suggests potential for sensory misperception rather than hallucination). Closely related, does the patient report increased negative thoughts and sensations under conditions of reduced stimulation (e.g., when the interview is conducted in a dimly lit room)? If so, this tends to suggest a relationship between external and internal sources of stimulation. Finally, Mrs. R.'s comment regarding memory testing on the Mental Status Examination ("this isn't interesting enough to remember . . . tell me a good sexy story instead") should alert the clinician to test other stimuli that are perhaps more salient or relevant and thus more meaningful to the patient. In this regard, I have used special memory stimuli consisting of word lists and story passages about such age-relevant topics as widowhood, social security, retirement, and geriatric sexuality. The Thorndike–Lorge (1944) word book can be used to choose test words which occur in the English language at a frequency comparable to that of more standardized test stimuli, thereby providing some measure of experimental control. Although only roughly analogous to standard stimuli, the use of age-relevant test stimuli sometimes generates dramatic differences in performance among older adults. In these cases, a "memory problem" washes out and becomes more an issue of stimulus saliency or task relevancy. This procedure would be quite appropriate in Mrs. R.'s case.

   Another related issue concerns execution of the neuropsychological screening examination. This phase of the interview is important in providing a cognitive data base from which to generate and test hypotheses. Repeated administrations of a brief screening battery adds regarding functional variability. In conducting this evaluation, a variety of instruments are available to the examiner, ranging from the standard mental status examination to various rating scales. The decision regarding which instrument to use is based upon presenting symptomatology, logistical constraints, the patient's educational and cultural idiosyncrasies, and the therapist's preference. Although limitations in geriatric testing have been described (see Albert, 1981), several instruments have been designed and developed specifically for older adults. Other methods, although representing more standard tests (e.g., Rey Auditory-Verbal Learning Test; Wechsler Memory Scale/Russell Recall Format), have nevertheless received sufficient research attention such that reasonable age-normative standards for these tests are available (see Bak & Green, 1980; Haaland, Linn, Hunt, & Goodwin, 1983; Query & Megran, 1983). Table 2 provides a selected listing of neuropsychological screening instruments and rating scales (see also Gallagher, Thompson, & Levy, 1980; Lezak, 1983).

Table 2. Geriatric Neuropsychological Screening: Selected Inventories, Rating Scales, and Ancillary Aids

Mental status-type inventories	
Mattis Organic Mental Syndrome Screening Examination	(Mattis, 1976)
Mattis Dementia Rating Scale	(Gardner et al., 1981; Mattis, 1976)
Mental Status Examination	(Simpson & Magee, 1973; Shrub & Black, 1977)
Mental Status Questionnaire	(Kahn & Miller, 1978; Kahn et al., 1960)
Mini-Mental State	(Folstein, Folstein, & McHugh, 1975)
Mental Status Checklist	(Lifshitz, 1960)
Geriatric Interpersonal Rating Scale	(Plutchik et al., 1971)
Short Portable Mental Status Questionnaire	(Pfeiffer, 1975)
Rating scales and observational measures	
Global Deterioration Scale for Primary Degenerative Dementia	(Reisberg et al., 1982)
Functional Dementia Scale	(Moore et al., 1983)
Dementia Rating Scale	(Coblentz et al., 1973)
Stockton Geriatric Rating Scale	(Meer & Baker, 1966)
Geratric Rating Scale	(Plutchik et al., 1970)
Sandoz Clinical Assessment—Geriatric	(Shader et al., 1974)
Ancillary rating scales	
Physical and Mental Impairment of Function Evaluation (PAMIE)	(Gurel et al., 1972)
Nurses' Observation Scale for In-patient Evaluation (NOSIE)	(Honigfeld, 1966)

Listing of Specific Problems. With completion of the initial interview phase of assessment, the geriatric clinician is now armed with a broad data base derived from many information sources and is therefore in a position to develop an initial list of specific problem areas. Each listed problem should be operationalized according to Meyer and Turkat (1979). In my own clinical work with older adults, the problem list represents a flexible, working model of the case which may undergo considerable revision and refinement as additional information is gathered and as hypotheses are either refuted or supported. The list also allows the clinician to begin making connections among problem areas, thus facilitating development of a tentative case formulation. Ultimately, the problem list will guide intervention planning, based upon the behavioral formulation.

To set the stage for execution of the problem list, I find it useful to begin by developing a brief asset list which is typically derived from interview observations. This brief list sometimes helps to rule out entire disorder classes, as well as to eliminate irrelevant problem areas and nonfruitful hypotheses. These data, therefore, help to clarify and sharpen the focus upon the subsequent problem list. Regarding Mrs. R., my asset list is as follows:

1. Keen awareness of difficulties and the ability to describe them in detail
2. Exquisite but not excessive attention to personal appearance, hygiene, etc.
3. Intact speech; no evidence of aphasic symptoms, dysfluency, perseveration, etc.
4. Conviviality and appropriate use of humor
5. No evidence of distrust or suspiciousness toward examiner

These data continue to rule out the possibility that presenting symptoms represent an organic mental disorder (OMD) such as primary degenerative dementia. In such cases, decreased awareness, speech disturbance, and decreased attention to personal hygiene would be more likely exhibited (See Schneck et al., 1982; Wells, 1979). It can be argued as well that the patient's use of humor and display of adequate social skills reflect well-retained abstraction and reasoning abilities which are also more consistent with a nonorganic mechanism for the presenting problems. These data, then, allow us (a) to continue to rule out degenerative brain state as the primary mechanism and (b) to execute a clinical search for another formulation of the case. It should be noted that data presented thus far are most consistent with a pseudodementia process. Pseudodementia is a recently popular descriptive term which says that the clinical picture of dementia-like symptoms is a "functional artifact" actually related to an intervening variable, the most popular of which has been depression (see Caine, 1981). Thus far, however, case data on Mrs. R. are not overwhelmingly in support of a depression-induced problem profile. Finally, the patient's general trust and acceptance of the examiner tend to speak against presence of a paranoid disorder; instead, a reality-based explanation for her seemingly paranoid comments ("these funny feelings that people were saying bad things about me and my husband") may be a more likely possibility.

In developing an initial list of clinical problems for a given geriatric case, I find Adams's (1981) response classification system to be a very useful organizational aid. Major response systems are delineated and defined within a behavioral framework, and the clinician is thus assisted in classifying the multitude of data which is so commonly abundant in geriatric cases. I use a two-step process in arriving at a final problem list. The first step is an exhaustive, overinclusive list of relevant organismic variables, clinical findings and impressions, and presenting problems. This helps to provide a complete and detailed picture of the patient. Step two represents a refinement of the initial list with primary emphasis on behavioral identification of targeted problem areas. The initial list for Mrs. R. is as follows:

A. Biological response system
   1. Mild cerebral atrophy as measured by CT scan
   2. Arthritis and mild hypertension
   3. Occasional sleep disturbance at home
   4. Questionable nutrition in home environment, in light of daily alcohol use
   5. Daily alcohol use and possible abuse
   6. Possible medication abuse
   7. Probable drug potentiation effect (alcohol + medication)
   8. Periodic nocturnal disorientation in hospital setting
B. Perceptual-motor response systems
   1. Significant hearing loss, necessitating use of hearing aid
   2. Significant vision loss; 70% right-eye vision loss
   3. Hallucinatory phenomena: auditory channel
C. Cognitive response system
   1. Periodic disorientation, noted only during evening hours
   2. Distractibility; high susceptibility to irrelevant cues
   3. Reported memory disturbance
   4. Possible referential thinking and quasi-paranoid statements
D. Emotional and social response systems
   1. Report of depression; crying episode noted by maid

2. Report of anxiety ("nerves")
3. Anger expressed toward daughter
4. Probable rumination ("I spend most of my time . . . thinking.")
5. Inadequate family supports
6. Inadequate social supports
7. Low level of social activity

For the purpose of case formulation, initial refinement can begin with an elimination of items one through four, listed under the biological response system. As noted earlier, the CT scan outcome of mild cerebral atrophy is not a significant finding in light of age-expected norms. Although arthritis restricts general mobility and access to certain activities (e.g., sewing), this health problem has only indirect relevance to the presenting complaints. A similar reason applies to mild hypertension since no data suggest use of antihypertensive medication; furthermore, no evidence exists regarding the possibility of a multiinfarct dementia. Data are lacking regarding sleep habits and nutritional intake while in the home environment. It could be speculated that since the patient's maid handled at least part of the cooking, access to adequate nutrition was available. Still, the well-known role of alcohol in promoting nutritional insufficiency (as well as sleep disturbance) cannot be dismissed. In any event, however, we will assume adequate nutritional status at the time of assessment.

Remaining problems within the biological response system therefore pertain to daily alcohol use and possible medication abuse and to nocturnal awakenings/disorientation in the hospital setting. Although information regarding home medication use is lacking, attention is drawn to Mrs. R.'s comment regarding her doctor's instructions on use of "several" prescription medications ("My doctor says to take one when I need it"). In light of earlier discussion on medication use in the elderly, this comment suggests likelihood of self-medication with potential for abuse. Mrs. R.'s daily alcohol intake is problematic, even though it represents one of the few pleasurable activities left to her. If one recalls age effects of alcohol metabolism (i.e., older adults reach higher blood alcohol levels), her daily consumption of 2–3 ounces is excessive. Therefore it is quite likely that some degree of alcohol–drug potentiation has occurred, and it is hypothesized that her first psychiatric admission was prompted by what was actually a toxic reaction. For current purposes, however, we will assume stabilization at the time of assessment. Regarding nocturnal disorientation, it would be important to know whether or not this behavior occurs in the home environment.

Although sleep does tend to be less sound in the later years, the absence or attenuation of such episodes at home would be consistent with a stimulus deprivation explanation.

Regarding the perceptual-motor response systems, it is hypothesized that significant vision and hearing impairments are exerting a critical influence upon presenting symptomatology. Hearing loss, in particular, has been strongly implicated in the development of hallucinatory and delusional experience (see Maher & Ross, 1984). Not only are sensory deficits eliminating access to activities (e.g., reading, radio), it is also probable that these losses have created a relatively deprived as well as distorted stimulus environment for Mrs. R. As a consequence, environmental disorientation is more likely to occur in unfamiliar settings and under conditions of reduced stimulus input (e.g., night-time in the hospital). The same holds true for auditory hallucinatory phenomena since incoming information (if lacking clarity in the first place) is more likely to be perceived in a distorted fashion (e.g., a running fan). Therefore, the patient's hallucinatory experience appears most consistent with a sensory misperception interpretation; quality and content of phenomena reported are consistent with this notion. It should also be noted that Mrs. R.'s complaint of "hearing funny things all the time" may actually reflect tinnitus (ear-ringing) which may accompany hearing loss, is more common among older adults, and is related to a variety of factors, such as medication, stress, and noise exposure (see Malatesta, Sutker, & Adams, 1980; Pulec, Hodel, & Anthony, 1978).

One may argue that the hypothesis of sensory misperception is strained when noting the quasi-paranoid quality attached to particular remarks made by Mrs. R. (e.g., "I even stopped going to church because I couldn't hear what they were saying and because I would get these funny feelings that people were saying bad things about me and my husband"). The most plausible explanation for these remarks, however, is (a) delusional experience induced by hearing loss (Maher & Ross, 1984) and (b) the reality of the widowhood experience. In this regard, people do tend to avoid widows out of discomfort, and people do talk—particularly if you were married to a powerful attorney and politician and were thus socially visible within a small southeastern community (see Adams, 1981, for a reality-based explanation for certain delusional beliefs).

Within the cognitive response system, periodic disorientation is listed a second time in order to draw attention to cognitive and perceptual aspects of this activity. Available data continue to converge on a sensory deprivation explanation. The patient displays no evidence of disorientation during normal waking hours when environmental input should be maximal. Moreover, Mrs. R.'s behavior during the interview did not appear to reflect disorientation. Rather, her two periods of apparent preoccupation during the interview (requiring that the interviewer call her name loudly and use physical touch to reestablish contact) appear more likely to be related to inappropriate attention to internally produced stimuli, that is, thoughts, and so forth.

Regarding the memory problems described, two data sources are provided: referral information citing memory disturbance during evening episodes of disorientation in the hospital, and the patient's complaints of forgetting names, addresses, telephone numbers, and her grandchildrens' names. On the first point, this is an expected finding, but not indicative of a memory problem. That is, since the process of information selection is impaired especially during periods of nocturnal disorientation, why would memory storage and retrieval for these episodes not be similarly affected? Regarding the second data source, a clue is provided by her statement, "not being concerned enough" to remember days or weeks. Although one may argue that this comment reflects apathic depression, it is more likely indicative of the relevancy or meaningfulness factor which is so important in memory functioning among older adults. Similarly, if it is assumed that she sees her grandchildren as frequently as she sees her daughter (i.e., once per year), it is not surprising that she experiences difficulty in recalling their names. Still, specific memory testing within this area is warranted.

A final issue regarding the cognitive response system concerns possible referential thinking and the quasi-paranoid statements made by Mrs. R. As noted above, these experiences are at least partially related to a reality-based explanation involving the widowhood experience (see Lopata, 1971; Malatesta, 1980b), which is exacerbated by hearing loss and sensory misperception. It is also possible that she is responding to internal cues in her description of people "saying bad things about me and my husband." If one hypothesizes a deprived or distorted external environment, it follows that internal sources of stimulation (particularly in light of her social isolation) would remain more salient. However, without external social feedback to correct and validate the meaning of these internally produced stimuli, the likelihood of distortion, along with a confusion of the internal and external environments, is considerably enhanced. Finally, the patient's report of increasing distrust (which was not displayed to the examiner) appears to represent an adaptive response by a sensorily impaired adult who lives alone and who holds an age-appropriate fear of victimization.

Information regarding the emotional response system is limited. Mrs. R. reports feeling depressed, although her interview behavior does not suggest mood disturbance. We also have no data suggestive of biological symptoms of depression (e.g., appetite loss, early morning awakenings). Perhaps the patient's report of depression, however, is related to her comment suggesting negative rumination ("I guess I spend most of my time just thinking"). Data are also lacking with regard to the possibility of maladaptive anxiety; our only piece of positive information is her report of occasional medication for "nerves" and "trouble sleeping." Still, anxiety feelings and agitation often are an immediate consequence of being disoriented; data nevertheless are lacking in this area.

The strongest emotional response presented in the case description is that of anger directed at her daughter (a) for instigating her first psychiatric hospitalization and, more important, (b) for restricting their contact to a single annual visit. Her expression points out her dissatisfaction with this arrangement, as well as the extreme lack of family supports in the patient's life. Although we have no information regarding siblings, no contact is noted, and, given her advanced age, it is possible that she has outlived other family members. Moreover, the case description clearly exemplifies the marked social and activity constrictions which typically follow widowhood and hearing loss. We also witness the loss of critical social supports provided by her widowed friends; it should be recalled that one woman was forced to move to a distant city, and Mrs. R.'s "best ladyfriend passed away." Clearly, these social losses precipitated the downward spiral to isolation and behavioral dysfunction. Finally, what remains socially is the maid who "visits" twice a week; here, one can appreciate the interpersonal urgency communicated by Mrs. R. in her use of the word "visit" to describe her relationship to the maid. It is also unfortunate that given her lack of family supports and informal social supports, Mrs. R. utilizes no community services specifically designed for older adults (senior center, geriatric companion, home health care, meals-on-wheels).

On the basis of the foregoing analysis and discussion, the revised problem list for Mrs. R is as follows:

1. Deprived and distorted stimulus environment
2. Sensory misperceptions: auditory channel
3. Distractibility
4. Episodic nocturnal disorientation
5. Inadequate discrimination between internal and external stimuli
6. Depressive feelings and negative rumination
7. Interpersonal isolation and inadequate social supports
8. Daily alcohol use
9. No utilization of community resources

Formulation

Meyer and Turkat (1979) define a behavioral formulation as a testable hypothesis that (a) interrelates all the patient's presenting difficulties through specification of a "mechanism" of the problem profile, (b) details the etiological variables giving rise to this hypothesized mechanism, and (c) offers predictions of the patient's behavior in different stimulus situations. Presumably, a treatment intervention based upon and guided by valid case formulation will prove most efficient as well as cost-effective in eliminating the patient's problems.

In the case of Mrs. R., it is hypothesized that an attention deficit identifies a behavioral mechanism of the presenting disorder. Viewed within this context, the hypothesis of attention deficit implies impairment in the process of information selection. This impairment is not viewed as a direct consequence of organic mediation, as is typically seen in cases of acute delirium and degenerative dementia. Although an organic factor, in principle, can never be ruled out, the behavioral mechanism of attention deficit describes a functional end point mediated by a specific sequence of etiological variables which is unique for a given geriatric case. In this situation, the sequence of variables is hypothesized as follows: (a) significant sensory loss with inadequate compensation, resulting in an altered and/or distorted stimulus environment; (b) age-expected decrement in the ability to suppress or ignore irrelevant stimuli (Botwinick, 1978; Layton, 1975); and (c) relative social isolation, resulting in unavailability of alternative, feedback-correcting external stimuli. The behavioral end point of attention deficit, therefore, is twofold: first, an acquired degree of inattention to appropriate external stimuli beyond that expected by sensory loss (attentional response atrophy) and second, a consequent but maladaptive focus on internally produced stimuli, such as thoughts, worries, and images (attentional response inversion).

The attention deficit hypothesis explains the problems of sensory misperception, distractibility, and nocturnal disorientation. Seemingly paranoid verbalizations, which appear to contain an element of truth by way of the widowhood experience, are exacerbated by confusion between internal and external sources of stimulation. Depressive feelings and negative rumination are thus viewed as consequences of the attention deficit. Although problems of interpersonal isolation and lack of social supports are realistic environmental components related to the experience of widowhood, the formulation of attention deficit would predict a degree of interpersonal avoidance which would tend to maintain isolation. Finally, the daily use of alcohol, although representing a life-long pattern and one of the few pleasurable activities left to Mrs. R., may also provide a solitary source of cognitive release by attenuating particular aspects of attention deficit (e.g., rumination, paranoid thoughts).

Clinical Experimentation. The purpose of clinical experimentation is to test specific predictions derived from the formulation, and the goal is to improve confidence in the validity of the hypothesized mechanism before embarking on a treatment plan. Miniexperiments may be designed and executed, and neuropsychological and psychodiagnostic techniques may be utilized as well. The decision regarding which procedures to employ in a given case, however, is determined by several factors, including (a) relevant patient variables, such as orientational status and degree and type of psychopathology; (b) the specific predictions deduced from the formulation; and (c) the preferences and creativity of the clinician. The end result, however, is that multiple response channels (behavioral observation, self-report, and neuropsychological indices) are examined and tested in an economical and empirical (*a priori*) fashion, and the data derived provide convergent validity for the formulation. The clinician is therefore in a position of confidence to employ the formulation in designing a treatment plan. Of course, if data do not converge in support of the formulation, it is likely that the conceptualization is inaccurate and in need of modification, in which case the process is repeated (see Carey, Flasher, Maisto, & Turkat, 1984, for a full discussion of this approach and its contrast to the standard psychodiagnostic test battery).

Regarding the case of Mrs. R., the formulation of an attention deficit leads directly to several predictions. First, if procedures can be devised or conditions arranged such that we can override or compensate for the attention deficit, then improvement should be observed in specific problem areas. On the other hand, if the attention deficit can be exacerbated through serendipitous conditions, we should anticipate increased symptom expression (e.g., increased distractibility, quasi-paranoid statements).

In the first case, the most obvious test would capitalize upon the assumption that if a stimulus exerts enough salience through meaningfulness or personal relevance, for example, then presentation of such a stimulus should be less susceptible to effects of attention deficit, thereby facilitating more accurate information encoding and subsequent processing. My previous example regarding special memory testing by use of relevant test words represents one experimental avenue. On a related level, a salient stimulus should also possess properties which will permit its use as an orientational anchor under conditions of reduced stimulus input when disorientation is more likely. For example, it will be recalled that the sundowning effect tends to be more common and more pronounced in unfamiliar environments where relevant and salient stimulus input is lacking. Therefore, to test minimization of attention deficit, I have used a variety of stimuli including different colored night-lights, large digital clocks (that display time and date), music, and objects brought from the patient's home environment (e.g., furniture, pictures, curtains). For instance, in one case, placement on the hospital room wall of two familiar paintings exerted enough specificity that later placement of unfamiliar pictures (unbeknownst to the patient) nearly eliminated the decrease in nocturnal disorientation observed under the first condition. In another case, a demented male patient who displayed evidence of an attention deficit showed marked change in orientational status when country-western music was provided by a radio which remained on throughout the night. Interestingly, other types of music tended to increase disorientation! These uncontrolled case findings cannot be explained by simple sensory effects since any kind of picture or kind of music should have exerted an identical effect had this been the case. These relatively simple manipulations, therefore, are in support of an attention deficit hypothesis and at the same time have important therapeutic implications which have been elaborated elsewhere (see Hussian, 1981; Lindsley, 1964; Skinner & Vaughan, 1983). Finally, the reader should be well aware that the above examples, although striking, are representative of only a small percentage of geriatric organic cases.

A second area of prediction derived from the formulation concerns the effects on relevant symptoms if the hypothesized attention deficit is somehow exacerbated through serendipitous conditions. For instance, if the attention deficit formulation is valid, we should observe an increase in sensory misperception and quasi-paranoid cognitions when Mrs. R. is exposed to environmental conditions which compound her difficulties in accurate information selection. Clinical experiments might include manipulation of extraneous room noise (e.g., use of running fan) or room lighting (e.g., fluorescent or nonfluorescent, dim or bright lighting). Symptom-related dependent variables could be measured in consequence (e.g., self-report and behavioral observation of anxiety level, distractibility, negative feelings). In one case, a patient's faulty hearing aid (which produced fluctuations in volume and background noise) provided a perfect vehicle for assessing changes in the frequency of paranoid statements and degree of interpersonal avoidance. Another patient, whose hearing aid was later found to have a defective battery, was experiencing relatively vivid "auditory hallucinations" until the malfunction was discovered. Finally, a male patient experienced regular periods of disorientation and confusion until his cataracts, which reduced and distorted visual input, were removed. These examples, although consistent with an attention deficit formulation, do not rule out the likely possibility that observed phenomena represent mere sensory effects. They also call attention to the acute need for availability of sensory assessments within the geriatric setting. Nevertheless, much investigative work remains to be accomplished within this intriguing area, and the above examples suggest viable experimental routes.

Therapeutic Implications. If the formulation of attention deficit is valid for particular geriatric organic cases, an intervention strategy presents itself. Besides therapeutic avenues suggested by clinical experimentation, the program developed by Adams and his colleagues (1981), for treatment of schizophrenia has direct relevance for remediation of attentional dysfunctions in selected organic cases. In essence, the patient is taught to attend, focus, and discriminate between relevant and irrelevant information (both internal and external) through an operant shaping procedure. Overlearning of such skills is a goal, and the program is specifically tailored to address the patient's unique difficulties in information selection. Initially, I employ highly salient stimuli and gradually fade in more nebulous cues. Orientational anchors are gradually faded out and the patient is taught to cope with onset of disorientation by focusing on environmental cues and by managing anxiety. To achieve these goals in an economical fashion while also fulfilling other patient needs (e.g., social interaction, maintenance of independent living), I have used trained nurse–therapists as well as the services of ancillary personnel (e.g., home health aids, geriatric companions, significant others) who are taught the above procedures.

The reader should bear in mind that the treatment approach outlined above represents but one component in the comprehensive management of geriatric organic syndromes. In the case of Mrs. R., for example, the role of social work would be important in helping the patient gain access to needed community services, including alcohol education and counseling. Medication assessment as well as complete sensory evaluations would also be warranted. The occupational therapist, whose title is somewhat of a misnomer in many repects, would collaborate with the psychologist in designing and/or recommending a "prosthetic environment" suitable for Mrs. R.'s unique needs and liabilities. Undoubtedly, the highest degree of independent living possible would be a realistic goal.

Finally, psychologists working with older adults have an ethical and professional responsibility to exercise both a firm knowledge of basic and clinical research in gerontology and related fields. The clinical geropsychologist must also maintain an empirical perspective in order to organize, evaluate, and modify his or her therapeutic efforts accordingly. Behavioral case formulation represents the most viable approach to achieve these objectives.

REFERENCES

Adams, H. E. (1981). *Abnormal psychology*. Dubuque, IA: Brown.

Adams, H. E., Malatesta, V., Brantley, P. J., & Turkat, I. D. (1981). Modification of cognitive processes: A case study of schizophrenia. *Journal of Consulting and Clinical Psychology, 49*, 460–464.

Albert, M. S. (1981). Geriatric neuropsychology. *Journal of Consulting and Clinical Psychology, 49*, 835–850.

American Psychiatric Association. (1968). *Diagnostic and Statistical Manual of Mental Disorders* (2nd ed.). Washington, DC: Author.

American Psychiatric Association. (1980). *Diagnostic and Statistical Manual of Mental Disorders* (3rd Ed.). Washington, DC: Author.

Arenberg, D. (1968). Concept problem solving in young and old adults. *Journal of Gerontology, 23*, 279–282.

Atchley, R. C. (1977). *The social forces in later life*. Belmont, CA: Wadsworth.

Bak, J. S., & Greene, R. L. (1980). Changes in neuropsychological functioning in an aging population. *Journal of Consulting and Clinical Psychology, 48*, 395–399.

Bakal, D. A. (1979). *Psychology and medicine: Psychobiological dimensions of health and illness*. New York: Springer.

Baltes, P. B. (1968). Longitudinal and cross-sectional sequences in the study of age and geration effects. *Human Development, 11*, 145–171.

Baltes, P. B., & Goulet, L. R. (1981). Exploration of developmental variables by manipulation and simulation of age differences in behavior. *Human Development, 14*, 149–170.

Baltes, P., & Schaie, W. (Eds.). (1973). *Life-span developmental psychology: Personality and socialization*. New York: Academic Press.

Barnes, E. K., Sack, A., & Shore, H. (1973). Guidelines to treatment approaches: Modalities and methods for use with the aged. *The Gerontologist, 13*, 513–527.

Barry, J. R. (1977). The psychology of aging. In J. R. Barry & C. R. Wingrove (Eds.), *Let's learn about aging: A book of readings*. New York: Halstead.

Benedict, R. C., & Ganikos, M. L. (1981). Coming to terms with ageism in rehabilitation. *Journal of Rehabilitation, 47*, 10–18.

Bergman, M. (1971). Changes in hearing with age. *The Gerontologist, 11*, 148–151.

Berry, R. G. (1975). Pathology of dementia. In J. G. Howells (Ed.), *Modern perspectives in the psychiatry of old age*. New York: Brunner/Mazel.

Birren, J. E., Butler, R. N., Greenhouse, S. W., Sokoloff, L., & Yarrow, M. R. (Eds.). (1971). *Human aging I: A biological and behavioral study* (U.S. Dept of Health, Education, and Welfare Publication No. ADM (74-122). Washington, DC: U. S. Government Printing Office.

Blanchard, E. B. (1982). Behavioral medicine: Past, present, and future. *Journal of Consulting and Clinical Psychology, 50*, 795–796.

Bondareff, W., Baldy, R., & Levy, R. (1981). Quantitative computed tomography in senile dementia. *Archives of General Psychiatry, 38*, 1365–1368.

Botwinick, J. (1978). *Aging and behavior* (2nd ed.). New York: Springer.

Botwinick, J. (1981). Neuropsychology of aging. In S. B. Filskov & T. J. Boll (Eds.), *Handbook of clinical neuropsychology*. New York: Wiley-Interscience.

Botwinick, J. (1977). Intellectual functions. In J. E. Birren & K. W. Schaie (Eds.), *Handbook of the psychology of aging*. New York: Van Nostrand.

Botwinick, J., & Storandt, M. (1974). *Memory, related functions, and age*. Springfield, IL: Thomas.

Brocklehurst, J. C. (1978). *Textbook of geriatric medicine* (2nd ed.). New York: Churchill Livingstone.

Brody, H., & Vijayashankar, N. (1977). Anatomical changes in the nervous system. In C. E. Finch & L. Hayflick (Eds.), *Handbook of the biology of aging*. New York: Van Nostrand Reinhold.

Butler, R. N., & Lewis, M. I. (1973). *Aging and mental health*. St. Louis: C. V. Mosby.

Butters, N., & Cermak, L. S. (1980). *Alcoholic Korsakoff's syndrome: An information-processing approach to amnesia*. New York: Academic Press.

Caine, E. D. (1981). Pseudodementia: Current concepts and future directions. *Archives of General Psychiatry, 38*, 1359–1364.

Carey, M. P., Flasher, L. V., Maisto, S. A., & Turkat, I. D. (1984). The a priori approach to psychological assessment. *Professional Psychology: Research and Practice, 15*, 515–527.

Carson, T. P., & Carson, R. C. (1984). The affective disorders. In H. E. Adams & P. B. Sutker (Eds.), *Comprehensive handbook of psychopathology*. New York: Plenum Press.

Cautela, J. R. (1966). Behavior therapy and geriatrics. *Journal of Genetic Psychology, 108*, 9–17.

Cautela, J. R. (1969). A classical conditioning approach to the development and modification of behavior in the aged. *The Gerontologist, 9*, 109–113.

Cautela, J. R., & Mansfield, L. (1977). A behavioral approach to geriatrics. In W. D. Gentry (Ed.), *Geropsychology: A model of training and clinical service*. Cambridge, MA: Ballinger.

Cleveland, W. P., & Gianturco, D. T. (1976). Remarriage probability after widowhood: A retrospective method. *Journal of Gerontology, 31*, 99–103.

Coblentz, J. M., Mattis, J., Zingesser, L. H., Kasoff, S. S., Wisniewski, H. M., & Katzman, R. (1973). Presenile dementia. *Archives of Neurology, 29*, 299–308.

Cohen, D. (1967). Research problems and concepts in the study of aging: Assessment and behavior modification. *The Gerontologist, 7*, 13–19.

Cohen, L. D., & Cooley, S. G. (1983). Psychology training programs for direct services to the aging (Status report: 1980). *Professional Psychology: Research and Practice. 14*, 720–728.

Coyle, J. T., Price, D. L., & DeLong, M. R. (1983). Alzheimer's disease: A disorder of cortical cholinergic innervation. *Science, 219*, 1184–1190.

Craik, F. I. M. (1977). Age differences in human memory. In J. E. Birren & K. W. Schaie (Eds.), *Handbook of the psychology of aging*. New York: Van Nostrand Reinhold.

Craik, F. I. M., & Trehub, S. (Eds.). (1982). *Aging and cognitive processes: Advances in the study of communication and affect*. New York: Plenum Press.

Cumming, E., & Henry, W. E. (1961). *Growing old: The process of disengagement*. New York: Basic Books.

Eisdorfer, C. (1969). Alternatives for the aging. *The Torch, 42*, 35–40.

Elliott, L. L. (1982). Effects of noise on perception of speech by children and certain handicapped individuals. *Sound and Vibration, 16*, 10–14.

Engel, G. L. (1977). The need for a new medical model: A challenge for biomedicine. *Science, 196*, 130–136.

Erikson, E. H. (1963). *Childhood and society (2nd ed.)*. New York: Norton.

Erikson, E. H., & Erikson, J. M. (1978). Introduction: Reflections on aging. In S. F. Spicker, K. M. Woodward, & D. D. Van Tassel (Eds.), *Aging and the elderly: Humanistic perspectives in gerontology*. Atlantic Highlands, NJ: Humanities Press.

Ernst, P., Beran, B., & Kleinhauz, M. (1979). Dr. Ernst and his colleagues reply. *The Gerontologist, 19*, 530–533.

Ernst, P., Beran, B, Safford, F., & Kleinhauz, M. (1978). Isolation and the symptoms of chronic brain syndrome. *The Gerontologist, 18*, 468–474.

Estes, E. H. (1977). Health experience in the elderly. In E. W. Busse & E. Pfeiffer (Eds.), *Behavior and adaptation in late life*. Boston: Little, Brown.

Fann, W. E. (1973). Interactions of psychotropic drugs in the elderly. *Postgraduate Medicine, 53*, 182–186.

Fauman, M. A. (1977). A diagnostic system for organic brain disorders: Critique amd suggestion. *Psychiatric Quarterly, 49*, 173–179.

Federal Council on Aging. (1981). *The need for longterm care: Information and issues*. DHHS No. (OHDS) 81-20704.

Filskov, S. B., & Boll, T. J. (Eds.). (1981). *Handbook of clinical neuropsychology*. New York: Wiley-Interscience.

Folstein, M. F., Folstein, S. E., & McHugh, P. R. (1975). "Mini-Mental State." *Journal of Psychiatric Research, 12*, 189–198.

Frolkis, V. V. (1977). Aging of the autonomic nervous system. In J. E. Birren & K. W. Schaie (Eds.), *Handbook of the psychology of aging*. New York: Van Nostrand Reinhold.

Gallagher, D., Thompson, L. W., & Levy, S. M. (1980). Clinical psychological assessment of older adults. In L. W. Poon (Ed.), *Aging in the 1980s: Psychological issues*. Washington, DC: American Psychological Association.

Gardner, R., Oliver-Munoz, S., Fisher, L., & Empting, I. (1981). Mattis Dementia Rating Scale: Internal reliability study using a diffusely impaired population. *Clinical Neuropsychology, 3*, 271–275.

Gentry, W. D. (Ed.). (1977). *Geropsychology: A model of training and clinical service*. Cambridge, MA: Ballinger.

Glenner, G. G. (1982). Alzheimer's disease (senile dementia): A research update and critique with recommendations. *Journal of the American Geriatric Society, 30*, 59–62.

Goethe, K. E., & Penberthy, A. R. (1980). *Drug use and the elderly: A review of the literature*. Richmond, VA: Virginia Commonwealth University Center on Aging.

Golden, C. J. (1981). *Diagnosis and rehabilitation in clinical neuropsychology (2nd ed.)*. Springfield, IL: Thomas.

Goldstein, G. (1979). Methodological and theoretical issues in neuropsychological assessment. *Journal of Behavioral Assessment, 1*, 23–41.

Goldstein, G., & Shelly, C. (1982). A multivariate neuropsychological approach to brain lesion localization in alcoholism. *Addictive Behaviors, 7*, 165–175.

Gonsalez, C. F., Grossman, C. B., & Palacios, E. (1979). *Computed brain and orbital tomography*. New York: Wiley.

Gottesman, L. E. (1977). Clinical psychology and aging: A role model. In W. D. Gentry (Ed.), *Geropsychology: A model of training and clinical service*. Cambridge, MA: Ballinger.

Goulet, L. R., & Baltes, P. B. (Eds.). (1970). *Life-span developmental psychology: Research and theory*. New York: Academic Press.

Gurel, L., Linn, M. W., & Linn, B. S. (1972). Physical and mental impairment of function evaluation in the aged: The PAMIE scale. *Journal of Gerontology, 27*, 83–87.

Haaland, K. Y., Linn, R. T., Hunt, W. C., & Goodwin, J. S. (1983). A normative study of Russell's variant of the Wechsler Memory Scale in a healthy elderly population. *Journal of Consulting and Clinical Psychology, 51*, 878–881.

Hamlin, R. M. (1967). A utility theory of old age. *The Gerontologist, 7*, 37–45 (Part II).

Hanaway, J., Scott, W. R., & Strother, C. M. (1979). *Atlas of the human brain and the orbit for computed tomography.* St. Louis: Warren Green.

Havighurst, R. J. (1968). A social-psychological perspective on aging. *The Gerontologist, 8*, 67–71.

Havighurst, R. J., Neugarten, B. L., & Tobin, S. S. (1968). Disengagement and patterns of aging. In B. L. Neugarten (Ed.), *Middle age and aging.* Chicago: University of Chicago Press.

Hayflick, L. (1975). Current theories of biological aging. In G. J. Thorbecke (Ed.), *Biology of aging and development.* New York: Plenum Press.

Hebb, D. O. (1955). The mammal and his environment. *The American Journal of Psychiatry, 111*, 826–831.

Hendricks, J., & Hendricks, C. D. (1977). *Aging in mass society: Myths and realities.* Cambridge, MA: Winthrop.

Heron, W. (1957). The pathology of boredom. *Scientific American, 196*, 52–56.

Hollister, L. E. (1977). Mental disorders in the elderly. *Drug Therapy, 7*, 128–135.

Honigfeld, G., & Klett, J. C. (1965). The Nurses' Observation Scale for Inpatient Evaluation. *Journal of Clinical Psychology, 21*, 65–69.

Horowitz, H. A. (1981). Psychiatric casualties of minimal brain dysfunction in adolescents. In: S. C. Feinstein, J. G. Looney, A. Z. Schwartzberg, & A. D. Sorosky (Eds.), *Adolescent psychiatry: Developmental and clinical studies* (Vol. 9). Chicago: Univ of Chicago Press.

Howard, M. E. (1983). *A handbook of behavior management strategies for traumatically brain-injured adults.* Kansas City, MS: Veterans Administration Medical Center. Unpublished manuscript.

Hoyer, W. J. (1973). Application of operant techniques to the modification of elderly behavior. *The Gerontologist, 13*, 18–22.

Hoyer, W. J., Mishara, B. L., & Riedel, R. (1975). Problem behaviors as operants. *The Gerontologist, 15*, 452–465.

Hulicka, I. M., & Grossman, J. L. (1967). Age-group comparisons for the use of mediators in paired-associate learning. *Journal of Gerontology, 22*, 46–51.

Hussian, R. A. (1981). *Geriatric psychology: A behavioral perspective.* New York: Van Nostrand Reinhold.

Jacoby, R. J., & Levy, R. (1980). Computerized tomography in the elderly. Senile dementia: Diagnosis and functional impairement. *British Journal of Psychiatry, 136*, 256–259.

Jaffee, C. C. (1982). Medical imaging. *American Scientist, 70*, 576–585.

Kahn, R. L. (1977). Perspectives in the evaluation of psychological mental health problems for the aged. In W. D. Gentry (Ed.), *Geropsychology: A model of training and clinical service.* Cambridge, MA: Ballinger.

Kahn, R. L., & Miller, N. E. (1978). Assessment of altered brain function in the aged. In M. Storandt, I. Siegler, & M. F. Elias (Eds.), *The clinical psychology of aging.* New York: Plenum Press.

Kahn, R. L., Goldfarb, A. L., Pollack, M., & Peck, A. (1960). Brief objective measures for the determination of mental status in the aged. *American Journal of Psychiatry, 117*, 326–328.

Lawton, M. P., & Gottesman, L. E. (1974). Psychological services to the elderly. *American Psychologist, 29*, 689–693.

Layton, B. (1975). Perceptual noise and aging. *Psychological Bulletin, 82*, 875–883.

Lazarus, R. S., & DeLongis, A. (1983). Psychological stress and coping in aging. *American Psychologist, 38*, 245–254.

Leber, W. R., & Parsons, O. A. (1982). Premature aging and alcoholism. *International Journal of the Addictions, 17*, 61–88.

Lehmann, H. E. (1972). Psychopharmacological aspects of geriatric medicine. In C. M. Gaitz (Ed.), *Aging and the brain*. New York: Plenum Press.

Lewinsohn, P. M., & Teri, L. (1983). *Clinical geropsychology*. New York: Pergamon.

Lewinsohn, P. M., Teri, L., & Hautzinger, M. (1984). Training clinical psychologists for work with older adults: A working model. *Professional Psychology: Research and Practice, 15*, 187–202.

Lezak, M. D. (1983). *Neuropsychological assessment* (2nd ed.). New York: Oxford University Press.

Lifshitz, K. (1960). Problems in the quantitative evaluation of patients with psychoses of the senium. *Journal of Psychology, 49*, 295–303.

Lindsley, O. R. (1964). Geriatric behavioral prosthetics. In R. Kastenbaum (Ed.), *New thoughts on old age*. New York: Springer.

Lopata, H. Z. (1971). Widows as a minority group. *The Gerontologist, 2*, 67–77.

Maher, B., & Ross, J. S. (1984). Delusions. In H. E. Adams & P. B. Sutker (Eds.), *Comprehensive handbook of psychopathology*. New York: Plenum Press.

Malatesta, V. J. (1980a). Female sexuality and aging: Issues and implications. *Journal of Women Studies, 2*, 16–27.

Malatesta, V. J. (1980b). The urban widow: A focus for gerontological study. In J. E. Montgomery & L. H. Walters (Eds.), *Presentations on aging*. Athens, GA: University of Georgia Press.

Malatesta, V. J. (1985). Differential diagnosis of geriatric depression and dementia: Clinical signs and symptoms. *Clinical Gerontologist, 3*, 42–43.

Malatesta, V. J., Sutker, P. B., & Adams, H. E. (1980). Experimental assessment of tinnitus aurium. *Journal of Behavioral Assessment, 2*, 309–317.

Malatesta, V. J., Chambless, D. L., & Pollack, M. (1983, May). *Sexual adaptations to widowhood: A life-span analysis*. Paper presented at the Sixth World Conference of Sexology: United States Consortium for Sexology, Washington, DC.

Marquez, J. (1983). Computerized tomography and neuropsychological tests in dementia. *Clinical Gerontologist, 2*, 13–22.

Mattis, S. (1976). Mental status examination for organic mental syndrome in the elderly patient. In L. Bellak & T. B. Karasu (Eds.), *Geriatric psychiatry*. New York: Grune & Stratton.

McAllister, T. W. (1983). Overview: Pseudodementia. *American Journal of Psychiatry, 140*, 528–533.

Meer, B. A., & Baker, J. A. (1966). The Stockton geriatric rating scale. *Journal of Gerontology, 21*, 622–626.

Meyer, V., & Turkat, I. D. (1979). Behavioral analysis of clinical cases. *Journal of Behavioral Assessment, 1*, 259–270.

Miller, N. C., & Cohen, G. D. (Eds.). (1981). *Aging. Vol. 15: Clinical aspects of Alzheimer's disease and senile dementia*. New York: Raven.

Mishara, B. L., & Kastenbaum, R. (1980). *Alcohol and old age*. New York: Grune & Stratton.

Moore, J. T., Bobula, J. A., Short, T. B., & Mischel, M. (1983). A functional dementia scale. *Journal of Family Practice, 16*, 499–503.

Mortimer, J., & Schumann, L. (Eds.). (1981). *The epidemiology of dementia*. New York: Oxford University Press.

National Institute on Alcohol Abuse and Alcoholism. (1982). *In brief: Alcohol and the elderly* (No. RPO-254). Rockville, MD: National Clearinghouse for Alcohol Information.

Neill, W. T. (1977). Inhibitory and facilitatory processes in selective attention. *Journal of Experimental Psychology: Human Perception and Performance, 3,* 444–450.

Nesselroade, J. R., & Reese, H. W. (Eds.). (1973). *Life-span developmental psychology: Methodological issues.* New York: Academic Press.

Neugarten, B. L. (1975). The future and the young-old. *The Gerontologist, 15,* 4–9 (Part 2).

Palmore, E. (1977). Facts on aging: A short quiz. *The Gerontologist, 17,* 315–320.

Parsons, O. A., & Hart, R. P. (1984). Behavioral disorders associated with central nervous system dysfunction. In H. E. Adams & P. B. Sutker (Eds.), *Comprehensive handbook of psychopathology.* New York: Plenum Press.

Patterson, R. L., & Jackson, G. M. (1981). Behavioral approaches to gerontology. In L. Michelson, M. Hersen, & S. M. Turner (Eds.), *Future perspectives in behavior therapy.* New York: Plenum Press.

Pease, R. A. (1974). Female professional students and sexuality in the aging male. *The Gerontologist, 14,* 153–157.

Pfeiffer, E. (1977). Psychopathology and social psychopathology. In J. E. Birren & K. W. Schaie (Eds.), *Handbook of the psychology of aging.* New York: Van Nostrand Reinhold.

Pfeiffer, E. (1975). SPMSQ: Short Portable Mental Status Questionnaire. *Journal of the American Geriatric Society, 23,* 433–441.

Pieper, H. G. (1977). Aged Americans: A profile of a growing minority. In J. R. Barry & C. R. Wingrove (Eds.), *Let's learn about aging: A book of readings.* New York: Halstead.

Plutchik, R., Conte, H., & Lieberman, M. (1971). Development of a scale (GIES) for assessment of cognitive and perceptual functioning in geriatric patients. *Journal of the American Geriatric Society, 19,* 614–623.

Plutchik, R., Conte, H., Lieberman, M. (1970). Reliability and validity of a scale for assessing the functioning of geriatric patients. *Journal of the American Geriatric Society, 18,* 491–500.

Poon, L. W. (Ed.). (1980). *Aging in the 1980s: Psychological issues.* Washington, DC: American Psychological Association.

Poon, L., Fozard, J., Cermak, L., Arenberg, D., & Thompson, L. (1980). *New directions in memory and aging.* Hillsdale, NJ: Erlbaum.

Pulec, J. L., Hodell, S. F., & Anthony, P. F. (1978). Tinnitus: Diagnosis and treatment. *Annals of Otology, Rhinology and Laryngology, 87,* 1–13.

Query, W. T., & Megran, J. (1983). Age-related norms for AVLT in a male patient population. *Journal of Clinical Psychology, 39,* 136–138.

Reichel, W. (Ed.). (1978). *Clinical aspects of aging.* Baltimore: Williams & Wilkins.

Reisberg, B., Ferris, S. H., DeLeon, M. J., & Crook, T. (1982). The global deterioration scale for assessment of primary degenerative dementia. *American Journal of Psychiatry, 139,* 1136–1139.

Richards, W. S., & Thorpe, G. L. (1978). Behavioral approaches to the problems of later life. In M. Storandt, I. C. Siegler, & M. F. Elias (Eds.), *The clinical psychology of aging.* New York: Plenum Press.

Rothchild, D. (1941). Poor correlation between pathologic and clinical findings in aged. *Diseases of the Nervous System, 2,* 49–54.

Salzman, C., Hoffman, S. A., & Schoonover, S. C. (1983). Geriatric psychopharmacology. In E. L. Bassuk, S. C. Schoonover, & A. J. Gelenberg (Eds.), *The practitioner's guide to psychoactive drugs* (2nd ed.). New York: Plenum Press.

Santos, J. F., & VandenBos, G. R. (Eds.). (1982). *Psychology and the older adult: Challenges for training in the 1980s.* Washington, DC: American Psychological Association.

Schaie, K. W. (1965). A general model for the study of developmental problems. *Psychological Bulletin, 64*, 92–107.

Schaie, K. W. (1967). Age changes and age differences. *The Gerontologist, 7*, 128–132.

Schneck, M. K., Reisberg, B., & Ferris, S. H. (1982). An overview of current concepts of Alzheimer's disease. *American Journal of Psychiatry, 139*, 165–173.

Schuckit, M. A. (1977). Geriatric alcoholism and drug abuse. *The Gerontologist, 17*, 168–174.

Schwartz, G. E. (1982). Testing the biopsychosocial model: The ultimate challenge facing behavioral medicine? *Journal of Consulting and Clinical Psychology, 50*, 1040–1053.

Seltzer, B., & Sherwin, I. (1978). Organic brain syndromes: An empircal study and critical review. *American Journal of Psychiatry, 135*, 13–21.

Shader, R. I., Harmatz, J. S., & Salzman, C. (1974). A new scale for clinical assessment in geriatric populations: Sandoz Clinical Assessment—Geriatric (SCAG). *Journal of the American Geriatric Society, 22*, 107–113.

Shock, N. W. (1962). The physiology of aging. *Scientific American, 206*, 100–110.

Simpson, J. F., & Magee, K. R. (1973). *Clinical evaluation of the nervous system.* Boston: Little, Brown.

Sinex, F. M. (1975). The biochemistry of aging. In M. G. Spencer & C. J. Dorr (Eds.), *Understanding aging: A multidisciplinary approach.* New York: Appleton-Century-Crofts.

Skinner, B. F. (1983). Intellectual self-management in old age. *American Psychologist, 38*, 239–244.

Skinner, B. F., & Vaughan, M. E. (1983). *Enjoy old age: A program of self-management.* New York: Norton.

Smyer, M. A., & Gatz, M. (1979). Aging and mental health: Business as usual? *American Psychologist, 34*, 240–246.

Solomon, J. R., Faletti, M. V., & Yunik, S. S. (1982). The psychologist as geriatric clinician. In T. Millon, C. Green, & R. Meagher (Eds.), *Handbook of clinical health psychology.* New York: Plenum Press.

Stachnik, T. J. (1980). Priorities for psychology in medical education and health care delivery. *American Psychologist, 35*, 8–15.

Steel, R., & Feldman, R. G. (1979). Diagnosing dementia and its treatable causes. *Geriatrics, 34*, 79–88.

Steuer, J. L., & Hammen, C. L. (1983). Cognitive-behavioral group therapy for the depressed elderly: Issues and adaptations. *Cognitive Therapy and Research, 7*, 285–296.

Storandt, M. (1983). Understanding senile dementia: A challenge for the future. *International Journal of Aging and Human Development, 16*, 1–6.

Storandt, M., Siegler, I. C., & Elias, M. F. (Eds.). (1978). *The clinical psychology of aging.* New York: Plenum Press.

Strub, R. L., & Black, F. W. (1977). *The Mental Status Examination in Neurology.* Philadelphia: Davis.

Strub, R. L., & Black, F. W. (1981). *Organic brain syndromes.* Philadelphia: Davis.

Terry, R. D., & Wisniewski, H. M. (1975). Structural and chemical changes of the aged human brain. In S. Gershon & A. Raskin (Eds.), *Aging* (Vol. 2). New York: Raven.

Thorndike, E. L., & Lorge, I. (1944). *The teacher's word book of 30,000 words.* New York: Teachers College, Columbia University Bureau of Publications.

Tollison, C. D. (1982). Chronic benign pain: An innovative program for South Carolina. *Journal of the South Carolina Medical Association, 78*, 379–383.

Tomlinson, B. E., Blessed, G., & Roth, M. (1970). Observations on the brain of demented old people. *Journal of Neurological Science, 11*, 205–211.

Traveras, J. M., & Wood, E. H. (1976). *Diagnostic neuroradiology* (2nd ed.). Baltimore: Williams & Wilkins.

Turkat, I. D., & Meyer, V. (1982). The behavior-analytic approach. In P. L. Wachtel (Ed.), *Resistence: Psychodynamic and behavioral approaches*. New York: Plenum Press.

Ullman, L. P., & Krasner, L. (1975). *A psychological approach to abnormal behavior* (2nd ed.). Englewood Cliffs, NJ: Prentice-Hall.

U. S. Department of Health and Human Services. (1980). *Facts about older Americans 1979* (HHS Publication No. 80-20006). Washington, DC: Office of Human Development Services, Administration on Aging.

VanderArk, G. D., & Kempe, L. G. (1973). *A primer of electroencephalography*. New Jersey: Rocom Press.

Vestal, R. E., McGuire, E. A., Tobin, J. D., Andres, R., Norris, A. H., & Mezey, E. (1977). Aging and ethanol metabolism. *Clinical Pharmacology and Therapeutics, 21*, 343–354.

Vital Statistics of the United States, 1970, Vol. 2, Mortality, Part A. Rockvilee, MD: U.S. Public Health Service, 1974.

Vogel, F. S. (1977). The brain and time. In E. W. Busse & E. Pfeiffer (Eds.), *Behavior and adaptation in late life*. Boston: Little, Brown.

Weingartner, H., Kaye, W., Smallberg, S. A., Ebert, M. H., Gillin, J. C., & Sitaram, N. (1981). Memory failures in progressive idiopathic dementia. *Journal of Abnormal Psychology, 90*, 187–196.

Wells, C. E. (1979). Diagnosis of dementia. *Psychosomatics, 20*, 517–522.

Wells, C. E., & Duncan, G. W. (1977). Danger of overreliance on computerized cranial tomography. *American Journal of Psychiatry, 134*, 811–813.

Wender, P. H., Reimherr, F. W., & Wood, D. R. (1981). Attention deficit disorder in adults. *Archives of General Psychiatry, 38*, 449–456.

Wershow, H. J. (1977). Reality orientation for gerontologists: Some thoughts about senility. *The Gerontologist, 17*, 297–302.

White, C. B. (1982). Sexual interest, attitudes, knowledge, and sexual history in relation to sexual behavior in the institutionalized aged. *Archives of Sexual Behavior, 11*, 11–21.

Wilson, G. T., Franks, C. M., Brownell, K. D., & Kendall, P. C. (1984). *Annual review of behavior therapy* (Vol. 9). New York: Guilford.

Wilson, W. P., Musella, L., & Short, M. J. (1977). The electroencephalogram in dementia. In C. E. Wells (Ed.), *Dementia* (2nd Ed.). Philadelphia: Davis.

Wohlwill, J. F. (1970). The age variable in psychological research. *Psychological Review, 77*, 49–64.

Zimbardo, P. G., Andersen, S. M., & Kabat, L. G. (1981). Induced hearing deficit generates experimental paranoia. *Science, 212*, 1529–1531.

Zubek, J. P. (Ed.). (1969). *Sensory deprivation: Fifteen years of research*. New York: Appleton-Century-Croft.

Zuckerman, M. (1979). *Sensation seeking: Beyond the optimal level of arousal*. Hillsdale, NJ: Erlbaum.

Author Index

309

Subject Index